LIBRARY
Institute of Cancer Research
15 Cotswold Road
Sutton
SM2 5NG

Institute of Cancer Research Library

Sutton

Please return this book by
the last date stamped below

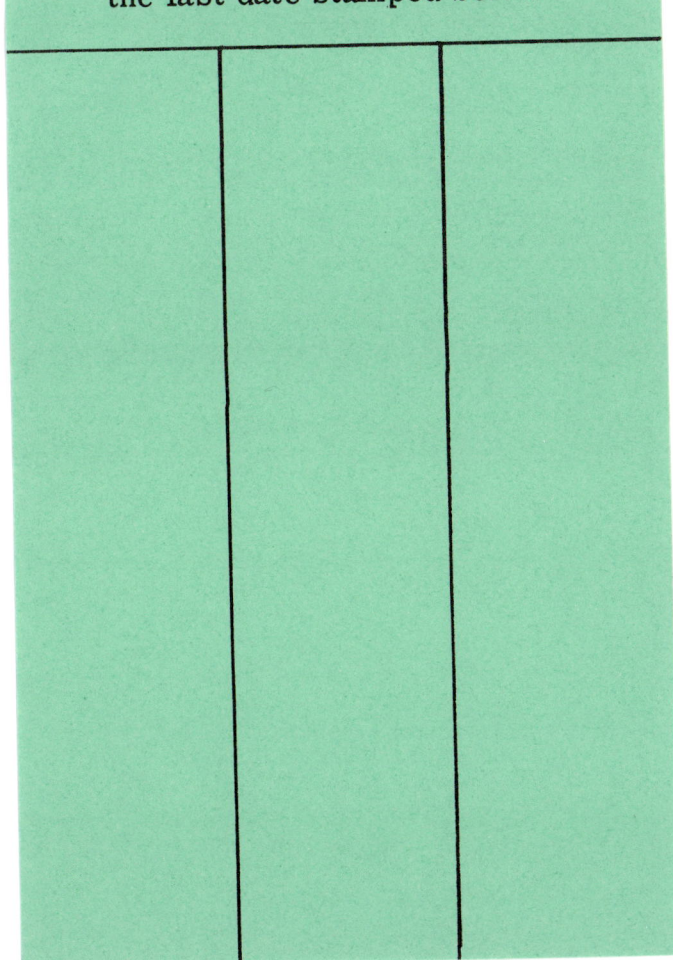

Rectal Cancer: Etiology, Pathogenesis and Treatment

Rectal Cancer: Etiology, Pathogenesis and Treatment

Paula Wells
and
Regina Halstead
Editors

Nova Biomedical Books
New York

Copyright © 2009 by Nova Science Publishers, Inc.

All rights reserved. No part of this book may be reproduced, stored in a retrieval system or transmitted in any form or by any means: electronic, electrostatic, magnetic, tape, mechanical photocopying, recording or otherwise without the written permission of the Publisher.

For permission to use material from this book please contact us:
Telephone 631-231-7269; Fax 631-231-8175
Web Site: http://www.novapublishers.com

NOTICE TO THE READER

The Publisher has taken reasonable care in the preparation of this book, but makes no expressed or implied warranty of any kind and assumes no responsibility for any errors or omissions. No liability is assumed for incidental or consequential damages in connection with or arising out of information contained in this book. The Publisher shall not be liable for any special, consequential, or exemplary damages resulting, in whole or in part, from the readers' use of, or reliance upon, this material. Any parts of this book based on government reports are so indicated and copyright is claimed for those parts to the extent applicable to compilations of such works.

Independent verification should be sought for any data, advice or recommendations contained in this book. In addition, no responsibility is assumed by the publisher for any injury and/or damage to persons or property arising from any methods, products, instructions, ideas or otherwise contained in this publication.

This publication is designed to provide accurate and authoritative information with regard to the subject matter covered herein. It is sold with the clear understanding that the Publisher is not engaged in rendering legal or any other professional services. If legal or any other expert assistance is required, the services of a competent person should be sought. FROM A DECLARATION OF PARTICIPANTS JOINTLY ADOPTED BY A COMMITTEE OF THE AMERICAN BAR ASSOCIATION AND A COMMITTEE OF PUBLISHERS.

LIBRARY OF CONGRESS CATALOGING-IN-PUBLICATION DATA

Rectal cancer : etiology, pathogenesis and treatment / [edited by] Paula Wells and Regina Halstead.
     p. ; cm.
  Includes bibliographical references and index.
  ISBN 978-1-60692-563-8 (hardcover)
  1. Rectum--Cancer. I. Wells, Paula. II. Halstead, Regina.
  [DNLM: 1. Rectal Neoplasms--etiology. 2. Colorectal Neoplasms, Hereditary Nonpolyposis--etiology. 3. Neoplasm Recurrence, Local. 4. Rectal Neoplasms--surgery. 5. Rectal Neoplasms--therapy. 6. Risk Factors. WI 610 R3103 2009]
  RC280.R37R427 2009
    616.99'435--dc22
                                                                                       2009010235

Published by Nova Science Publishers, Inc. ✢ New York

Contents

Preface vii

Research and Review Studies

Chapter I	Surgical Treatment of Rectal Cancer – Current Controversies *I. D. Vilcea and I. Vasile*	1
Chapter II	The Effect of Adjuvant Therapy on Surgical Treatment of Rectal Cancer *Luca Stocchi and Victor W. Fazio*	41
Chapter III	Three-Dimensional Endorectal Ultrasonography in Rectal Cancer Staging *G.A. Santoro, S. Magrini and L. Cancian*	65
Chapter IV	Transanal Endoscopic Micsrosurgery (TEM) in Early Rectal Cancer *A. Suppiah and J. R. T. Monson*	95
Chapter V	Staging and treatment of early rectal cancer *G. Baatrup and P. Pfeiffer*	113
Chapter VI	Transanal endoscopic microsurgery of rectal tumor. A review *Damian Casadesus*	145
Chapter VII	Correlation between Metabolic Enzymes of Nucleic Acid in Colorectal Cancer Patients and FRNA/TSIR, Prognostic Factors *Kenji Katsumata, Tetsuo Sumi, Daisuke Matsuda, Shoji Suzuki, Masayuki Hisada, Yasuharu Mori, Tatehiko Wada, Akihiko Tuchida and Tatsuya Aoki*	159
Chapter VIII	Germline and Somatic Mutations in Colorectal Cancers from Patients with Hereditary Nonpolyposis Colorectal Cancer *Michiko Miyaki, Tatsuro Yamaguchi and Takeo Mori*	173
Chapter IX	Women and Colorectal Cancer *Samantha Hendren*	191

Chapter X	Dietary Fatty Acids and Acyl-CoA Synthetases in the Modifier Concept of Colorectal Carcinogenesis *Nikolaus Gassler, Elke Kaemmerer, Christina Klaus and Andrea Reinartz*	211

Short Communications

A	Risk factors of local recurrence after curative resection in patients with middle and lower rectal carcinoma *Wu Ze-yu, Wan Jin, Zhao Gang, Peng Lin, Du Jia-lin, Yao Yuan, Liu Quan-fang, Wang Zhi-du, Huang Zhi-ming and Lin Hua-huan*	223
B	CT-Guided Interstitial Brachytherapy as an Innovative Adjunct to Current Therapeutic Strategies in the Treatment of Colorectal Liver Metastases *Christian Grieser, Dirk Schnapauff and Timm Denecke*	233
Index		241

PREFACE

Current controversies about rectal cancer treatment are examined and discussed in this book. In particular, oncologic outcomes, which claim an aggressive approach over the primary tumor, lymph nodes and distant metastasis. Also, the functional outcome, whose important objective is to preserve the anal sphincter and the preservation of the pelvic nervous plexus. Radical resection with total mesorectal excision is the mainstay of rectal cancer treatment. However, it is associated with significant surgical morbidity/mortality, possible stoma surgery/complications and long-term gastrointestinal dysfunction with deterioration in quality of life. This book also explores the risk factors of local recurrence after curative resection in patients with middle and lower rectal carcinoma. The relationships between mesorectal metastasis and local recurrence and the possible correlations between circumferential resection margin status and local recurrence were identified. The relationships between local recurrence and clinicopathologic characteristics of middle and lower rectal carcinoma were also evaluated.

Chapter I - It has been over 100 years since the first resection for rectal cancer, and many points of debate still exist; probably the main controversy is determined by the two most important objectives for rectal cancer treatment:

- oncologic outcomes, who claim an aggressive approach over the primary tumor, lymph nodes and distant metastasis;
- functional outcome, whose most important objective is to preserve the anal sphincter (and sometimes the reservoir role of the rectum), and the preservation of the pelvic nervous plexus, with good postoperative urinary and genital function.

These objectives are somehow contradictorily but compromises have been made in both directions:

- the inferior rectal resection limit was lowered to 2 cm, permitting an increase in sphincter-saving resection, without compromising oncologic results; there were also developed techniques that permit the construction of a reservoir through an ileal or colonic pouch;

- the oncologic outcome has been improved, at least in terms of reducing local recurrences, by developing the total mesorectal excision technique, in combination with a preoperative chemoiradiation protocol;
- the instrumental dissection of mesorectum permits the identification and the preservation of hypogastric nerves and pelvic nervous plexus, whose damage is responsible for urinary and genital postoperative disturbances;

The possibility to combine these two objectives to obtain the best possible results in each case depends especially on the tumor stage, but also on the tumor topography on the rectum (for example, the tumor location in the upper rectum has much less problems than those in the middle and lower rectum); in locally advanced cases the oncologic objectives become more important than the functional outcome, therefore, the complete resection of the tumor must be achieved without many concerns about the functional outcome (anyway, in these cases preexist lesions of internal genitalia or urinary involvement, that imply extended resection of these organs).

Another problem regarding the surgical treatment of the rectal cancer is lymphadenectomy, and especially the level of nodal resection: is there always necessary ligation of the inferior mesenteric artery at the origin, or below of the left colic artery origin? There is also lateral pelvic nodes dissection necessary and, if it is, in which circumstances and what will the benefit be in this case?

Other problems concerning the rectal cancer surgical treatment are:

- is local treatment truly beneficial from the oncologic point of view in early stages of rectal cancer, and which is the best modality to perform it: by classic approach or by transanal endoscopic microexcision technique?
- which is the role of the surgical treatment in advanced cases of disease (locally extended tumors), and how this approach improved the patient survival and the quality of life?
- in the era of miniinvasive approach, which is the place of laparoscopic surgery in rectal cancer?

Chapter II - Surgery is the most widely used modality in the treatment of rectal cancer with curative intent and has achieved rates of local recurrence in the order of 10% or less.

However, the results for surgery alone in locally advanced rectal cancer remain suboptimal as a significant percentage of patients are at risk of systemic failure and local recurrence albeit rare remains a devastating event. Therefore, multimodality treatment including not only surgery but also radiotherapy and chemotherapy has been gradually recognized as the most effective treatment for locally advanced rectal cancer. While multimodality treatment is widely accepted, there is a variety of different opinions regarding the timing, sequence, dosages and agents to be used.

The aim of this presentation is to illustrate some of the current issues, controversies and future directions of adjuvant treatment for rectal cancer and its influence on surgical approach with curative intent on the primary disease.

Chapter III - Management of rectal cancer is influenced by local factors such as depth of rectal wall invasion, presence of mesorectal lymph node metastases and status of circumferential resection margin (CRM). Accurate preoperative staging plays a decisive role in selecting patients suitable to local resection, radical surgery with total mesorectal excision or neoadjuvant chemoradiotherapy (CRT). Imaging modalities used for local staging include computed tomography, two-dimensional endorectal ultrasonography (2D-ERUS) and magnetic resonance.

The new technique of high-resolution three-dimensional ERUS, constructed from a synthesis of standard 2D cross-sectional images, promises to further improve the accuracy in rectal cancer staging. This tool seems to offer best information on early tumoral invasion into the rectal wall, presence of mesorectal lymph node metastases, prediction of surgical CRMs, restaging rectal carcinomas after neoadjuvant CRT and detection of local recurrence after primary treatment. It has also the advantage of being an office-based procedure, well tolerated, with fast acquisition times and relatively low cost.

Chapter IV - Radical resection with total mesorectal excision is the mainstay of rectal cancer treatment. However, it is associated with significant surgical morbidity/mortality, possible stoma surgery/complications and long-term gastrointestinal dysfunction with deterioration in quality of life. Re-assessment of surgical treatment is required in view of new cancer trends. There is an observable stage migration towards early stage cancer due to cancer screening and increased patient awareness, especially in the West. Simultaneously, better health care provision leads to an increasingly elderly population. The result is an elderly population group with significant co-morbidity and the probability of non-cancer related death which have early stage cancers with low recurrence rates. Radical resection risks over-treatment in these patients by attempting to achieve lowest recurrence rates but at the risk of non-cancer related death or deterioration in quality of life.

Transanal endoscopic microsurgery (TEM) is relatively new method of local excision without the morbidity associated with radical resection. It is superior to other local excision techniques. Published long-term outcomes in selected cancers appear to be comparable to radical resection although this is unproven in the context of randomised control trial. TEM may be an acceptable surgical alternative with minimal morbidity and gastrointestinal dysfunction but with acceptable compromise in recurrence rates. This chapter discusses the role of TEM in modern oncological surgery where the aim of oncological surgery should not just emphasise lowest recurrence rates but rather a balance of surgical risk, an acceptable post-operative quality of life and the possibility of non-cancer related death. TEM appears to balance all this areas and in selected cancers groups, TEM may well prove to be the treatment of choice in the future.

Chapter V - Accurate preoperative staging of early rectal cancers is necessary in order to select those patients who will benefit from local resection or non-surgical treatment. Staging should combine inspection, digital examination, biopsy and transanal endoluminal ultrasonography. The patients' age and physical performance may also influence the decision.

Major surgery for early rectal cancer is followed by a long term cancer-specific survival of more than 90%. The overall mortality is largely due to the surgical trauma or causes other than the cancer disease. Some patients with high age or co-morbidity and rectal cancers of T stage 1 and 2, sometimes even 3 can be offered local resection without compromising long term survival.

The low risk T1 cancers can safely be treated with transanal endoscopic microsurgery. The long term results match those of major surgery. The long term results for high risk early cancers treated with radiotherapy and transanal endoscopic microsurgery may match those of major surgery, but prospective randomized trials are needed for a firm conclusion.

Local resection of high risk, early rectal cancers should be reserved for those with high age or co morbidity or it should be combined with preoperative radiotherapy. In cases of possible oncological compromise, the patient should decide how to prioritize short and long term survival, risk of complications and quality of life. The patient and the surgeon should be prepared for early rescue surgery after transanal surgery in case of staging errors.

The oncological safety of colonoscopic submucosal dissection is not clear and transanal endoscopic microsurgery is currently recommended for local resection of early rectal cancers.

Non-surgical treatment of early rectal cancers has gained renewed interest. The rate of complete oncological response is increasing as external radiotherapy is combined with modern chemotherapy and possible endocavitary radiotherapy. Combined oncological treatment induces a complete pathological response in 30% or more of the early cancers.

The frequency of early rectal cancers is low in areas without population screening programmes and the decision and planning of the treatment should be handled by a multidisciplinary team of dedicated specialists.

Chapter VI - In 1984, G. Buess introduced transanal endoscopic microsurgery (TEM). Since this time the frequency of such procedure has been increasing for rectal adenoma resection and selected cases of rectal cancer. For the purposes of this review, Medline literature search was performed in order to locate articles on the indications, clinical and functional results of TEM. Emphasis was placed on reports from the past decade. Perusal of the literature reveals that TEM is a safe technique in the treatment of rectal adenomas with better outcomes compared with other techniques. TEM appears to be an effective method of excising selected T1 carcinomas of the rectum. The place of this technique in the resection of advanced carcinomas has yet to be properly evaluated; however its use has produced better results compared with radical techniques. In conclusion, TEM is a safe procedure and can achieve good results in terms of local tumor resection, with lower recurrences rates, fewer complication and higher survival rates than those of radical techniques.

Chapter VII - This study examined metabolic pathway of 5-fluorouracil (5-FU) in cancer and non-cancer sites of colorectal cancer patients including: 16 patients who received 500 mg/day 5-FU drip infusion for 3 days (group R), and 19 patients who received 500 mg/day 5-FU continuous venous injection (groupC). The metabolic pathway was examined in both groups as non-cancerous group (No) and cancerous group (Ca), focusing on the relationship between nucleic acid metabolizing enzymes and 5-FU incorporation into RNA (FRNA) as well as tymidylate synthetase inhibition rate (TSIR). Of the enzyme concentrations in non-cancer and cancer sites, no difference was observed with dyhydropyridine (DPD) at the either site, whereas significantly higher concentrations were detected with orotate phosphoribosyl transferase (OPRT), thymidine phosphorylase (TP), uridine phosphorylase (UP), and tymidine synthetase (TS) free at cancerous than non-cancerous sites ($p<0.0005$). Among the enzymes, correlations were found between TP and UP in No ($p=0.01$), and, in Ca, correlations were seen TP and UP ($p=0.01$) and between DPD and TS free ($p=0.05$). There was no correlation between the enzymes in group R-No, whereas in group R-Ca, correlations were found between FRNA and OPRT (p=0.01), and between TSIR and OPRT as well as TS free (p=0.05); in group C-No, correlations were seen between FRNA and UP as well as TS free (p=0.05), and TSIR and TS free (p=0.05); and, in group C-Ca, correlations were observed between FRNA and DPD (p=0.05), and between TSIR and TS free (p=0.05). These findings indicated that 5-FU metabolism in the large intestine differed at non-cancer or cancer sites and by different 5-FU administration methods.

And we examined the correlation among immunostaining metabolic enzyme of nucleic acid and clinicopathologic factors, prognosis. Result showed TP staining positive cases had a higher incident of progression (p=0.0403) and those with TS staining (p=0.0324). These cases had lower 5-year survival rates. But DPD had no incidence of these factors. These findings suggested that TP and TS are prognostic factors of colorectal cancer patients.

Chapter VIII - Hereditary nonpolyposis colorectal cancer (HNPCC) is one of the most common hereditary colon cancer syndromes. The causative genes of HNPCC are DNA mismatch repair genes, and inactivation of these genes triggers HNPCC tumors.

We detected germline mutations of the hMSH2, hMLH1 and hMSH6 genes in Japanese HNPCC families. These mutations included single-base substitutions and frameshifts, both resulting in truncated proteins, a mutation at the splice donor site of exon 5, and a 2kb genomic deletion encompassing exon 5. The coexistence of germline and somatic mutations of DNA mismatch repair genes was observed in colorectal and extracolorectal cancers. The majority of somatic mutations were frameshift, one was a mutation at the splice donor site of exon 5, and two were loss of the normal allele. All HNPCC cancers exhibited high microsatellite instability. Sixty-four % of HNPCC colorectal cancers included somatic mutations of either the APC or ß-catenin gene, whereas only 13% of the cancers had p53 mutations and none of the cancer cases showed the BRAF mutation. The loss of heterozygosity at tumor suppressor regions (chromosomes 5q, 8p, 17p, 18q and 22q) was not observed. We also detected frequent somatic frameshift mutations of growth-related genes with coding repeats in HNPCC colorectal cancers. Mutation frequencies at these repeats were 77% at TGFßRII(A)$_{10}$, 55% at hMSH3(A)$_8$, 52% at CASP5(A)$_{10}$, 48% at BAX(G)$_8$, 48% at RIZ(A)$_8$ and (A)$_9$, 45% at RAD50(A)$_9$, 45% at MBD4(A)$_{10}$, 36% at hMSH6(C)$_8$, 23% at BLM(A)$_9$, 19% at IGFIIR(G)$_8$ and 19% at PTEN(A)$_6$.

The present data have the following implications: Inactivation of DNA mismatch repair genes through germline and somatic mutations causes genetic instability resulting in somatic mutations in various growth-related genes. Disruption of the WNT signaling pathway by mutations of the APC or ß-catenin gene and disruption of the TGF-ß signaling pathway by alteration of the TGFßRII gene seem to largely contribute to the development of HNPCC colorectal cancer via adenomas. Moreover, inactivation of apoptosis-related genes, such as the BAX, CASP5 and RIZ genes, may also contribute to the development, and inactivation of the IGFIIR and PTEN genes play a role in the progression of HNPCC colorectal cancer.

Chapter IX - Colorectal cancer deaths are equally distributed among women and men. Prevention is possible using risk-stratified screening strategies and healthy lifestyle. Good outcomes are possible if the disease is discovered and treated at an early stage. Quality of life can be preserved but in rectal cancer patients, sexual function and changes in body image occur.

Chapter X - Epidemiological studies confirm a strong association between intake of saturated fatty acids and colon cancer risk. Fatty acids have been especially shown to be involved in gene expression and cellular reactivity mediated by several signaling cascades. However, the molecular pathways determining this phenomenon are not well elucidated. Here we discuss a putative pathway by which fatty acids could be able to modify the behaviour of intestinal epithelia via acyl-CoA synthetase isoform 5 (ACSL5), a mitochondrial located enzyme preferentially catalyzing the synthesis of long chain acyl-CoA derivatives. In enterocytes, strong association of ACSL5 over-expression and susceptibility for apoptosis has been shown. This physiological mechanism probably facilitates maturation and shedding of enterocytes along the crypt-plateau axis in normal intestinal mucosa. On the molecular level, ACSL5 synthesized acyl-CoA derivatives might interfere with ceramide synthesis, membrane composition, protein lipidation, activity of intramitochondrial enzymes, and finally gene transcription. Disturbances in this complex system are suggested to modify enterocyte behaviour promoting intestinal carcinogenesis.

Short Commmunication A - *AIM:* To explore the risk factors of local recurrence after curative resection in patients with middle and lower rectal carcinoma.

Materials and Methods: Cancer specimens from 56 patients with middle and lower rectal carcinoma who received total mesorectal excision at the Department of General Surgery of Guangdong Provincial People's Hospital were studied. A large slice technique was used to detect mesorectal metastasis and evaluate circumferential resection margin status. The relationships between mesorectal metastasis and local recurrence and the possible correlations between circumferential resection margin status and local recurrence were identified. The relationships between local recurrence and clinicopathologic characteristics of middle and lower rectal carcinoma were also evaluated.

Results: Local recurrence after curative resection occurred in 12.5 percent (7 of 56 cases) of patients with middle and lower rectal carcinoma. Local recurrence was significantly associated with family history ($P=0.047$), high CEA level ($P=0.026$), cancerous perforation ($P=0.004$), tumor differentiation ($P=0.009$) and vessel cancerous emboli ($P=0.001$). Conversely, No significant correlations were found between local recurrence and other variables such as age ($P=0.477$), gender ($P=0.0.749$), tumor diameter ($P=0.516$), diameter of tumor infiltration ($P=0.168$), Ming's classification ($P=0.727$), depth of tumor invasion ($P=0.101$), lymph node metastases ($P=0.055$) and TNM staging system ($P=0.152$). 21.4 per cent (12 of 56 cases) of patients with middle and lower rectal carcinoma had positive circumferential resection margin. Local recurrence rate of patients with positive circumferential resection margin was 33.3%(4/12), whereas it was 6.8%(3/44) in those with negative circumferential resection margin. The difference between these two groups was statistically significant ($P=0.014$). 64.3 per cent (36 of 56 cases) of patients with middle and lower rectal carcinoma were detected mesorectal metastasis. Local recurrence occurred in 16.7 per cent (6 of 36 cases) of patients with mesorectal metastasis, and in 5.0 per cent (1 of 20 cases) of patients without mesorectal metastasis. However, the difference between these two groups was not statistically significant ($P=0.206$).

Conclusion: Our results demonstrate that family history, high CEA level, cancerous perforation, tumor differentiation, vessel cancerous emboli and circumferential resection margin status are significant risk factors of local recurrence after curative resection in patients with middle and lower rectal carcinoma. Local recurrence may be more frequent in patients with mesorectal metastasis, compared with patients without mesorectal metastasis. Larger sample investigations are helpful to draw a further conclusion.

Short Communication B - Beside surgical resection and systemic chemotherapy locally ablative treatment has gained a broad acceptance in multimodal treatment concepts of colorectal liver metastases over the past decade. Limitations of the thermodestructive ablation modalities such as radiofrequency ablation and laser induced thermotherapy are number, size, and location of target lesions. Combining technical features derived from locally ablative treatment in interventional radiology and from radiation therapy, these limitations can be overcome to a great part. After CT-guided percutaneous implantation of catheters into the hepatic tumor, the irradiation is performed via afterloading following a 3D-radiation plan based on CT images. This minimally invasive procedure allows circumscriptive high dose rate irradiation of the target lesion in a single session, independent of breathing motion or potential cooling effects of neighboring vessels. By modifying the dwell locations and dwell times of the radiation source (Iridium-192), the ablation zone can be adjusted to the shape and size of the lesion without repositioning of catheters. This enables sufficient dosing even of large tumors or lesions close to risk structures, such as liver hilum or adjacent bowel, in which thermoablation is not favored. Good local control rates have been achieved in colorectal liver metastases, and promising clinical indications are currently elaborated. This article gives an overview of the application technique and the possible fields of indication in the multimodal treatment setting of patients with colorectal liver metastases.

In: Rectal Cancer: Etiology, Pathogenesis and Treatment
Editors: Paula Wells and Regina Halstead

ISBN 978-1-60692-563-8
© 2009 Nova Science Publishers, Inc.

Chapter I

SURGICAL TREATMENT OF RECTAL CANCER – CURRENT CONTROVERSIES

I. D. Vilcea and I. Vasile
Emergency Hospital of Craiova, Romania.

ABSTRACT

It has been over 100 years since the first resection for rectal cancer, and many points of debate still exist; probably the main controversy is determined by the two most important objectives for rectal cancer treatment:

- oncologic outcomes, who claim an aggressive approach over the primary tumor, lymph nodes and distant metastasis;
- functional outcome, whose most important objective is to preserve the anal sphincter (and sometimes the reservoir role of the rectum), and the preservation of the pelvic nervous plexus, with good postoperative urinary and genital function.

These objectives are somehow contradictorily but compromises have been made in both directions:

- the inferior rectal resection limit was lowered to 2 cm, permitting an increase in sphincter-saving resection, without compromising oncologic results; there were also developed techniques that permit the construction of a reservoir through an ileal or colonic pouch;
- the oncologic outcome has been improved, at least in terms of reducing local recurrences, by developing the total mesorectal excision technique, in combination with a preoperative chemoiradiation protocol;
- the instrumental dissection of mesorectum permits the identification and the preservation of hypogastric nerves and pelvic nervous plexus, whose damage is responsible for urinary and genital postoperative disturbances;

The possibility to combine these two objectives to obtain the best possible results in each case depends especially on the tumor stage, but also on the tumor topography on the rectum (for example, the tumor location in the upper rectum has much less problems than those in the middle and lower rectum); in locally advanced cases the oncologic objectives become more important than the functional outcome, therefore, the complete resection of the tumor must be achieved without many concerns about the functional outcome (anyway, in these cases preexist lesions of internal genitalia or urinary involvement, that imply extended resection of these organs).

Another problem regarding the surgical treatment of the rectal cancer is lymphadenectomy, and especially the level of nodal resection: is there always necessary ligation of the inferior mesenteric artery at the origin, or below of the left colic artery origin? There is also lateral pelvic nodes dissection necessary and, if it is, in which circumstances and what will the benefit be in this case?

Other problems concerning the rectal cancer surgical treatment are:

- is local treatment truly beneficial from the oncologic point of view in early stages of rectal cancer, and which is the best modality to perform it: by classic approach or by transanal endoscopic microexcision technique?
- which is the role of the surgical treatment in advanced cases of disease (locally extended tumors), and how this approach improved the patient survival and the quality of life?
- in the era of miniinvasive approach, which is the place of laparoscopic surgery in rectal cancer?

INTRODUCTION

It is never enough emphasized that a good oncologic and even functional result in rectal cancer, as in any other topography of neoplasic disease, is achieved only by a complex therapy, comprising surgery, as central therapeutic modality, radiation therapy, chemotherapy and other oncologic treatments. The sequence in which these modalities are combined depends on the possibility to explore preoperatively the patient, and also on the best possibly pathologic report.

The good preoperative staging plays a major role in the type of surgery that may be performed, especially in early tumor stages, in which the local treatment may be discussed, without compromising the oncologic results.

The most important factor, which dictates the type of surgical operation is the tumor topography: a tumor located in the upper rectum or rectosigmoid junction is almost always resolved through a rectosigmoidian resection, followed by a colorectal anastomosis and only in few complicated cases (occlusive or perforated upper rectal cancers, or too frail patients) resection will be followed by a terminal colostomy and closure of the rectal stump (Hartmann's procedure).

A lower rectal cancer (located just above the anal verge) will be resolved through an abdominoperineal excision (Miles procedure), and in some selected cases through a local procedure.

The most debated topography from surgical point of view is middle and some lower rectal cancers, in which all of the aforementioned surgical procedures could be, theoretically, performed.

LOCAL TREATMENT IN RECTAL CANCER

The term *local treatment* refers to several therapeutic methods that address to the primary tumor, without the possibilities of removing the lymphatic territory that drains the tumor, and may contain involved lymph nodes; these techniques remove or destroy only the primary tumor, without a major rectal resection.

Some of these methods realize destruction of the primary tumor (cryosurgery, laser, electrofulguration or irradiation), thus it is difficult or even impossible to obtain a specimen for the pathologic assessment; because of this major disadvantage they are extremely rare used as a curative procedure, being reserved only for palliation in some selected cases [1].

Usually, the local treatment is made surgically: conventional surgery or transanal endoscopic microsurgery technique (TEM); both of them assume that the tumor is surgically removed with apparent healthy surrounding tissue (at least 1 cm), offering a full-thickness specimen for pathologic analysis, mandatory if the local therapy is to be performed for cure; an adjuvant or neoadjuvant treatment may be applied in order to consolidate surgical results.

Primary tumor may be approached surgically through a transanal approach (the usual way) or by transphincteric (Mason) or transsacral (Kraske) route; these are highly surgeon-dependent with some advantages and disadvantages, but their problems are similar from the oncologic point of view, problems which will be discussed later.

Local treatment in rectal cancer is the most debatable procedure in nowadays medical literature; many surgeons also performed it on some patients, there are no prospective data to sustain this kind of approach, at least on a suitable patient for a more radical procedure. Local excision of a rectal cancer is recommended for its lower morbidity compared to radical excision, but the main problem in discussion is the important percentage of locoregional recurrences. Therefore, if local excision could be performed safely as a palliative procedure or even curative intent on some patients with limited life span (other terminal diseases), its indication as a curative procedure in a suitable patient for major surgery is debatable for at least two reasons: failing to deal with lymphatic spread of cancer and risk of incomplete resection; both of them concur to a higher risk of locoregional recurrence after the excision.

There are several factors that determine if a tumor is suitable or not for transanal excision: the tumor must be located in the lower rectum, so its superior border to be accessible (for conventional transanal excision the maximum limit is established to 10 cm from the anal verge); the macroscopic height of tumor must not exceed 3-4 cm; favorable histology (well or moderate grade of differentiation, absence of lymphovascular and perineural invasion) (later condition may be established only after the pathologic examination of a biopsy specimen or after the removal of the tumor).

The main disadvantages of local excision in rectal cancer may be grouped in several clinical, pathologic and oncologic problems. All of these are determined by the aforementioned aspects of a local procedure:
- a local procedure fail to deal with lymphatic spread of cancer, which is known to occur in very early studies, as demonstrated by numerous retrospective studies, some of them already analyzed in a series of reviews; [2-5]
- the bigger the tumor is the higher is the risk to perform an incomplete local excision (difficulties to remove the superior pole of the tumor with enough surrounding healthy tissue to ensure a safe oncologic procedure).

Clinical Problems of Local Excision in Rectal Cancer

Maybe the most troublesome aspects of an indication for local excision as a curative treatment is lack of prospective studies that could demonstrate comparable results with local excision versus radical resection in terms of cure, reported to the same tumor stage.

As already analyzed in many reviews, all studies referring to local treatment in rectal cancer are the retrospectives ones, therefore, all of them carry some biases in selecting the cases, emphasized in all mentioned reviews. Moreover, most studies are in fact a case-based studies, and the statistical significance is doubtfully due to the small number of cases included (one hundred cases studies may lead to an apparently significant result, but from a statistically point of view, the number of cases necessary to determine an actually statistically significant result may be much more) [2-5].

We can conclude that, at least for the moment, there is no significant study that has the ability to claim that local excision in rectal cancer is a safe procedure in terms of oncologic results (similar rates of local recurrences or similar survival rates when comparing to radical rectal resection for the same stage).

Another clinical problem of local excision as a curative procedure in rectal cancer is determined by the difficulties in preoperative selection of the cases that may benefit from this procedure; this is related to the inability of present preoperative assessment imagistic techniques to accurate stage the primary tumor, and especially their inability to predict nodal status with great accuracy. As a consequence, a number of cases considered suitable for local excision will have residual mural or nodal disease, which will lead to recurrence and, eventually, will compromise long term results.

In order to establish the local treatment indication for a rectal tumor, a good preoperative staging is mandatory, altogether with the patient's informed consent; the absence of any of these two conditions impose a major surgical resection.

Digital rectal examination offers many details for a trained specialist, but establishing the local excision indication only after such procedure may be hazardous. Anyway, nowadays several preoperative imagistic methods could perform a good preoperative staging: endorectal ultrasound, computed tomography (CT), or magnetic resonance imaging (MRI).

Endorectal ultrasound is essential in the assessment of the depth of tumor penetration in the rectal wall; as already discussed, this is a very important aspect in establishing the indication for local treatment in rectal cancer, therefore it must be performed in any case in which such treatment is attempted. Although its accuracy in determining mural tumoral penetration is very good (between 82-93%), the endorectal ultrasound has limitations in determining nodal status, which leads to an increased risk of residual nodal disease after local excision [6, 7].

Separate analysis depending on T stage revealed almost 100% accuracy for 3D endorectal ultrasound in T1 tumors, but only 75% accuracy in T2 tumors (many cases are over-staged), tumors otherwise suitable for local excision [7].

Main problems appear to be related to nodal status characterization on endosonography, in this case accuracy being too low to be a reliable method in establishing the indication for a local procedure (only 48% accuracy in predicting nodal status for T1 tumors and only 67% for T2 tumors, with a specificity of 67% and 75% respectively) [6].

Therefore, establishing the indication for local surgery based only on the results of endosonography is too risky, a great number of cases being left with residual disease.

Magnetic resonance imaging has a similar accuracy in staging tumor and nodal status; in the study of Chun et al., the accuracy of T stage and lymph nodes involvement was similar between MRI and endorectal ultrasound (63.6% accuracy in detecting lymph node involvement with MRI and 57.6% with endorectal ultrasound) [8].

The advantage of MRI results in a better assessment of circumferential rectal margin and mesorectal fascia involvement over the endorectal ultrasound but, regarding local excision, there are no significant differences between those two imaging modalities; therefore, applying a local excision based on each of these two procedures may lead to an important percentage of local nodal residual disease, which imply subsequently an important number of locoregional recurrences [9].

Using CT for staging mural and nodal involvement has even worse consequences, the accuracy of this imaging modalities being inferior to those discussed previously, as it was emphasized in all reviews analyzed, and in the study of Vliegen et al. (an overall accuracy of only 54-66% in determining T stage and approximately 60% accuracy in determining nodal involvement) [2,3,9].

In conclusion, there are no reliable preoperative method to detect both mural and nodal involvement, thus permitting a local excision only on the basis of these imagistic modalities; preoperative staging remains only orientative, surgery and postoperative pathologic examination, being the best methods to accurately assess tumoral extent.

Pathologic Considerations Regarding Local Excision in Rectal Cancer

The pathologic examination results represent the most important factors, after which a local excision may be performed or a more radical approach becomes necessary. It is the pathologic exam which must demonstrate some tumoral characteristics associated with an increased risk of local recurrence after local excision (so called high-risk cases).

Pathologic evaluation must report the involvement of resection margins (residual disease at the local excision margin) and circumferential radial excision margins, and the risk factors for nodal involvement, since the nodal status cannot be predicted in a local excision specimen.

Tumor diameter is one of the most important parameters in establishing an indication for local excision; to be considered suitable for local excision tumor it must be smaller than 3-4 cm in diameter, or it must have a maximum 40% of rectal circumference. As it has been already demonstrated, there is no relation between tumor dimension and degree of penetration through rectal wall, or nodal involvement [10]. Still, in the study of Takano et al., a colorectal tumor bigger than 2 cm carries a higher risk of nodal involvement (93% versus 80%), but this was not an independent prognostic factor [11].

Therefore a maximum diameter of 3 cm was established after analysing a lot of articles, already analyzed in some reviews, which demonstrate that the bigger the tumor is, the higher the risk is to perform an incomplete local excision, and leaving residual local disease; this is mainly because of the difficulties of removing the superior pole of tumor with enough surrounding healthy tissue to ensure a safe oncologic procedure [1,2].

Another reason for this is because removing a larger tumor with at least 1-2 cm surrounding tissue will result in a large rectal defect, very difficult to close (although it is not always necessary to do this) [1,2].

Tumor location on rectal wall may also play a role in establishing the local excision indication; thus, the tumor must be located below 10 cm if it is located on the anterior rectal wall, because of the risk of vaginal or prostate and bladder lesion through a full-thickness excision; location on the side rectal wall or on the posterior surface permits to extend the limit to 15, respectively 20 cm from the anal verge, but the excision in such situations is accessible only to transanal endoscopic technique, in such cases tumors being too high for a conventional transanal approach [1,2].

Tumor's macroscopic appearance. The macroscopic appearance of tumor (pedunculated, ulcerated or infiltrative) does not represent a major criterion in selecting a rectal cancer for local excision. Even so, a careful approach must be given to ulcerated tumors which have a tendency to quickly invade through the rectal wall, and to metastasis to the local lymph nodes [1].

Tumor penetration in the rectal wall represents a very important pathologic aspect in performing a local excision; now it is accepted that only Tis, low-risk T1 tumor and in selected cases low-risk T2 tumors can be approached through local excision. This is mainly due to the increased risk of lymphatic spread with the degree of penetration in the rectal wall, as demonstrated in many studies.

The study of Fang et al., showed a 14.3% of nodal involvement in T1 rectal cancer, and a 18.4% nodal metastasis in T2 lesions; still, not only the degree of rectal wall penetration was important, but also other pathologic factors, such as lymphovascular invasion and a higher grade of differentiation (G3 tumors) [12].

The study of Sitzler et al. revealed a 5.7% lymphatic involvement in T1 tumors and 19.6% in T2, respectively; lymphovascular invasion have had a positive predictive value of 98%. The percentage of lymph node metastasis was much higher in younger than 45 years patients (33.3%, and 30% respectively for T1 and T2 tumor). As a result, only T1 tumors in patients older than 45 years were considered to bear an acceptable low-risk of nodal dissemination [13].

The study of Blumberg et al. showed a risk of 10% for T1 tumors and 17% for T2 tumors for nodal metastasis; a separate analysis demonstrates a risk of 7% and 14% of nodal involvement in low-risk T1 and T2 rectal cancers. Poor differentiation, lymphatic vessels invasion and blood vessel invasion were significant predictors for lymph node metastasis in this cases. The tumor size was not a significant predictive factor for lymphatic metastasis [14].

A detailed study of lymphatic metastasis in T1 stage was performed by Choi et al.; they found an overall 14.3% of lymph node involvement in submucosal invasive colorectal cancer. Significant predictors were sm3 (invasion of the lower third of submucosa), poorly differentiated cancer, tumor cell dissociation and (only in univariate analysis) lymphovascular invasion [15].

As already mentioned, other microscopic factors are related to a high-risk nodal involvement in rectal cancer: lymphovascular invasion, poor differentiation, perineural and vascular invasion, tumor cell dissociation. Regarding these factors, it is very important to emphasize that many of them are established only after tumor removal, and it is very difficult or even impossible to have a complete pathologic report only on preoperative biopsy specimen.

Once the aforementioned high-risk factors of rectal cancer are discovered, local excision must be followed by a radical excision, or at least by an adjuvant chemoradiation protocol, in order to consolidate the results and to prevent locoregional recurrence. In these cases, the so-called "local excision" becomes actually an excisional biopsy.

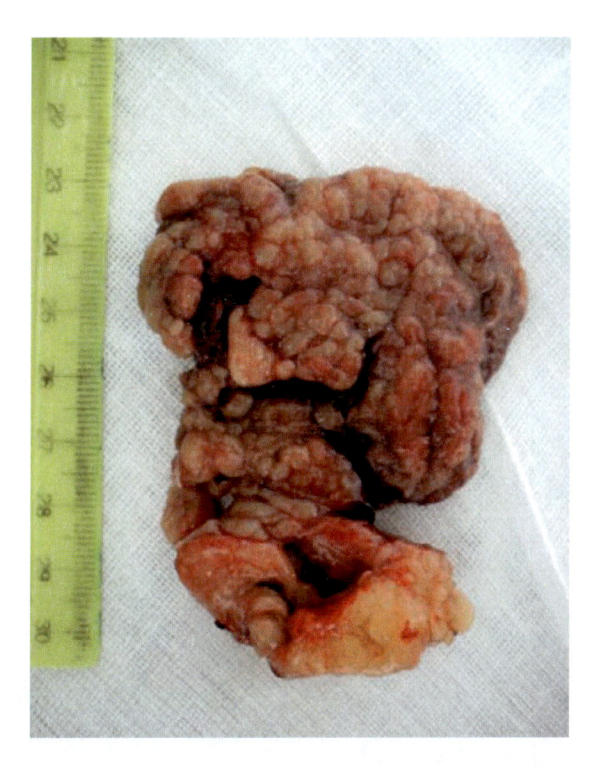

Figure 1. Rectal pedunculated tumor fitted for local excision (macroscopic aspect of fresh resection specimen).

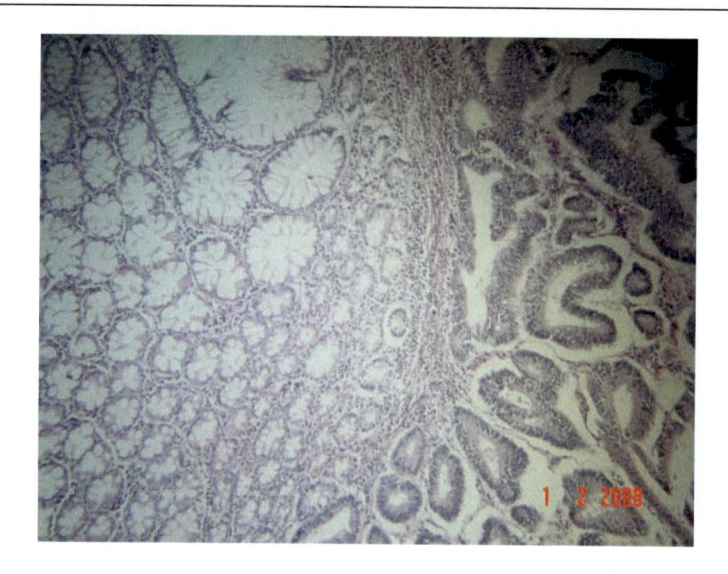

Figure 2. Pathologic examination revealed area of well differentiated adenocarcinoma (Van Gieson staining, 200x).

Oncologic Considerations Regarding Local Excision in Rectal Cancer

The major oncologic concern is related to a higher local recurrence rates after local excision in T1 or T2 rectal cancers, reported in all published articles. This situation is determined by the lack of lymph nodes excision and by the local residual disease in local excision.

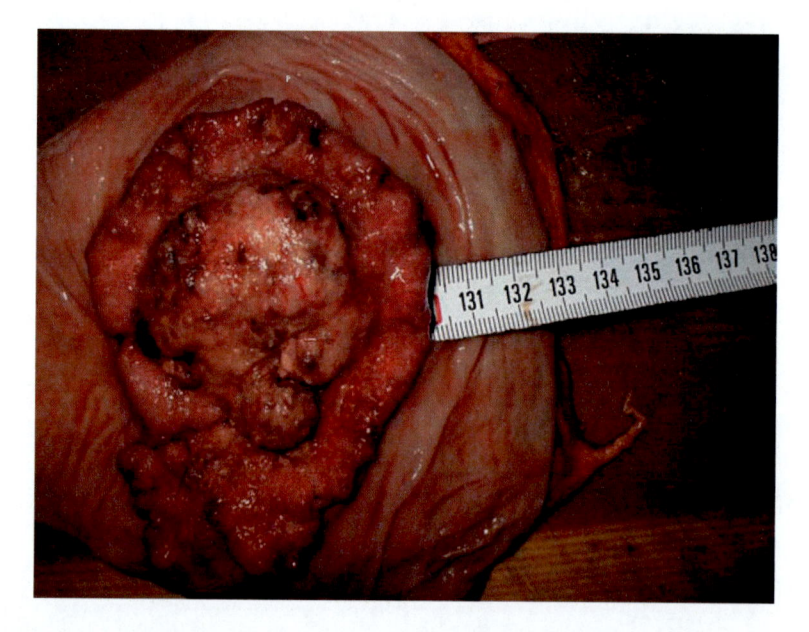

Figure 3. Large ulcero-exofitic tumor, extended over 50% of rectal wall circumference; absolute contraindication for local excision (macroscopic aspect of fresh resection specimen).

Several articles have examined the oncologic results of local excision, with or without neoadjuvant or adjuvant treatment, with the same oncologic end-point: a higher recurrence rates in local excision group versus radical excision, regardless of the depth of the tumor penetration through the rectal wall. The same studies have also demonstrated a lower survival rates in cases submitted to radical surgery for locoregional recurrence after local excision.

The main oncologic concern results also from the lack of prospective studies that analyze this approach in rectal cancer.

According to Tepetes et al., the locoregional recurrence rate for T1 tumors ranges from 4%-29%, thus the risk of local recurrence being 2 to 5-fold higher in local excision group versus radical resection [4].

Miyamoto et al., in their study, have reported excellent results in local treatment for Tis and for T1 with less than 1000μm vertical submucosal invasion [16].

Analyzing only low-risk T1 rectal cancer, Ptok et al., found a 5-year recurrence rate of a 6% in local excision, significantly different from 2% in radical resection group, and concluded that, even if local excision has a much lower morbidity, it still remains an oncologic compromise [17].

Min et al., demonstrate in their retrospective study that local excision alone may not be sufficient, even for T1 cancers, in terms of oncologic results, but these results could be alleviate through an adjuvant chemoradiation protocol, with 100% local recurrence-free survival rate at 89 month of follow-up, compared to 76% in those patients who did not received adjuvant treatment [18].

A similar conclusion had the study of Chakravarti et al., who recommend adjuvant chemoirradiation for all patients undergoing local excision for T2 cancers and T1 cancers with adverse pathologic features [19].

Moreover, the study of Chen et al., brings in discussion another point of debate related to local excision and adjuvant chemoradiation protocol in T3 rectal cancers, but the small number of cases (9) and the follow-up period of only 17.9 month make difficult to apply their results in general practice; they recommend such an attitude for patients with T3 rectal cancers otherwise unfitted for a more aggressive surgery or patients who deny a rectal resection, especially when is followed by a permanent colostomy [20].

Another study, that assesses the possibility to perform local excision in more advanced rectal cancers, was conducted by Kim et al.; their patients underwent a neoadjuvant chemoradiation protocol, after which local excision was attempted. The results were very good in patients who achieved a complete pathologic response, but for the others they recommend a radical resection; an indication for local excision was also established only for patients unfit for major surgery [21].

At the same conclusion reached Borschitz et al., in their review, in which they conclude that indication of local excision after a neoadjuvant chemoradiation protocol is feasible in cT2-cT3 rectal cancers, the strongest prognostic parameter being completeness of response to neoadjuvant treatment (ypT0 or ypT1), on the excised specimen [22].

Transanal endoscopic microsurgery (TEM) represents a relatively new developed technique that permits to combine the advantages of local excision with those of endoscopic approaches in rectal cancers: a lower rate of postoperative morbidity and mortality, a decreased number of patients with local residual disease at the resection margin, and an increased number of cases in which local treatment may be attempted [2,3].

TEM offers the possibility to extend the indication of local surgical treatment in rectal cancer for tumors located in the mid-upper rectum, 10-12 cm for anterior tumors, 15 cm for laterally developed tumors, and 20 cm for posterior located rectal tumors.

After TEM exists the risk of specific complication, and especially the risk of anal incontinence, mainly due to the endoscope caliber and the duration of procedure, but it has been demonstrated that this complication tends to decrease in incidence 6 month after the operation, making this procedure an attractive method.

A recent study also suggested that complications after TEM are related to location of the tumor on the lateral rectal wall and with diameter of the excised tumor, but these conclusions need to be further evaluated and confirmed [23].

Another disadvantage of the procedure is represented by the necessity of initial financial investment for equipment (estimated 50,000 GBP) and the learning curve, but after these the indication for local procedures in rectal cancers may be extended as mentioned for upper tumors, and even for some bigger tumors (especially as palliative measures) since the 1-2 cm healthy tissue may be achieved with TEM in selected cases [2].

In terms of oncologic results, there are little possibilities to obtain better results compared to those obtained through a conventional transanal excision technique, while the TEM procedure had the same oncologic disadvantage: impossibility to interfere and assess with the lymphatic spread of rectal cancer.

Both methods are actually the same oncologic indication: as palliative measures in unfit patients for major rectal resection, and in patients who refuse the surgical resection. A true benefit from both surgical and oncologic point of view may be achieved only in a relatively small number of cases: Tis and T1 rectal cancers without adverse pathologic features (lymphovascular invasion, blood vessel or perineural invasion, poor tumoral differentiation, tumor cell dissociation), but an aggressive postoperative follow-up is recommended to early discover an eventual recurrence.

In more advanced cases, usually discovered after the local procedure was employed, the adverse outcome may be prevented through an early (the first 30 days after the procedure) rectal major resection, since the salvage operation underwent at the time of recurrence is possible only for a few cases, and the results may be worse than expected because of a more advanced locoregional disease.

Maybe the most comprehensive study on the usage and the results of local excision (conventional or TEM) in rectal cancer, also retrospective, was performed by the Nancy You et al., and revealed the increase trend in incidence of these procedures over the last years. Still, the results clearly demonstrate that, even in the cases most selected for local procedures (T1 cases without pathologic adverse features), it is a three-fold increased risk for local recurrence; the risk is much higher in advanced tumors, therefore it is even difficult to recommend it in such cases [25].

Until the results of a prospective randomized large trial will be available, to establish the indication for local procedure as a curative one in rectal cancer remains a debatable problem, especially in young patients, fitted for radical conventional surgery; the problem of correct indication and multimodality treatment in such cases remains unsolved.

A local procedure (conventional or TEM) may, however, be the best choice as a palliative measure for a patient unfit for major surgery, with limited life-span or a patient who denies a permanent colostomy. To reduce the risk of recurrence, an adjuvant treatment is necessary to be employed.

As final considerations regarding local treatment, for the present, the real beneficial of local excision is a too lower rectal cancer to permit an anastomosis (it cannot respect the 2 cm limit below the tumor), in a Tis or T1 lesion without adverse pathologic features; an upper lesion may be solved with a rectal resection with total mesorectal excision, followed by a coloanal anastomosis, or a transanal pull-through technique, or colorectal anastomosis for lesion located in the middle rectum. Morbidity in terms of anal incontinence or urinary and sexual dysfunction is comparable with risk of local recurrence after local excision.

On the other hand, local excision preceded or followed by chemoradiation to reduce the risk of locoregional recurrence may lead to an unexpected number of functional disturbances, in terms of anal continence or sexually or urinary dysfunction (radiation sphincter or pelvic nerve damage), therefore the functional results over time may not be as good as initially believed.

Studies which suggest a good outcome of local excision technique have a lot of biases due to next objectives facts: there are no prospective randomized trials to compare local excision (with or without adjuvant or neoadjuvant treatment) versus radical rectal resection; all studies published have a small number of retrospective cases, usually selected because the patients denied other forms of treatment; an increased number of locoregional recurrences noticed even in the most optimistic retrospective studies, some of them truly oncologic failures.

As a result, the option of local procedure in virtually curative cases of rectal cancer has to be a matter of informed consent from the patient, correctly informed about the risk of the adverse oncologic outcome.

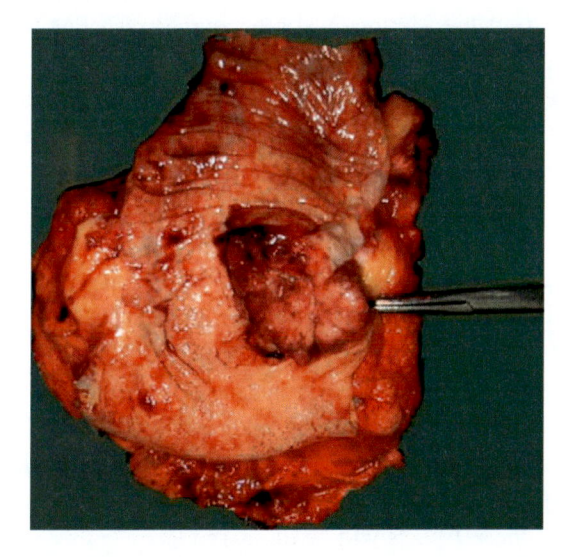

Figure 4. Locally recurrent rectal cancer 23 month after incomplete local excision (fresh resection specimen, macroscopic appearance).

A method that seems to combine the advantage of local procedures with a rectal resection (the possibility to remove and assess lymphatic tumoral drainage) was recently described by Tarantino et al.; the primary tumor local excision was followed by an endoscopic posterior mesorectal resection for T1 rectal cancer. Even if the median number of lymph node removed through this procedure is smaller than after a low anterior resection, this kind of approach could be the next step in rectal cancer surgical treatment, but the feasibility of it remains to be confirmed by future studies [26].

MAJOR RECTAL RESECTIONS IN RECTAL CANCER

The first objective for a surgeon who treats a rectal cancer is to ensure the best chance for the patient's cure; this means the surgeon will have to perform an operation that leads to the best possible locoregional disease control. This objective could only be reached, at least at the actual level of knowledge, only through a standard rectal resection, which includes en block the tumor and the portion of the rectum that includes it, along with the adjacent mesentery, which is known to carry the lymph nodes possible invaded by cancer.

In locally advanced rectal cancers an en block resection of adherent or invaded adjacent organs will give the chance for cure in many cases.

In particular, another objective in rectal cancer is to be reached by the surgeon: anal sphincter preserving, in order to maintain a proper function, and avoid a colostomy whenever is possible.

Nowadays, there are two major procedures that could accomplish the first objective: an abdominoperineal excision of the rectum and anterior resection of the rectum, followed by a restoration procedure of bowel continuity.

Another type of procedures, performed only in some cases of rectal cancer, usually the complicated ones, is the so-called Hartmann's procedures: resection of the sigmoid and rectum along with the tumor, followed by a terminal colostomy and closure of the rectal stump; the bowel continuity could be restored in some cases, several months later.

It is obvious that the second objective in rectal cancer could be achieved only through a rectal resection that maintains distal part of the rectum and the anus; in these cases the continuity of the digestive tract could be obtained through a colorectal anastomosis or a coloanal anastomosis, with or without a reservoir. A better quality of life is to be expected after rectal resection with continuity restoration, but this is not always the case, and anyway, this must not interfere with the patient's chance for cure [27,28].

As already mentioned, a rectal resection for cancer must include the lymphatic territory that drains the tumor, in order to ensure the best possible local control; in rectal cancer, in order to obtain this objective is mandatory to perform a *mesorectal excision*; to complete the lymph node excision it is sometimes necessary to perform high ligation of the primary feeding vessel at the origin of the inferior mesenteric artery, and sometimes to perform a lateral pelvic dissection, but these aspects will be discussed latter in this chapter.

Mesorectal Excision

The mesorectum was first described by Heald in 1981 as the lymphovascular, fatty and neural perirectal tissue; dissecting in the exact vascular plan, it is possible to remove pelvic visceral fascia intact, along with mesorectal tissue, also the parietal pelvic fascia remaining intact [30].

In the mesorectal tissue, Heald was the first who described deposits of tumoral cells, independent of the lymph nodes, distal to the rectal tumor, thus becoming a possible source of local recurrence; therefore, the technique of mesorectal excision was developed, and led to a dramatically decrease of local recurrences after a curative rectal cancer resection, to 6% at 5 years and 8% at 10 years after a curative resection [30,31].

The same study was one of the first which described better results in terms of local recurrences after an anterior resection (5% at 5 years) when compared with abdominoperineal resection (17% recurrence rate at 5 years and 36% at ten years) [31].

The mesorectum starts at the sacral promontory, where the superior hemorrhoidal vessel divides into the right and left branches, then tapers and diminishes below the Waldayer's fascia, around the levator ani muscles. Later studies have demonstrated that it is not always necessary to remove the entire mesorectum, a 4 cm length below the inferior margin of the tumor being sufficient [27,29].

This means that for the cancers located in the upper rectum only a partial mesorectal excision is necessary, while for the mid-lower rectal cancers the total mesorectal excision technique, as described by Heald, is mandatory to be performed.

The value of total mesorectal excision in rectal cancer was confirmed afterwards by other numerous studies, all of them showing a better locoregional control achieved using this technique.

In the study performed by Tocchi et al., the recurrence rate was 9% after a 68.9 month mean period of follow-up; none of the patients received neoadjuvant treatment. The same study confirmed the existence of non-nodal metastasis in the mesorectum, in 24 out of 53 consecutive cases, which emphasizes the value of a correct mesorectal excision technique [32].

The main issue that has been brought into question regarding the total mesorectal excision technique was the increased length of operative time; the average time reported by Heald for a complete mesorectal excision was initially of four hours; yet, the study of Tocchi showed a reduction in the operative time at a mean period of 156 minutes. Thus, the length operative time inconvenient was surpassed; there also become more evident other major advantages of the total mesorectal excision technique: the dissection is performed into an areolar avascular plan, an increased rate of resections followed by anastomosis, compared to the classic approach, the possibility to avoid hypogastric nerve damage, thus maintaining a better genital and urinary postoperative function [31,32].

In a study published in 1992 [33], Heald reaffirmed the validity of the initial results of total mesorectal excision, in terms of local recurrence rates: a 2.6% rate of local recurrence, with a cumulative risk of local recurrence at 5 years of only 3.5%, with surgery alone; therefore, he concluded that preoperative radiotherapy, and even chemotherapy may be unjustified in such lower rate of recurrences.

Another important aspect of the study was that of the distal mural spread of rectal cancer, which rarely exceeded 1 cm; thus, an important percent of cases may benefit from a rectal resection followed by anastomosis, and it was necessary to perform an abdominoperineal resection in only 9.8% of the cases [33].

A very similar report was made by Brenann et al.; analysis of the available literature at that time (2002) clearly demonstrated the lower rate of local recurrence obtained through the total mesorectal excision technique alone (without neoadjuvant radiation therapy), and also an increased number of rectal resections with colorectal or coloanal anastomosis [34].

In a more recent study, Andreoni et al. have evaluated the surgical morbidity and long-term results in colorectal cancer, over 10 years period. Among 406 rectal cancers the authors performed 18% abdominoperineal resection and 2.9% local excisions; in this study also neoadjuvant radiation therapy was used in high risk cases (T3, T4 or N+ cases), but it was not clearly demonstrated the benefit of neoadjuvant over postoperative radiation therapy in terms of overall survival. Local recurrence rate after rectal cancer resection in this study was 10.8%. Overall morbidity after rectal cancer surgical treatment was 37.2%, with anastomotic leakage present in 10.4% of cases [35].

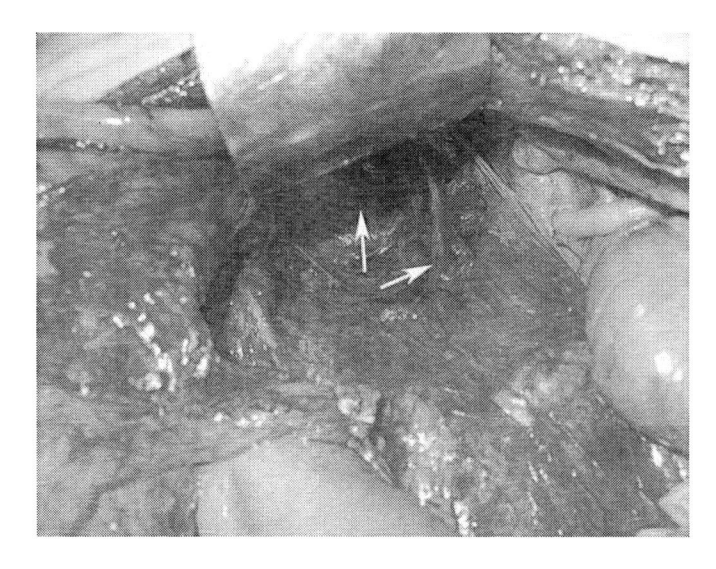

Figure 5. Retrorectal areolar space after mesorectal excision; is visible the right hipogastric nerve (upper arrow) and also, the shiny surface of mesorectal fascia (lower arrow) (intraoperative aspect).

The main advantage, in terms of oncologic results, offered by the total mesorectal excision, as presented by Heald, is that of permitting a much better clearance and analysis of radial margins of clearance in rectal cancer; it has already been demonstrated that involved radial margins, or even "close" radial margin correlates with poorer prognosis and a high recurrence rate after surgical treatment of rectal cancer [36].

In fact, the involvement of radial resection margins represents a very important predictive factor of locoregional recurrence after rectal surgery.

The rate of radial resection margin involvement varies between 12-25% of the cases; the risk of local recurrence in cases of involved radial resection margin is significantly higher than in cases without it [36]. Therefore, these patients need more postoperative oncologic approach.

In case of mesorectal tumor invasion, in T3 rectal cancer patients, the deeper the invasion is, the greater the risk of local recurrence is (when the tumor invasion in the mesorectum exceeds 7-8 mm). Also, mesorectal invasion by a T3 rectal tumor over 6 mm correlates with significant decrease in 5-years overall survival: 37-50% overall survival when the tumor invades the mesorectum more than 6 mm, compared to 59-72% 5-year overall survival in case of less than 6 mm invasion [37].

As a consequence, the quality of surgical mesorectal excision and a careful pathologic assessment of the specimen have an important role in establishing the need for adjuvant treatment, and in the patient's prognosis.

For the assessment of the quality of mesorectal excision a classification has been made, that contains three categories: complete mesorectal excision (intact mesorectum with minor irregularities, no defect lager than 5 mm, no coning, smooth circumferential margin on transverse slicing; nearly complete mesorectal excision (irregular surface of mesorectum, but no muscularis propria visible); incomplete mesorectal excision (defects down onto the muscularis propria, very irregular circumferential resection margin or marked coning). In the first case, the surgical excision is considered "good", in the second case, "moderate", and in the latter, "poor" [38,39].

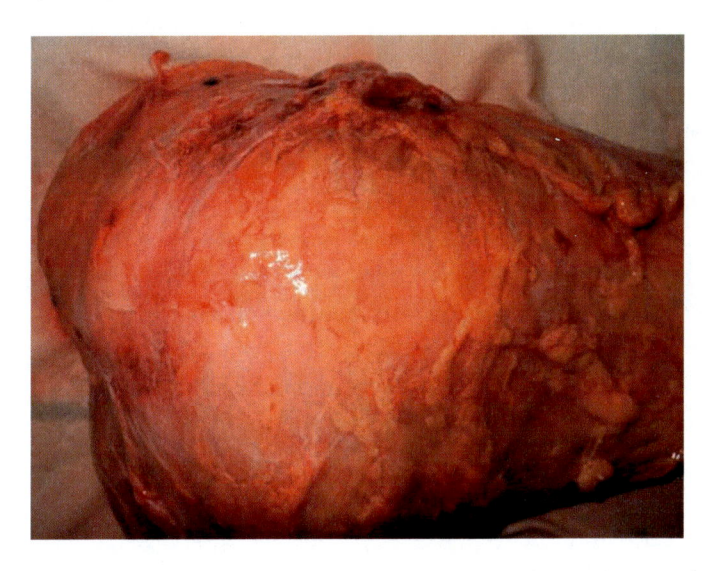

Figure 6. Rectal resection specimen with shiny mesorectal fascia attached to it (fresh resection specimen, macroscopic appearance).

The most important critique brought to total mesorectal excision technique is the increased anastomotic leakage compared to conventional rectal resection; all studies signal a percentage of 10.4-17% anastomotic failure, which led to an increased number of protective, defunctioning colostomies or ileostomies.

The most important cause of this risk of anastomotic failure after total mesorectal excision correlates with a grade of ischemia in the rectal anastomotic partner, but also, a pelvic haematoma or abscess draining spontaneously thorough anastomosis was advocated.

Other risk factors for postoperative anastomotic leakage were male gender, the level of the anastomosis (below 7 cm from the anal verge leads to an increased risk of leakage), and old age [41,42].

The presence of a defunctioning stoma reduces the clinical significance of anastomotic leakage and favors the closure of it, but remains the controversy of poor long-term results in patients with anastomotic failure after rectal cancer resection. In the study of Jung et al., the incidence of local recurrence rates in patients who developed postoperatively an anastomotic leakage was higher than in others (9.6 versus 2.2%), but it did not reach the statistical significance [41].

In a randomized multicenter trial Matthiessen et al., have been demonstrated that the presence of a defunctioning stoma after a rectal resection with total mesorectal excision (loop ileostomy or loop transversostomy) has had a good impact on outcome: a significant lower leakage rate (10.3 versus 28%), and a lower rate for urgent abdominal reoperation (8.6 versus 25.4%) in patients with defunctioning stoma [42].

In order to reduce the need of a second operation for stoma-closure, Tschmelitsch et al., have performed a study that demonstrated the feasibility of tube-cecostomy in protecting low rectal anastomosis; they obtain the similar rate of postoperative complications with loop ileostomy or loop colostomy, but a reduced number of reoperation needed for stoma closure, and a shorter hospital stay [43].

The local control in rectal cancer seems to be significantly improved with a protocol of preoperative irradiation, such as that proposed by the Swedish rectal cancer trial. In one study, Kapitejin et al., have demonstrated a significant decrease in local recurrence, at 2 years, if rectal resection with mesorectal excision is preceded by neoadjuvant irradiation (2.4% local recurrence in preoperative irradiated patients versus 8.2% if surgery was the only method of treatment), but there was no improvement in overall survival; the effect was also significant for mid and lower rectal tumors in stage II or III [44].

A more recent study of Folkesson et al., showed the same results, but after 13 years of follow-up a improvement in overall survival rate was noticed in irradiated rectal cancer patients: 38% versus 30% [45].

Therefore, even though total mesorectal excision improved local control, by decreasing the local recurrence rates, it seems that there is place for improvement for rectal cancer treatment.

According to Strassburg et al., using preoperative high-resolution MRI, the indication for preoperative radiotherapy may be established in high-risk cases, as follows: T4 tumors; mobile tumor in which MRI showes the tumor to be 1 mm or less from the mesorectal fascia (circumferential radial positive margins); tumors extending below the levator origin and infiltrating beyond the muscularis propria [39].

However, the need for preoperative radiotherapy must be very well weighted, since this is not a harmless procedure, especially on anal sphincter function, as revealed by the study of Hassan et al., and Gervaz et al.: internal anal sphincter permanent damage, with increased need for a reoperation and a permanent colostomy [46,47].

Types of Resections

The type of rectal resection performed in rectal cancer dependents on tumor topography on the rectal wall, tumor stage and patient's general status (age, co-morbidities, and life-span expectancy).

A tumor located in the upper rectum will generally be resolved with an anterior rectal resection followed by restoration of bowel continuity through a colorectal anastomosis.

Tumors located in the mid and lower rectum have the most difficult problems in terms of surgical intervention, restoration of continuity with respect to oncologic and functional outcomes: a lower local recurrence rate and a good long-distant survival rate, with as better as possible quality of life.

ABDOMINOPERINEAL EXCISION

Abdominoperineal excision was first developed by Miles one hundred years ago; for many years in the past century it was considered the gold standard in rectal cancer.

In the latest years, the development of total mesorectal technique by Heald had an important impact on diminishing the rate of abdominoperineal resections, in conjunction with the development of the stapling devices, neoadjuvant treatment (this also has no conclusive results on sphincter preservation, as mentioned above). Another important factor was ascertained by rare distal spread beyond 1 cm from the lowest tumor edge through the rectal wall, but more frequent and more distal spread within the mesorectum [27,29,48].

As a consequence, the number of abdominoperineal resections decreased significantly over the last years, as it is demonstrated by numerous studies in Europe, England, and United States [49,50].

The study of Tilney et al. has shown a decreased in abdominoperineal resection incidence between 1996 to 2004, from 29.4% to 21.2%, significant statistically; in the study of Nagtegaal et al., the incidence of abdominoperineal excision was 30.6%, and it included patients randomized to neoadjuvant radiotherapy protocol [49,50].

These decreases in incidence were stimulated by the low quality of life after abdominoperineal resection, mainly due to the permanent colostomy, but other specific complications may also occur, such as an increased percent of urinary and sexual dysfunctions, an increased incidence of postoperative bowel obstruction and perineal wound related complications [51].

Some studies have shown an increased morbidity and mortality after abdominoperineal resection when compared to anterior resection, but the most surprisingly observation is that abdominoperineal resection has a higher incidence of local recurrence (22.3% versus 13.5%) and a lower survival rates (52.3% versus 65.8%) than modern anterior resection, though this was not demonstrated by all studies [49,50,52].

Thus, the study of Chiappa et al., showed a higher incidence in local recurrence for double stapling technique versus abdominoperineal excision (25% versus 5%), but no significant difference in overall survival [53].

Di Betta et al., have shown in their review no difference in terms of local control and survival between the abdominoperineal resection and low anterior resection for distal rectal cancer, and they also noticed no difference in terms of postoperative morbidity and mortality between those two procedures. They concluded that sphincter saving resection may be the standard procedure for low rectal cancer [54].

Nakagoe et al., in their multivariate analysis, did not find a significant difference between low anterior resection and abdominoperineal resection for distal rectal cancer, with regard to local recurrence (9.5% versus 10.3%) and 5-years disease specific survival rates (78.3% versus 71.5%); still, an increased number of recurrences were found after abdominoperineal excision, and a shorter 5-year disease free survival [55].

These facts could be explained partially through a greater proportion of lymphatic invasion, and a higher number of cases with more advanced depth of penetration in the group of abdominoperineal excision, but also by the extended lateral lymphadenectomy performed in stage III of disease [55].

Considered for many years the most radical surgical procedure in rectal cancer, surprisingly, with the development of total mesorectal excision, the abdominoperineal excision of the rectum not only decreased in incidence, but has also proved to be inferior to low rectal excision in terms of circumferential margin involvement and oncologic outcome.

In the abdominoperineal excision, the incidence of positive circumferential margin was significantly higher in the study of Nagtegaal et al. (26.5% versus 12.6%), and the study of Marr et al. (41% versus 12%) [50,52].

This fact may have several reasons: a better mesorectal excision in anterior resection, difficulties in mesorectal excision at the lower level of the levator ani, more advanced tumor in which abdominoperineal excision is attempted, or a different way of lymphatic spread for cancer of the lower third of the rectum.

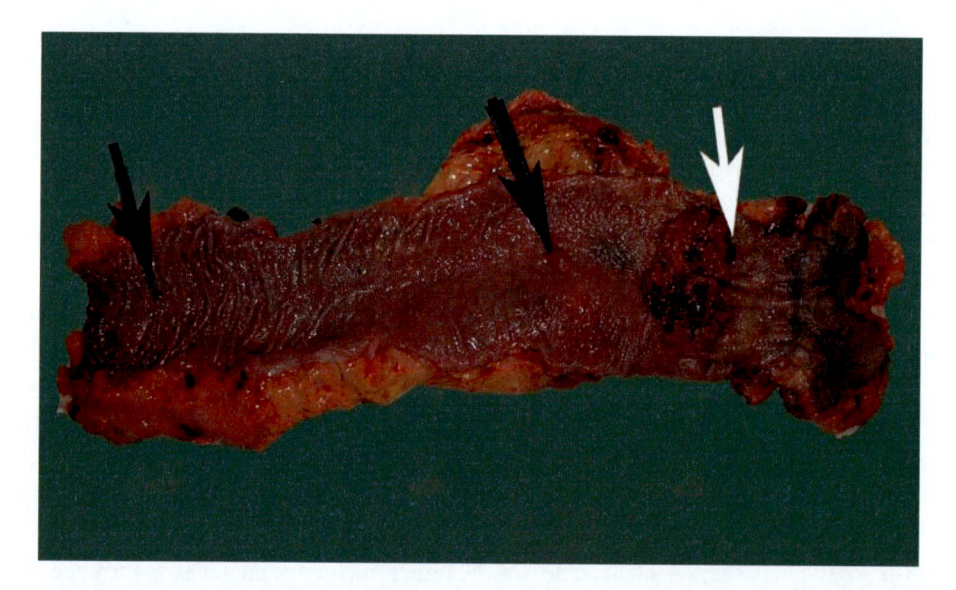

Figure 7. A too lower rectal cancer, just above the anal sphincter, in order to perform a sphincter-preservation resection. White arrow shows the limit between lower edge of tumor and anal sphincter; black arrows show small polyps on the resection specimen. (fresh specimen, macroscopic appearance).

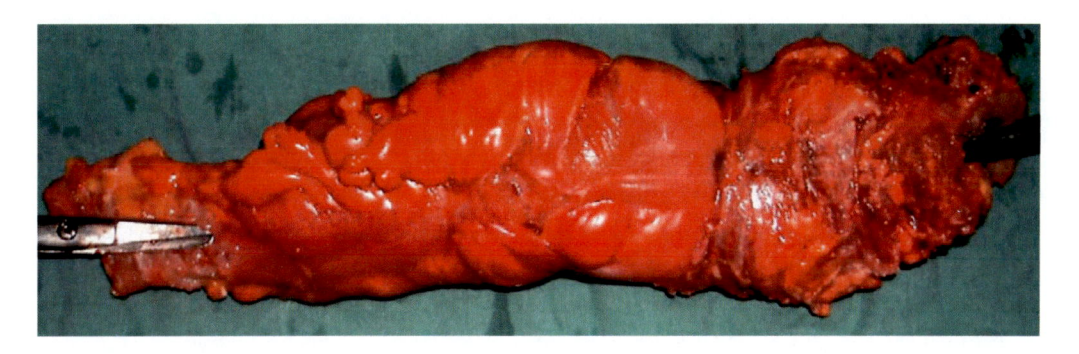

Figure 8. A resection specimen after abdominoperineal excision of the rectum (fresh specimen).

Regarding these reasons, a concern is raised by the results of abdominoperineal excision, since an important number of cases of rectal cancer will continue to be treated through this procedure; this is especially the case of a too lower rectal cancer to permit at least 1 cm distal uninvolved margin, even after a careful dissection of the mesorectum, and for the cancers that invade the anal sphincter or to bulky to permit subtumoral resection at a convenient level of oncologic certainty, especially in men with narrow pelvis.

An assessment of the quality of abdominoperineal resection with regard to the levator ani and anal canal must differentiate grade 3 (complete: parts of the levator ani resected over the entire circumference), grade 2 (moderate: resection line at the muscularis propria, no parts of the levator ani included on the specimen), and grade 1 (poor: parts of the muscularis propria are absent from the specimen or iatrogenic perforation of the tumor) [39].

The complete grade of resection must be achieved through an extended dissection to include a circumferential portion of the levator ani, fat of the ischiorectal fossa, as in the originally described Miles procedure, but also through a better surgical training and rectal cancer surgery specialization [50,52].

ANTERIOR RESECTIONS OF THE RECTUM

The first attempt to perform an anastomosis between colon and rectal stump after resection for rectal cancer was made by Kraske, who described the transsacral approach; the subsequent faecal fistula formation was difficult to close and make the quality of the patient's life even lower than after a colostomy [27,28].

The "father" of modern anterior resection technique with colorectal anastomosis was Dixon (1939, 1940), who demonstrated that an anastomosis after a rectal resection is feasible through abdominal approach [27,28].

At the beginning, at least 5-6 cm macroscopic healthy tissue distal to cancer was considered necessary in order to achieve a good oncologic outcome; still, with new research, that proved a distal mural invasion is less than 2 cm for most rectal cancers, and with developing of total mesorectal excision and stapling devices, the number of anterior resection increased significantly. Thus, nowadays, anterior resection with colorectal or coloanal anastomosis may be achieved in over two thirds of rectal cancer resections.

The distance from lower edge of tumor to the excision margin of the specimen is recommended to be measured on fresh specimen, immediately after resection, through eversion and not section of the specimen, in order to allow to pathologist the possibility to assess the circumferential resection margin.

The results seem to be similar, or even better, to those obtained through abdominoperineal excision, in terms of oncologic outcome, but the quality of life is much better in the anterior resection group, as it has already been demonstrated [33,35,48-55].

Once trust in colorectal or coloanal anastomosis has been gained, other problems have been raised, regarding especially low anterior resection (below the peritoneal reflection): which is the best method to ensure the best results in terms of postoperative morbidity, oncologic outcome, and also the best functional results.

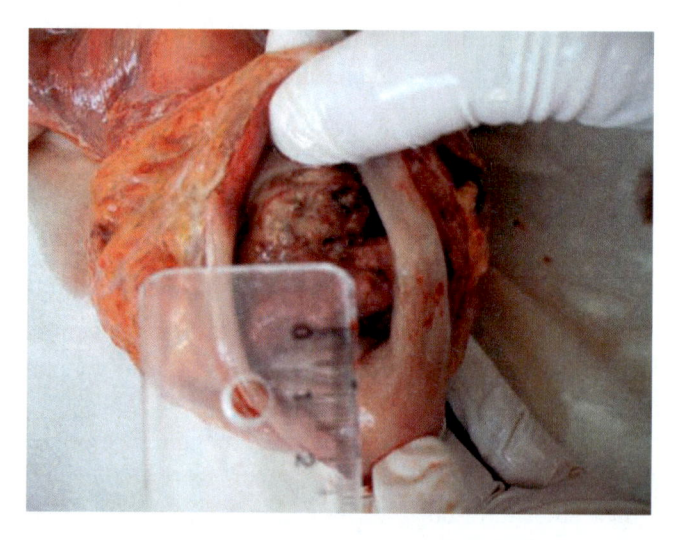

Figure 9. Everted tumor and 2 cm security margin between the lower edge of the tumor and margin of the resection specimen.

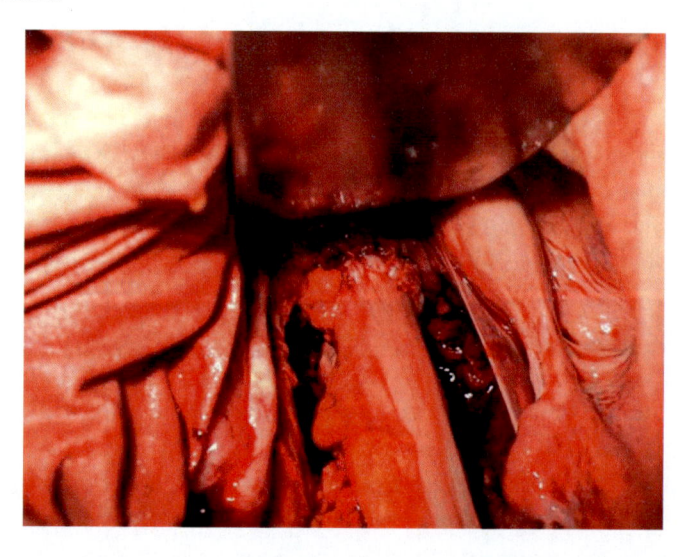

Figure 10. A low colorectal anastomosis after a low rectal resection for cancer, hand-sutured (intraoperative detail).

As it has already been discussed, the rate of anastomotic failure is much higher in low colorectal or coloanal anastomosis than in the conventional one; risk factors and modality of solving these problems has already been exposed.

In terms of oncologic outcomes it seems that it is no difference in local recurrence rate and cancer specific survival among the colorectal anastomosis and coloanal anastomosis, with or without reservoir, if an adequate distal resection margin is granted [56].

There are also no significant differences between hand-sewn versus stapled colorectal anastomosis, but usage of the stapling devices allows a much easier and a much lower anastomosis, even in men with narrow pelvis.

In terms of functional outcome, there is an important aspect to be discussed: regardless of the type of anastomosis (an end-to-end or side-to-end colorectal or coloanal anastomosis, or anastomosis with reservoir), a damaged anal sphincter (preoperatively or in the course of surgical intervention, or through the radiation therapy) will lead to a poor quality of life, even compared to a permanent colostomy, after abdominoperineal excision. Therefore, when a preoperative dysfunction of the anal sphincter is suspected, a manometry test should be obtained, and, if results are unsatisfactorily, the abdominoperineal resection could be a better alternative to a postoperative anal incontinence. The same is valid for those cases in which dissection process may result in sphincter damage, and the same outcome is to be expected. With these condition submitted numerous studies have tried to analyze the best method to achieve a good functional outcome in terms of postoperative continence, urgency, bowel movements.

Oya et al., have demonstrated through a scintigraphic assessment that poor neorectal evacuation is a cause of impaired defecatory function after low anterior resection with straight colorectal anastomosis; the same situation is in the case of reconstruction, using a colonic J pouch (the bigger the J-pouch is the severe is defecatory impairment) [57]. The defecatory impairment has two possible reasons: limitations in rectal motility due to perirectal fibrosis, after mesorectal dissection, or hypogastric nerve damage [57].

A very good functional result in terms of functional outcome was obtained by Berger et al. with a coloanal anastomosis with colonic reservoir, 7 cm long, with satisfactory continence in 96% of patients after one year. Postoperative morbidity and mortality were similar to the anterior resection with straight anastomosis; the main problem of this type of reconstruction was represented by the evacuating difficulties, but that was relatively easy to solve with an evacuating suppository or a small enema [58].

The same favorable results were obtained by Hida et al. when they compared colonic J-pouch with straight coloanal anastomosis; at five years patients in the J-pouch group had fewer bowel movements, less urgency, and less soiling than those in the straight anastomosis group [59].

When they compared colonic J-pouch to a side-to-end anastomosis after low rectal resection, the results were very similar after 6 months, with no difference in continence status; a slight tendency to constipation was noticed in colonic J-pouch group, while a higher stool frequency was observed in the side-to-end group for the first six months [59].

A superiority of a colonic J-pouch over the straight coloanal anastomosis, or even over a coloplasty has been demonstrated by the randomized study of Fazio et al.; in terms of functional outcome, the colonic J-pouch was superior to coloplasty at 24 months, with fewer bowel movements, less clustering, fewer pad usage, and a lower fecal incontinence severity index. On the other hand, coloplasty did not seem superior to a straight anastomosis in terms of functional outcome [61].

Sometimes, in advanced stages, after a neoadjuvant chemoradiation protocol, it is possible to downsize the tumor, and perform a R0 anal sphincter preserving resection, as suggested in some studies. However, in these advanced cases, sphincter-preservation does not really represent an objective for the chemoradiation protocol, the real objective being always the oncologic one (to downstage or downsize the tumor in order to achieve a curative resection) [62,63].

There are several protocols, but to draw a conclusion after a limited number of articles it may be hasty; larger, prospective randomized trials, with an established objective of sphincter-preservation resections are necessary to be employed.

HARTMANN'S PROCEDURE

There are several situations in which it is not possible to perform a sphincter-preserving surgery, neither an abdominoperineal excision: [27]
- occlusive rectal tumors with severe comorbidities or in advanced stage of disease, making the anastomosis to risky;
- perforated rectal carcinoma, in which to perform a resection to remove the source of contamination of peritoneal cavity is mandatory, but an anastomosis is largely contraindicated;
- palliation in locally advanced tumor or advanced stages of cancer (inoperable metastasis), in which resection is expected to be followed by a local recurrence in short time; performing an abdominoperineal excision is far too excessively in these cases, and also if possible to construct an anastomosis, this could be comprised by the recurrence in short time.

In all these situations, Hartmann's procedure is the "ideal" choice because it assures primary tumor removal (and palliation of symptoms related to it), but avoids an anastomosis, source of almost sure severe postoperative complications.

The rectal stump is usually closed with suture (manually or with stapler device), but sometimes may be left open, with a drain within, exteriorized transanally.

In some cases (in which Hartmann's procedure were employed for an occlusive or perforated cancer, but otherwise in an acceptable stage of disease), 6 months or a year later, the colostomy may be undone, and an anastomosis performed [27].

EXTENDED RESECTIONS

It is now well established that, in a fitted patient, a rectal cancer invading a neighboring organ, without distant metastasis may safely be resected with excellent surgical and oncological outcome. Many studies have been made the object of such attitude [64-68].

Even if the cancer did not really invade the adjacent organ, the resection is preferable to dissection between invaded organs because of the risk of tumor dissemination; en block resection to achieve negative resection margin is mandatory to be performed even if the real percentage of cancer invasion varies between 40-70% [64-68].

Usually, a preoperative chemoradiation protocol is performed for these locally advanced cancers (T4 rectal cancer) in an attempt to downsize the tumor and achieve a better local control [66].

From the surgical point of view, the high ligation of inferior mesenteric artery is recommended because of the large number of lymph node involvement in these advanced cases (57-66.7%, and 18% of lateral lymph node involvement) [64,67].

Frequently, the involved organ is bladder in men and internal genitalia in women; if an en block rectal resection with resection of internal female genitalia could be performed safely by any well trained surgeon, removal of the bladder and especially reconstruction recommend close collaboration with an urologist.

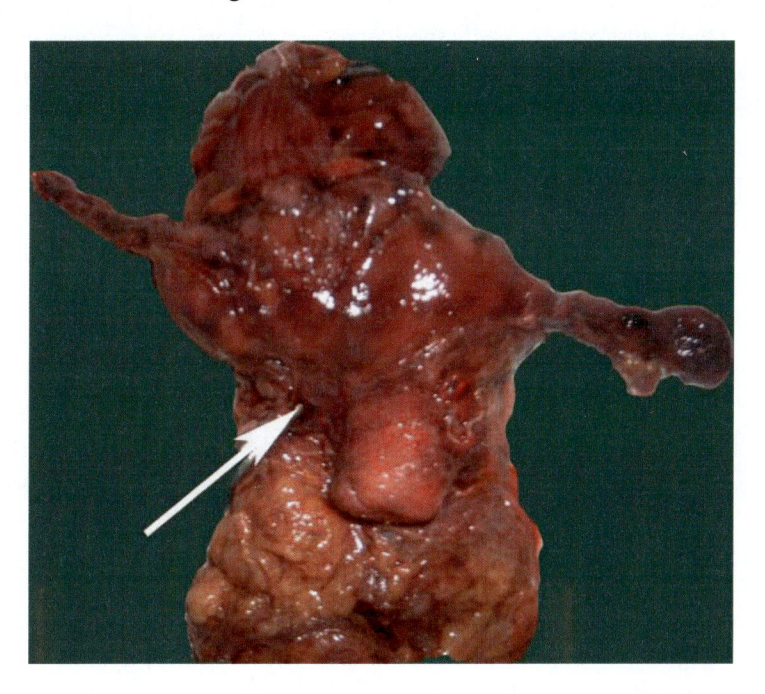

Figure 11. En block resection of the rectum and the uterus imposed by tumor adherence (white arrow).

If bladder is only partially involved, outside the trigonal area, a partial cystectomy, performed at the beginning of rectal resection could be performed in order to achieve negative resection margin [63-65].

Involvement of the trigonal area imposes a more aggressive approach, in these cases a pelvic exenteration being the procedure of choice, in selected cases [65,67,68].

Practically, there is no controversy in establishing the indication for multiorgan resection in locally advanced rectal cancer, it only has to be emphasized that a highly trained surgeon in pelvic reconstruction techniques and close collaboration between different specialties is mandatory to achieve the best results in terms of postoperative morbidity and mortality, and oncologic outcome.

The locally recurrent rates varies between 21.6% to 40%, and overall 5-year survival could reach 44-57%, which along to an acceptable rate of postoperative morbidity (27-54%) and mortality (1-4%) have been imposed multiorgan resection and even pelvic exenteration as the unique therapeutic procedure that gives to such patients a chance for cure [63-68].

LAPAROSCOPIC APPROACH IN RECTAL CANCER

Minimally, invasive surgery gained a well motivated popularity over the past twenty years, becoming the gold standard for cholecistectomy and antireflux surgery; yet, even the first laparoscopic colectomy has been performed in 1991, the laparoscopic approach for large bowel cancer has not become much more popular since then.

Laparoscopic approach in rectal cancer remains only a second choice, for selected cases, gold standard for the moment being considered open surgery.

Still, more and more surgeons trained in both open rectal cancer surgery and laparoscopic surgery become aware of the advantages of laparoscopic approach in rectal cancer, and more and more studies are published with the objective of defining the role of miniinvasive approach in rectal cancer.

A review performed by the Lourenco et al,. has extracted some points of debate from literature: laparoscopic approach in rectal cancer has the same advantages over the classic surgery, with less blood loss during the surgery, less postoperative pain and shorter hospital stay, more rapid return to usual activities. The results are similar in terms of postoperative morbidity and mortality, and the quality of life between laparoscopic and open surgery for rectal cancer is quite similar [69].

There were some concerns about the oncologic outcome of this procedure, but the same analysis has demonstrated comparative results with open surgery in terms of local recurrence, overall survival, and disease free survival [69,70].

In terms of oncologic results, there are some problems related to the possibility to perform a correct resection of the mesorectum, and the number of lymph nodes retrieved after laparoscopic surgery; the same study, and others, have shown that with adequate training and experience the mesorectum may be safely resected, and the number of lymph node retrieved are similar to open surgery [69-73].

Laparoscopic resections for rectal cancer, nevertheless, present some specific problems, that the surgeon must surpass in order to achieve similar results with open surgery.

One of the problems is training in laparoscopic colorectal surgery which represents an advanced laparoscopic technique, accessible only for well trained surgeons in open rectal cancer surgery and in laparoscopic techniques.

A greater duration of the laparoscopic operation, with subsequent influences on immune response, was a frequent reproof (a mean operating time of 240-278 minutes). Nevertheless, it has to be mentioned that a good total mesorectal excision in open surgery necessitates at least the same time (at the beginning of the total mesorectal excision technique over 4 hours were necessary to perform the resection!). Therefore, we could say that in terms of operative time, open surgery and laparoscopic rectal surgery are very similar, without a significant difference [69,71].

Another problem concerning laparoscopic rectal resection is related to the narrow operative field, especially in men with obese infiltration of the mesentery that obstructs the access to the pelvis. With good training and a good preoperative bowel preparation, the operative field may become acceptable, and the laparoscopic operation could be performed. However, greater difficulties must be expected when the stapling device must be inserted, in order to transect the rectum below the tumor, and then when performing the anastomosis [69,70].

With regard to these last aspects, concerns may arise related to distal margin clearance in laparoscopic resection for rectal cancer; in this problem, and even more important than narrow operative field, there is the impossibility to palpate the tumor and its lower edge; a rigid rectoscopic exploration on the operating table before and during the operation (just before the time of distal rectal transaction), and marking with clips the lower edge of tumor will permit an oncologic and surgical safe distal resection [70].

Another problem in laparoscopic resection for rectal cancer concerns the circumferential margin, which was found involved in some studies, after pathologic examination; this fact could lead to an increased rate of local recurrences. Nevertheless, local recurrence rate has proved to be similar between laparoscopic and open surgery [70-73].

In the study performed by Bianchi et al., the local recurrence rate, after a mean follow-up period of 35.8 months, was only of 0.95 (one local recurrence out of 107 laparoscopic resection for rectal cancer); 5-year survival rates and disease free survival were estimated to 81.4% and 79.8% [70].

Naitoh et al., found a 95.7% survival rate and 80.3% disease free survival rate in their study about rectal cancer, but they did not analyze separately the local recurrence rate after laparoscopic rectal resection [72].

Nakamura et al., in their comparative study between open and laparoscopic resection for rectal and rectosigmoid cancers, found no differences in terms of local recurrence rates, with a recurrence-free survival rate of 96.7% in laparoscopic resection versus 82.4% in open surgery; cumulative 5-year survival rates were 91.6% in laparoscopic group and 92.7% in open surgery group (no significant difference) [71].

The results of laparoscopic resection are encouraging, and with development of the new stapling and transecting devices, miniinvasive approach may become more often offered to patients; some restriction will still remain related to some contraindications for laparoscopic surgery in rectal cancer: locally advanced lesions, invading the adjacent organs, general contraindication for laparoscopic approach, previous major pelvic surgery, and especially previous sepsis or peritonitis involving the pelvis [27].

SURGERY ADDRESSED TO LYMPH NODES IN RECTAL CANCER – IMPLICATIONS

The importance of nodal involvement in rectal cancer was demonstrated for the first time by Dukes, who included all cases with nodal involvement by a rectal cancer as a separate category from tumoral mural invasion: C stage.

Since then, the staging system in rectal cancer has proved to be a dynamic and complex one, with multiple changes over time, changes that tried to adapt to clinical and pathological necessity.

Over time it has been demonstrated that the involvement of lymph nodes correlates with a poorer prognostic, lymphatic invasion by cancer being the most important predictive factor of recurrence and poor survival; as an argument, 5-year survival in rectal cancer without nodal involvement exceed 75-80%, while with nodal involvement 5-year survival drops to below 50%.

Recently, AJCC adapted its TNM classification according to the new discoveries in the field of rectal cancer nodal involvement in three subcategories, which independently correlates with the patient's prognosis: [75, 76]

- stage IIIA is represented by tumor confined to the rectal wall (T1 or T2) with limited nodal involvement (below three lymph nodes invaded), which correlates with a relatively good prognosis (59.8% 5-year survival);
- stage IIIB means tumor extended through the rectal wall into the perirectal tissue (T3) or directly adhere or invade adjacent organs (T4), also with limited nodal involvement (below three lymph nodes invaded), which correlates with a poorer prognosis (42% 5-year survival);
- stage IIIC is the worst, with cancer invading more than three lymph nodes, regardless of primary tumor depth of penetration through the rectal wall, with a survival of only 27.3% at 5-years.[76]

In order to assure the best possible postoperative staging, an accurate and complete pathologic evaluation must be performed; for the moment, the only pathologic accepted technique is hematoxilin-eosin staining of lymph node, the significance of micrometastasis, detected with more advanced techniques such as imunohistochemistry or polymerase chain reaction, being insufficient established [75,76].

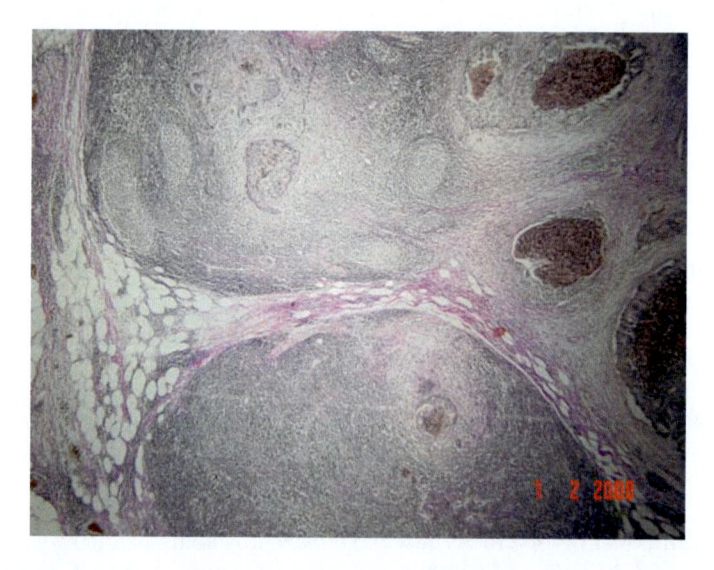

Figure 12. Pathologic evaluation of invaded lymph nodes: metastasis (upper node) and micrometastasis (lower lymph node) from a rectal cancer (Van Gieson staining, 100x).

Over the last ten years, many debates were about the number of lymph nodes necessary to be examined in order to define non-nodal involvement, thus classifying a stage I or II [74-83].

Yoshimatsu et al., have found that if less than 9 lymph nodes were examined in a presumable Dukes B stage, cumulative 5-year survival was similar to Dukes C stage, while in more than 9 lymph nodes examined group, cumulative 5-years survival was significantly better (86.7% versus 66.7%) [78].

However, with the new AJCC classification, a number of at least 12 lymph nodes are mandatory to be examined, which has been proved by many articles as sufficient to avoid understaging; moreover, if this number of lymph nodes examined could not be accomplished, the patient must be considered at risk for residual disease and, therefore, must follow a postoperative chemoradiation protocol [29,74-83].

There are many factors that affect the number of lymph nodes harvested and pathologically examined; one of the most important is the quality of surgery, being known that the surgeon dedicated to rectal cancer treatment is able to retrieve more lymph nodes on the resection specimen (on reverse, the number of lymph node resected is a measure of the quality of surgical department). The same finding is available also for the pathologist (a rectal cancer study dedicated one will seek and analyze much more lymph nodes on the resected specimen than the usual) [81].

Horzic and Kopljar have found in their study that in multiple regression analysis male gender, better tumor differentiation and bigger tumor size, and the presence of acute inflammation were independent predictors of the increased number of lymph node examined, but the report was not confirmed by others [79].

Wijesuriya et al., have demonstrated in their study that neoadjuvant therapy may be responsible in rectal cancer by the reduced number in lymph nodes examined; the median number of lymph nodes examined in the neoadjuvant group was 4 versus 9 in non-preoperatively treated patients. This may be explained through a decrease in nodal size after neoadjuvant chemoradiation, but more important, they raise an important problem related to the real effect of preoperative neoadjuvant treatment: it really induces a down-staging, or is, actually, an under-staging determined by the significantly decrease in the number of lymph nodes examined? [77, 80]

An important factor, already mentioned, that influences the number of harvested lymph nodes in rectal cancer is nodal morphology: invaded lymph nodes have proved to be smaller than 5 mm in 50-70% of cases, and 90% of invaded lymph nodes are smaller than 1 cm. This might explain the difficulties in lymph node retrieval from an abundant, fatty infiltrated specimen, but also interfere with preoperative nodal evaluation (difficulties to detect such smaller lymph node with imagistic available methods) [77,81].

A population-based study, conducted by Baxter et al., between 1988 and 2001, revealed a concerning conclusion: only 37% of the patients received adequate lymph node evaluation, but the adequacy increased over time (from 32% in 1988 to 44% in 2001); in 6.5% of the patients no lymph node was pathologically assessed [81].

Advanced stage of disease, younger patients and poorly differentiated cancers were more likely to receive adequate lymph node analysis. Also, rectal topography correlates with a decreased number of lymph nodes examined, when compared to other colic sites [81,82].

Some studies suggested that at least 14 lymph nodes should be examined, in order to improve staging accuracy; however, it is recognized that the many lymph nodes retrieved and submitted to analysis from the pathological specimen, the better chance to improve the accuracy of staging [82].

There are several methods to improve lymph nodes retrieval from a rectal cancer resection specimen: extended lymphadenectomy in order to include more lymph nodes, fat-clearance technique, lymphatic mapping and sentinel node analysis. Out of these, fat-clearance has a well established benefit, but it is costly and time consuming, therefore it is applied only in some medical centers, and is not largely available [79,82].

A simple method seems to have been discovered by Märkl et al., which allow identification of more lymph nodes on the resection specimen, through the injection of methylene blue in the superior rectal artery, ex vivo. This permits to highlight the lymph nodes, and makes them visible for pathologist, increasing the number of lymph nodes retrieved to 27±7 versus 14±4 in the control group. The technique seems simple and easily applicable, but the results need further confirmation [83].

Lymphatic mapping and sentinel node analysis seem to be a promising technique in gastrointestinal neoplasm, as it was demonstrated in malignant melanoma and breast cancer. Injecting a radioactive tracer or a vital colorant in peritumoral rectal wall, this will migrate through the lymphatic channels into the lymph nodes, which become more easily identifiable and submitted to analysis [84,85].

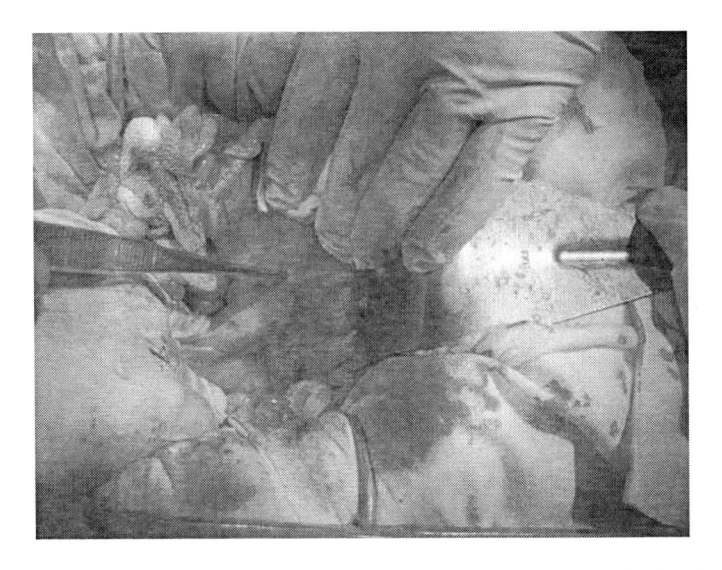

Figure 13. Lymphatic mapping in upper rectal cancer (the clamp show the sentinel node topography).

Sentinel lymph node is considered primary lymph node to which the tumor drains; also at the beginning, one lymph node was considered as sentinel node, in gastrointestinal neoplasm usually more lymph nodes become evident after the tracer was administered, and it is recommended for all to be submitted for pathologic analysis.

Initially, sentinel lymph node was considered as an alternative to lymphadenectomy (if sentinel node was negative on pathologic examination, lymphadenectomy became unnecessary, thus avoiding related complication).

However, this is not the case for colorectal cancers, in which resection techniques include lymph node excision; nevertheless, sentinel node technique may improve accuracy of nodal staging, and if negative, sentinel node may avoid extensive search for other lymph nodes: it may become unnecessary to analyze 12 or more lymph nodes since the chance for a positive node if sentinel node is negative, is less than 0.5-0.6% with a positive predictive value of 93-100% [84-86].

In case of positive sentinel node, it is necessary to search for a large number in order to establish the N grade (N1 – less than three lymph nodes involved or N2 – four or more lymph nodes involved).

Usually, sentinel node is detected after injecting a blue dye (isosulfan blue or methylene blue) subserosally, around the tumor, and expecting for 1 minute for tracer to diffuse through the lymph channels into the sentinel lymph node(s); this node is marked, and submits for conventional pathologic analysis. Imunohistochemistry staining can detect micrometastasis that escapes to conventional staining, but the significance of it remains to be established [84,85].

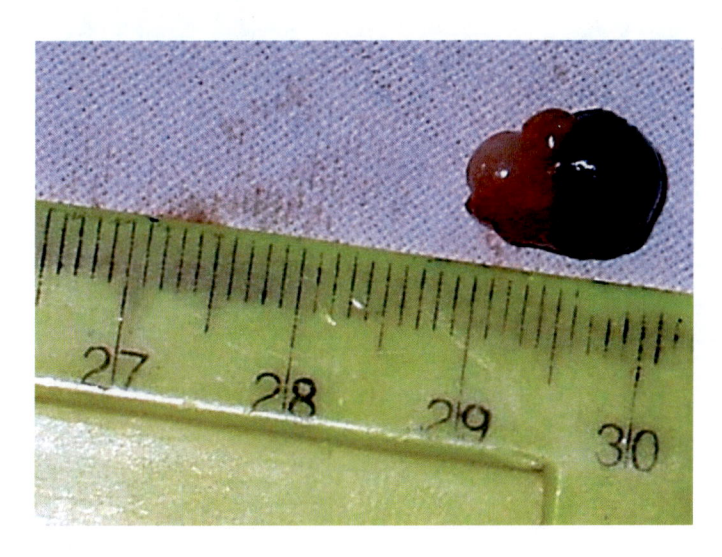

Figure 14. Blue methylene stained, 1 cm long sentinel node (postoperative fresh specimen).

In rectal cancers located below the peritoneal reflection, it is difficult to perform this technique without disruption of the peritoneum and because of the thickness of the mesorectum; a transanal approach with injection of the tracer submucosal around the tumor was less successful, with only 50% of nodal identification. Therefore, sentinel node technique in rectal cancer it is recommended to be approached with caution since standard resection includes mesorectal excision [85,86].

With in vivo technique being difficult to realize, ex vivo technique become more attractive; Baton et al. reported good results, with 97% feasibility, and a 13% upstaging rate [86].

Published articles, even though optimistic, do not permit to adopt yet any definitive conclusion on this matter.

In rectal cancer, the sentinel node may have another important role: to establish the indication for lateral pelvic dissection (extended lymphadenectomy).

A preliminary study trying to identify retroperitoneal and lateral pelvic lymph nodes susceptible to be invaded by rectal cancer, has failed to detect with accuracy the sentinel node [87].

The study of Funahashi permits identification of two major lymphatic spread ways: upwards, through the mesorectum, and along superior rectal artery and inferior mesenteric artery, and laterally, towards lateral pelvic wall, with a percentage of metastasis of 13% in lateral pelvic nodes [88].

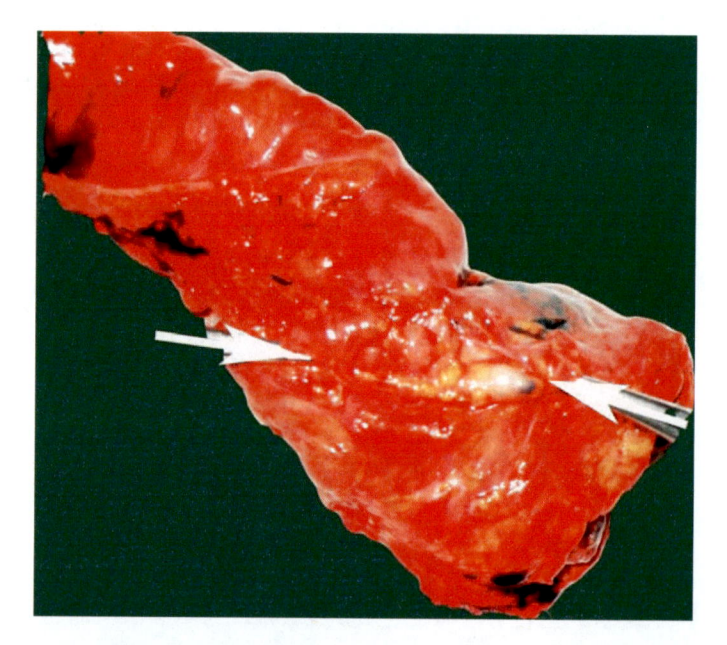

Figure 15. Ex vivo sentinel lymph nodes (fresh resection specimen) (arrows indicate the site of at least two lymph nodes stained with blue methylene).

The importance of this conclusion is the fact that these lateral pelvic nodes do not enter in the field of usual rectal resection with mesorectal excision, thus, an important number of patients with presumably curative resections being left with residual nodal disease; the consequence is the high risk of locoregional recurrence with the origin in those lymph nodes.

Kim et al., have evaluated the risk of locoregional recurrence due to lateral pelvic nodes involvement, after rectal resection with total mesorectal excision and neoadjuvant treatment, in advanced lower rectal cancers. They found that 82.7% of recurrences were determined by the lateral pelvic node involvement; 41.6% of these cases had no distant metastasis, therefore, an extended lateral pelvic dissection had been curative for these patients [89].

A benefit for some patients submitted to lateral pelvic dissection was also reported by the Shiozawa et al.; in their study 33.3% of the patients submitted to lateral pelvic dissection in advanced lower rectal cancer had lateral lymph node metastasis, yet they remain disease-free at 5 years. Even though, the local recurrence rate and disease free survival did not differ between patients who underwent pelvic dissection and those who did not [90].

The same lack of benefit in terms of disease free survival and recurrence rate at 5 years, between patients who underwent and those that did not underwent extended pelvic dissection, was found out by Hasdemir et al., in their study [91].

The most fervent sustainers of lateral pelvic dissection are Asian researchers (from Japan, China and Korea), who reported better results with this approach in rectal cancer [92-95].

Sugihara et al., found a significantly increased incidence of lateral lymph node involvement in females, lower rectal cancers, high grade cancers, T3-T4 tumors with over 4 cm diameter. The incidence of lateral nodal involvement in these cases varies between 13.9% and 23.5% (in case of mesorectal involvement the percentage of lateral lymph node involvement reaches the maximum value). In case of positive lateral nodal involvement, the most beneficial were cases in stage II, while in stage III of disease, the lateral node-positive patients had a worse prognosis (5-year survival rate of 45.8% in case of positive lateral lymph nodes, versus 71.2% in node negative cases) [92].

The same optimistic results are published by Dong et al.; they found an incidence of 11% lateral pelvic nodal involvement, and the 5-year and 10-year survival rate after extended resection (including lateral pelvic nodes, second and third upper groups) was significantly better (68% and 47%) after extended resection, when compared to conventional surgery (42.9% and 25.3% respectively) [93].

Wu et al., found a 14.6% incidence of lateral node metastasis in advanced lower rectal carcinoma, but the incidence rose to 30% in poorly differentiated carcinomas. The recurrence rate was significantly higher in node-positive group (64.3% in node-positive group versus 11% in node-negative group). Therefore, positive lateral lymph node found during extensive nodal dissection has a great impact on local recurrence in advanced lower rectal cancer [94].

Ueno et al., found 17% incidence of lateral lymph node involvement in advanced lower rectal cancer; the 5-year survival rate in patients having positive lateral lymph nodes was 41.6%. The most suggestive risk factor for lateral lymph node involvement was nodal diameter, over 5 mm (16.1%), and especially over 10 mm (34% nodal involvement).

This observation may be a starting point for the indication of lateral pelvic dissection in cases in which such enlarged lymph nodes are discovered preoperatively, or intraoperatively. This study also raised another problem: the significance of high ligation of inferior mesenteric artery at the origin has a much lower prognostic value than lateral pelvic dissection [95].

Generally, most surgeons will perform ligation of the inferior mesenteric artery at the origin in locally advanced cases (T3, T4) and in the case of nodal involvement.

With regard to lateral pelvic dissection, no evidence exists of a truly benefit from it, compared with its morbidity, in terms of urinary and sexual dysfunctions. Removal of positive lateral lymph nodes not always correlates with improvement in local control and distance survival, the main role remaining rather as a prognostic indicator.

Still, almost a quarter of patients with rectal cancer are at risk of lateral nodal metastasis, though reported improvements in survival and local control after lateral pelvic dissection impose further study to select the most appropriate cases with the greatest benefit from an extended lymphadenectomy.

FINAL CONSIDERATIONS

Surgical treatment in rectal cancer continues to represent a challenge for any surgeon who performs it; many controversies are still present, related to the aggressively surgical approach and low functional results which reflects in lower quality of life in survivors.

Local treatment, applied in highly selected cases may play an important role in functional outcome improvements, but remains the oncological outcome which may be severely affected.

In inappropriate cases for local approach, sphincter-preserving surgery is the best option.

In case of locally advanced tumors (T4), with involvement of adjacent organs, it has been proved that they could be solved successfully from the oncologic point of view, with an acceptable postoperative morbidity and mortality and good long distance outcome. Still, the quality of life for these patients may be low due to aggressive surgery they underwent (pelvic exenteration with both, definitive colostomy and ureterostomy).

In the matter of extended lymphadenectomy, further studies are necessary to permit a better selection of cases, in which this approach could be truly beneficial.

In the end what matters in the selection of surgical treatment is the patient's survival and his informed consent.

No comments in this chapter were made regarding the surgery of stage four of disease; this is mainly because little controversies exist in this field.

It was already well established the role of hepatectomy and even repeated hepatectomy in hepatic metastasis of rectal cancer; in the case of operable liver metastasis, rectal surgery will have the same curative intent as usual.

In other metastasis, the role of surgery is limited, usually as palliation of symptoms or treatment of acute tumoral complications, with the only purpose to prolonge survival and alleviates the patient's quality of life.

REFERENCES

[1] Lasser, Ph. Traitements locaux du cancer du rectum. *J. Chir. (Paris)*, 1996, 133(1), 23-26.
[2] Nastro, N; Beral, D; Hartley, J; Monson, JRT. Local Excision of Rectal Cancer: Rewiev of Literature. *Dig Surg*, 2005, 22, 6-15.
[3] Balch, GC; De Meo, A; Guillem, JG. Modern management of rectal cancer: A 2006 update. *World J Gastroenterol*, 2006, 12(20), 3186-3195.
[4] Tepetes, K; Spyridakis, ME. Local Excision for Early Rectal Cancer in the Era of Neoadjuvant Strategies. *Hepato-Gastroenterology*, 2007, 54, 1689-1693.
[5] Nano, M; Ferronato, M; Solej, M; D'Amico, S. T1 Adenocarcinoma of the Rectum: Transanal Excision or Radical Surgery? *Tumori*, 2006, 92, 496-473.
[6] Landmann, R; Wong, D; Hoepfl, J; Shia, J; Guillem, J; Temple, L; Patty, Ph; Weiser, M. Limitation of early rectal cancer nodal staging may explain failure after local excision. *Dis Colon Rectum*, 2007, 50(10), 1520-1525.

[7] Vysloužil, K; Cwiertka, K; Zbořil, P; Kučerova, L; Klementa, I; Starý, L; Skalický, P; Duda, M. Endorectal sonography in rectal cancer staging and indication for local surgery. *Hepato-Gastroenterology*, 2007, 54, 1102-1106.

[8] Chun, HK; Choi, D; Kim, MJ; Lee, J; Yun, SH; Kim, SH; Lee, SJ; Kim, CK. Preoperative staging of rectal cancer: comparison of 3-T high-field MRI and endorectal sonography. *AJR*, 2006, 187, 1557-1562.

[9] Vliegen, R; Dresen, R; Beets, G; Daniels-Gooszen, A; Kessels, A; van Engelshoven, J; Beets-Tan, R. The accuracy of multi-detector row CT for the assessment of tumor invasion of the mesorectal fascia in primary rectal cancer. *Abdom Imaging*, 2008, 33, 604-610.

[10] Wolmark, N; Fisher, E; Wieand, S; Fisher, B. The relationship of depth of penetration and tumor size to the number of positive nodes in Dukes C colorectal cancer. *Cancer*, 1984, 53, 2707-2712.

[11] Takano, S; Kato, J; Yamamoto, H; Shiode, J; Nasu, J; Kawamoto, H; Okada, H; Shiratori, Y. Identification of risk factors for lymph node metastasis of colorectal cancer. *Hepato-Gastroenterology*, 2007, 54, 746-750.

[12] Fang, WL; Chang, SC; Lin, JK; Wang, HS; Yang, SH; Jiang, JK; Chen, WC; Lin, TC. Metastatic potential in T1 and T2 colorectal cancer. *Hepato-Gastroenterology*, 2005, 52, 1688-1691.

[13] Sitzler, PJ; Seow-Choen, F; Ho, YH; Leong, APK. Lymph node involvement and tumor depth in rectal cancers. *Dis Colon Rectum*, 1997, 40(12), 1472-1475.

[14] Blumberg, D; Patty, Ph; Guillem, J; Picon, A; Minsky, B; Wong, WD; Cohen, A. All patients with small intramural rectal cancers are at risk for lymph node metastasis. *Dis Colon Rectum*, 1999, 42(7), 881-885.

[15] Choi, P; Yu, CS; Jang, S; Jung, S; Kim, H; Kim, J. Risk factors for lymph node metastasis in submucosal invasive colorectal cancer. *World J Surg*, 2008, (online first)

[16] Miyamoto, M; Nishioka, M; Kurita, N; Natagawa, T; Yoshikawa, K; Higashijima, J; Miyatani, T; Shimada, M. Usefulness of local excision for early lower rectal cancer. *Hepato-Gastroenterology*, 2007, 54, 736-739.

[17] Ptok, H; Marusch, F; Meyer, F; Schubert, D; Koeckerling, F; Gastinger, I; Lippert, H. Oncological outcome of local vs radical resection of low-risk pT1 rectal cancer. *Arch Surg*, 2007, 142(7), 649-655.

[18] Min, BS; Kim, NK; Ko, YT; Lee, KY; Baek, SH; Cho, CH; Sohn, SK. Long-term oncologic results of patients with distal rectal cancer treated by local excision with or without adjuvant treatment. *Int J Colorectal Dis*, 2007, 22, 1325-1330.

[19] Chakravarti, A; Compton, CC; Shellito, PC; Wood, WC; Landy, J; Machuta, SR; Kaufman, D; Ancukiewicz, M; Willett, CG. Long-term follow-up of patients with rectal cancer managed by local excision with and without adjuvant irradiation. *Ann Surg*, 1999, 230(1), 49-54.

[20] Chen, CC; Leu, SY; Liu, MC; Jian, JJM; Chen, CM. Transanal local wide excision for rectal adenocarcinoma. *Hepato-Gastroenterology*, 2005, 52, 460-463.

[21] Kim, CJ; Yeatman, TJ; Coppola, D; Trotti, A; Williams, B; Barthel, JS; Dinwoodie, W; Karl, RC; Marcet, J. Local excision of T2 and T3 rectal cancers after downstaging chemoradiation. *Ann Surg*, 2001, 234(3), 352-359.

[22] Borschitz, T; Wachtlin, D; Möhler, M; Schmidberger, H; Junginger, Th. Neoadjuvant chemoradiation and local excision for T2-3 rectal cancer. *Ann Surg Oncol*, 2008, 15(3), 712-720.

[23] Kreisssler-Haag, D; Schuld, J; Lindemann, W; König, J; Hildebrandt, U; Schiling, M. Complications after transanal endoscopic microsurgical resection correlate with location of rectal neoplasms. *Surg Endosc*, 2008, 22, 612-616.

[24] Duek, S; Issa, N; Hershko, D; Krausz, M. Outcome of transanal endoscopic microsurgery and adjuvant radiotherapy in patients with T2 rectal cancer. *Dis Col Rectum*, 2008, 51, 379-384.

[25] You, N; Baxter, N; Stewart, A; Nelson, H. Is increasing rate of local excision for stage I rectal cancer in the United States Justified? *Ann Surg*, 2007, 245, 726-733.

[26] Tarantino, I; Hetzer, FH; Warschow, R; Zund, M; Stein, HJ; Zerz A. Local excision and endoscopic posterior mesorectal resection versus low anterior resection in T1 rectal cancer. *Br J Surg*, 2008, 95(3), 375-380.

[27] Keighley, M; Williams, N. Management of carcinoma of the rectum. In: Keighley M, Williams N, editors, *Surgery of the anus, rectum and colon*, third edition. Philadelphia, Saunders Elsevier, 2008, 1115-1262.

[28] Ross, H; Mahmoud, N; Fry, R. The current management of rectal cancer. *Current Problems in Surgery*, 2005, 42(2), 67-132.

[29] Nelson, H; Petrelli, N; Carlin, A; Couture, J; Fleshman, J; Guillem, J; Miedema, B; Ota, D; Sargent, D. Guidelines 2000 for colon and rectal surgery. *J Nat Cancer Instit*, 2001, 93(8), 583-594.

[30] Heald, R; Husband, E; Ryall, R. The mesorectum in rectal cancer surgery – the clue to pelvic recurrence? *Br J Surg*, 1982, 69, 613-616.

[31] Heald, R; Moran, B; Ryall, R; Sexton, R; MacFarlane, J. Rectal cancer – the Basingstoke experience of total mesorectal excision, 1978-1997. *Arch Surg*, 1998, 133, 894-899.

[32] Tocchi, A; Mazzoni, G; Lepre, L; Liotta, G; Costa, G; Agostini, N; Micini, M; Scucchi, L; Frati, G; Tagliaccozo, S. Total mesorectal excision and low rectal anastomosis for the treatment of rectal cancer and prevention of pelvic recurrences. *Arch Surg*, 2001, 136, 216-220.

[33] Heald, R; Karanija, N. Results of radical surgery for rectal cancer. *World J Surg*, 1992, 16, 848-857.

[34] Brennan, T; Lipshutz, G; Gibbs, V; Norton, J. Total mesenteric excision in the treatment of rectal carcinoma: methods and outcomes. *Surg Oncol*, 2002, 10, 171-176.

[35] Andreoni, B; Chiappa, A; Bertani, E; Bellomi, M; Orrechia, R; Zampino, MG; Fazio, N; Venturino, M; Orsi, F; Sonzogni, A; Pace, U; Monfardini, L. Surgical outcomes for colon and rectal cancer over a decade: results from a consecutive monocentric experience in 902 unselected patients. *World J Surg Oncol*, 2007, 5, 73-83.

[36] Haas-Kock, D; Baeten, C; Jager, J; Langendijk, J; Schouten, L; Volovics, A; Arends, J. Prognostic significance of radial margins of clearance in rectal cancer. *Br J Surg*, 1996, 83, 781-785.

[37] Miyoshi, M; Ueno, H; Hashiguchi, Y; Mochizuki, H; Talbot, I. Extent of mesorectal tumor invasion as a prognostic factor after curative surgery for T3 rectal cancer patients. *Ann Surg*, 2006, 243, 492-498.

[38] Quirke, P; Durdey, P; Dixon, MF; Williams, NS. Local recurrence of rectal adenocarcinoma due to inadequate surgical resection. Histopathological study of lateral tumor spread and surgical excision. *Lancet*, 1986, 1, 996-998.

[39] Strassburg, J; Lewin, A; Ludwig, K; Kilian, L; Linke, J; Loy, V; Knuth, P; Püttcher, O; Ruehl, U, Stöckmann, F; Hackenthal, M; Hopfenmüller, W; Huppertz, A. Optimised surgery (so-called TME surgery) and high-resolution MRI in the planning of treatment of rectal carcinoma. *Lagenbecks Arch Surg*, 2007, 392, 179-188.

[40] Law, WI; Chu, KW; Ho, J; Chan, CH. Risk factors for anastomotic leakage after low anterior resection with total mesorectal excision. *Am J Surg*, 2000, 179, 92-96.

[41] Jung, SH; Yu, CS; Choi, PW; Kim, DD; Park, IJ; Kim, HC; Kim, JC. Risk factors and oncologic impact of anastomotic leakage after rectal cancer surgery. *Dis Colon Rectum*, 2008, 51, 902-908.

[42] Matthiessen, P; Hallböök, O; Rutegård, J; Simert, G; Sjödahl, R. Defunctioning stoma reduces symptomatic anastomotic leakage after low anterior resection of the rectum for cancer – a ranomized multicenter trial. *Ann Surg*, 2007, 246, 207-214.

[43] Tschmelitsch, J; Wykypiel, H; Prommegger, R; Bodner, E. Colostomy versus tube cecostomy for protection of a low anastomosis in rectal cancer. *Arch Surg*, 1999, 134, 1385-1388.

[44] Kapiteijn, E; Marijnen, C; Nagtegaal, I; Putter, H; Steup, W; Wiggers, T; Rutten, H; Pahlman, L; Glimelius, B; van Krieken, H; Leer, J; van de Velde, C. Preoperative radiotherapy combined with total mesorectal excision for respectable rectal cancer. *N Engl J Med*, 2001, 345, 638-646.

[45] Folkesson, J; Birgisson, H; Pahlman, L; Cedemark, B; Glimelius, B; Gunnarsson, U. Swedish rectal cancer trial: long lasting benefits from radiotherapy on survival and local recurrence rate. *J Clin Oncol*, 2005, 23(24), 5644-5649.

[46] Gervaz, P; Coucke, Ph; Gillet, M. Irradiation du petit basin et fonction ano-rectale: plaidoyer pour une radiothérapie d'épargne sphinctériénne. *Gastroenterol Clin Biol*, 2001, 25, 457-462.

[47] Hassan, I; Larson, D; Wolff, B; Cima, R; Chua, H; Hahnloser, D; O'Byrne, M; Larson, D; Pemberton, J. Impact of pelvic radiotherapy on morbidity and durability of sphincter preservation after coloanal anastomosis for rectal cancers. *Dis Colon Rectum*, 2008, 51, 32-37.

[48] Phillips, R. Adequate distal margin of resection for adenocarcinoma of the rectum. *World J Surg*, 1992, 16, 463-466.

[49] Tilney, H; Heriot, A; Purkayastha, S; Antoniou, A; Aylin, P; Darzi, A; Tekkis, P. A national perspective on the decline of abdominoperineal resection for rectal cancer. *Ann Surg*, 2008, 247(1), 77-84.

[50] Nagtegaal, I; van de Velde, C; Marijnen, C; van Krieken, J; Quirke, Ph. Low rectal cancer: a call for a change in approach in abdominoperineal resection. *J Clin Oncol*, 2005, 23(36), 9257-9264.

[51] Rothenberger, D., Wong, D. Abdominoperineal resection for adenocarcinoma of the low rectum. *World J Surg*, 1992, 16, 478-485.

[52] Marr, R; Birbeck, K; Garvican, J; Macklin, C; Tiffin, N; Parsons, W; Dixon, M; Mapstone, N; Sebag-Montefiore, D; Scott, N; Johnston, D; Sagar, P; Finan, P; Quircke, Ph. The modern abdominoperineal excision: the next challenge after total mesorectal excision. *Ann Surg*, 2005, 242(1), 74-82.

[53] Chiappa, A; Biffi, R; Zbar, A; Bertani, E; Luca, F; Pace, U; Biela, F; Grassi, C; Zampino, G; Fazio, N; Pruneri, G; Poldi, D; Venturino, M; Andreoni, B. The influence of type of operation for distal rectal cancer: survival, outcomes, and recurrence. *Hepato-Gastroenterol*, 2007, 54, 400-406.

[54] di Betta, E; D'Hoore, A; Filez, L; Penninckx, F. Sphincter saving rectum resection is the standard procedure for low rectal cancer. *Int J Colorectal Dis*, 2003, 18, 463-469.

[55] Nakagoe, T; Ishikawa, H; Sawai, T; Tsuji, T; Tanaka, K; Hidaka, S; Nanashima, A; Yamaguchi, H; Yasutake, T. Survival and recurrence after a sphincter-saving resection and abdominoperineal resection for adenocarcinoma of the rectum at or below the peritoneal reflection: a multivariate analysis. *Surg Today*, 2004, 34, 32-39.

[56] Nakagoe, T; Ishikawa, H; Sawai, T; Tsuji, T; Takeshita, H; Nanashima, A; Akamine, S; Yamaguchi, H; Yasutake, T. Oncological outcome of ultra-low anterior resection with total mesorectal excision for carcinoma of the lower third of the rectum: comparison of intrapelvic double-stapled anastomosis and transanal coloanal anastomosis. *Hepato-Gastroenterol*, 2005, 52, 1692-1697.

[57] Oya, M; Sugamata, Y; Komatsu, J; Ishikawa, H; Nozaki, M. Poor neorectal evacuation as a cause of impaired defecatory function after low anterior resection: a study using scintigraphic assessment. *Surg Today*, 2002, 32, 111-117.

[58] Berger, A; Tiret, E; Parc, R; Frileux, P; Hannoun, L; Nordlinger, B; Ratelle, R; Simon, R. Excision of the rectum with colonic J pouch-anal anastomosis for adenocarcinoma of the low and mid rectum. *World J Surg*, 1992, 16, 470-477.

[59] Hida, J; Yoshifuji, T; Matsuzaki, T; Hattori, T; Ueda, K; Ishimaru, E; Tokoro, T; Yasutomi, M; Shiozaki, H; Okuno, K. Long-term functional changes after low anterior resection for rectal cancer compared between a colonic J-pouch and a straight anastomosis. *Hepato-Gastroenterol*, 2007, 54, 407-413.

[60] Huber, F; Herter, B; Siewert, JR. Colonic pouch vs side-to-end anastomosis in low anterior resection. *Dis Colon Rectum*, 1999, 42, 896-902.

[61] Fazio, V; Zutshi, M; Remzi, F; Parc, Y; Ruppert, R; Fürst, A; Celebrezze, J; Galanduik, S; Orangio, G; Hyman, N; Bokey, L; Tiret, E; Kirchdorfer, B; Medich, D; Tietze, M; Hull, T; Hammel, J. A randomized multicenter trial to compare long-term functional outcome, quality of life, and complications of surgical procedures for low rectal cancers. *Ann Surg*, 2007, 246(3), 481-490.

[62] Gambacorta, MA; Valentini, V; Coco, C; Manno, A; Doglietto, G; Ratto, C; Cosimelli, M; Miccichè, F; Maurizi, F; Tagliaferi, L; Matini, G; Balducci, M; La Torre, G; Barbaro, B; Picciocchi, A. Sphincter preserving in four consecutive PHASE II studies of preoperative chemoradiation: analysis of 247 T3 rectal cancer patients. *Tumori*, 2007, 93, 160-169.

[63] Synglarewicz, B; Matkowski, R; Kasprzak, P; Sydor, D; Forgacz, J; Pudelko, M; Kornafel, J. Sphincter-preserving R0 total mesorectal excision with resection of internal genitalia combined with pre- or postoperative chemoradiation for T4 rectal cancer in females. *World J Gastroenterol*, 2007, 13(16), 2339-2343.

[64] Moriya, Y; Akasu, T; Fujita, S; Yamamoto, S. Aggressive surgical treatment for patients with T4 rectal cancer. *Colorectal Dis*, 2003, 5, 427-431.

[65] Carne, PW; Frye, JN; Kennedy-Smith, A; Keating, J; Merrie, A; Dennett, E; Frizelle, FA,. Local invasion of the bladder with colorectal cancers: surgical management and patterns of local recurrence. *Dis Colon Rectum*, 2004, 47, 44-47.

[66] Kurt, M; Ozkan, L; Ercan, I; Kahraman, S; Zorluoglu, A; Gurel, S; Memik, F; Engin, K. Preoperative chemoradiotherapy in patients with locally advanced rectal cancer. *Hepato-Gastroenterol*, 2005, 52, 1095-1100.

[67] Takeuchi, H; Ueo, H; Haraoka, M; Maehara, Y. Surgical results of total pelvic exenteration for locally advanced colorectal adenocarcinoma. *Hepato-Gastroenterol*, 2005, 52, 90-93.

[68] Law, WL; Chu, KW; Choi, HK. Total pelvic exenteration for locally advanced rectal cancer. *J Am Col Surg*, 2000, 190, 78-83.

[69] Lourenco, T; Murray, A; Grant, A; McKinley, A; Krukowski, Z; Vale, L. Laparoscopic surgery for colorectal cancer: safe and effective? – A systematic review. *Surg Endosc*, 2008, 22, 1146-1160.

[70] Bianchi, PP; Rosati, R; Bona, S; Rottoli, M; Elmore, U; Ceriani, C; Malesci, A; Montorsi, M. Laparoscopic surgery in rectal cancer: a prospective analysis of patient survival and outcome. *Dis Colon Rectum*, 2007, 50, 2047-2053.

[71] Nakamura, T; Kokuba, Y; Mitomi, H; Onozato, W; Hatate, K; Satoh, T; Ozawa, H; Ihara, A; Watanabe, M. Comparison between the oncologic outcome of laparoscopic surgery and open surgery for T1 and T2 rectosigmoidal and rectal carcinoma: matched case-control study. *Hepato-Gastroenterol*, 2007, 54, 1094-1097.

[72] Naitoh, T; Tsuchiya, T; Honda, H; Oikawa, M; Saito, Y; Hasegawa,Y. Clinical outcome of the laparoscopic surgery for stage II and III colorectal cancer. *Surg Endosc*, 2008, 22, 950-954.

[73] Fukunaga, Y; Higashino, M; Tanimura, S; Takemura, M; Osugi, H. Laparoscopic colorectal surgery for neoplasm. A large series by a single surgeon. *Surg Endosc*, 2008, 22, 1452-1458.

[74] Melinda M; Khatri, V; Bennet, J; Petrelli, N. Total mesorectal excision and pelvic node dissection for rectal cancer: an appraisal. In: Khatri V, Petrelli N, editors, *Lymphadenectomy in surgical oncology: staging and therapeutic role*. Philadelphia, WB Saunders, 2007, 16(1), 177-198.

[75] Greene, FL; Page, DL; Fleming, ID (eds). AJCC cancer staging manual, sixth edition. New York, Springer, 2002, 12-1 – 12-3.

[76] Compton, C; Greene, F. The staging of colorectal cancer: 2004 and beyond. *CA Cancer J Clin*, 2004, 54, 295-308.

[77] Charbit, L; Peschaud, F; Penna, Ch. Ganglions et cancer du rectum. *J Chir*, 2005, 142(2), 85-91.

[78] Yoshimatsu, K; Ishibashi, K; Umehara, A; Yokomizo, H; Yoshida, K; Fujimoto, T; Watanabe, K; Ogawa, K. How many lymph nodes should be examined in Dukes' B colorectal cancer? Determination on the basis of cumulative survival rates. *Hepato-Gastroenterol*, 2005, 52, 1703-1706.

[79] Horzic, M; Kopljar, M. Minimal number of lymph nodes that need to be examined for adequate staging of colorectal cancer – factors influencing lymph node harvest. *Hepato-Gastroenterol*, 2005, 52, 86-89.

[80] Wijesuriya, R; Deen, K; Hewavisenthi, J; Balawardana, J; Perera, M. Neoadjuvant therapy for rectal cancer down-stages the tumor but reduces lymph node harvest significantly. *Surg Today*, 2005, 32, 442-445.

[81] Baxter, N; Virnig, D; Rothenberger, D; Morris, A; Jessurun, J; Virnig, B. Lymph node evaluation in colorectal cancer patients: a population-based study. *J Natl Cancer Instit*, 2005, 97, 219-225.

[82] Wong, J; Johnson, S; Hemmings, D; Hsu, A; Imai, T; Tominaga, G. Assessing the quality of colorectal cancer staging. *Arch Surg*, 2005, 140, 881-887.

[83] Märkl, B; Kerwel, T; Wagner, T; Anthuber, M; Arnholdt, H. Methylene blue injection into the rectal artery as a simple method to improve lymph node harvest in rectal cancer. *Modern Pathol*, 2007, 20, 797-801.

[84] Chen, S; Iddings, M; Scheri, R; Bilchick, A. Lymphatic mapping and sentinel node analysis: current concepts and applications. *CA Cancer J Clin*, 2006, 56, 292-309.

[85] Tsioulias, G; Wood, T; Morton, D; Bilchick, A. Lymphatic mapping an focused analysis of sentinel lymph nodes upstage gastrointestinal neoplasms. *Arch Surg*, 2000, 135, 926-932.

[86] Baton, O; Lasser, Ph; Sabourin, JC; Boige, V; Duvillard, P; Elias, D; Malka, D; Ducreux, M; Pocard, M. Ex vivo sentinel lymph node study for rectal adenocarcinoma: preliminary study. *World J Surg*, 2005, 29, 1166-1170.

[87] Quadros, CA; Lopes, A; Araújo, I; Fahel, F; Bacellar, MS; Dias, CS. Retroperitoneal and lateral pelvic lymphadenectomy mapped by lymphoscintigraphy and blue dye for rectal adenocarcinoma staging: preliminary results. *Ann Surg Oncol*, 2006, 13(12), 1617-1621.

[88] Funahashi, K; Koike, J; Shimada, M; Okamoto, K; Goto, T; Teramoto, T. A preliminary study of the draining lymph node basin in advanced lower rectal cancer using a radioactive tracer. *Dis Colon Rectum*, 2006, 49(10S), S53-S58.

[89] Kim, TH; Jeong, SY; Choi, DH; Kim, DY; Jung, KH; Moon, SH; Chang, HJ; Lim, SB; Choi, HS; Park, JG. Lateral lymph node metastasis is a major cause of locoregional recurrence in rectal cancer treated with preoperative chemoradiotherapy and curative resection. *Ann Surg Oncol*, 2007, 15(3), 729-737.

[90] Shiozawa, M; Akaike, M; Yamada, R; Godai, T; Yamamoto, N; Saito, H; Sugimasa, Y; Takemiya, S; Rino, Y; Imada, T. Lateral lymph node dissection for lower rectal cancer. *Hepato-Gastroenterol*, 2007, 54, 1066-1070.

[91] Hasdemir, O; Çöl, C; Yalçin, E; Tunç, G; Bilgen, K; Kuçukpinar, T. Local recurrence and survival rates after extended systematic lymph-node dissection for surgical treatment of rectal cancer. *Hepato-Gastroenterol*, 2005, 52, 455-459.

[92] Sugihara, K; Kobayashi, H; Kato, T; Mori, T; Mochizuki, H; Kameoka, S; Shirouzu, K., Muto, T. Indication and benefit of pelvic sidewall dissection for rectal cancer. *Dis Colon Rectum*, 2006, 49, 1663-1672.

[93] Dong, XS; Xu, HT; Yu, ZW; Liu, M; Cui, BB; Zhao, P; Wang, XS. Effect of extended radical resection for rectal cancer. *World J Gastroentrol*, 2003, 9(5), 970-973.

[94] Wu, ZY; Wan, J; Li, JH; Zhao, G; Yao, Y; Du, JL; Liu, QF; Peng, L; Wang ZD; Huang, ZM; Lin HH. Prognostic value of lateral lymph node metastasis for advanced low rectal cancer. *World J Gastroenterol*, 2007, 13(45), 6048-6052.

[95] Ueno, H; Mochizuki, H; Hashiguchi, Y; Ishiguro, M; Miyoshi, M; Kajiwara, Y; Sato, T; Shimazaki, H; Hase, K. Potential prognostic benefit of lateral pelvic node dissection for rectal cancer located below the peritoneal reflection. *Ann Surg*, 2007, 245(1), 80-87.

In: Rectal Cancer: Etiology, Pathogenesis and Treatment
Editors: Paula Wells and Regina Halstead

ISBN 978-1-60692-563-8
© 2009 Nova Science Publishers, Inc.

Chapter II

THE EFFECT OF ADJUVANT THERAPY ON SURGICAL TREATMENT OF RECTAL CANCER

Luca Stocchi and Victor W. Fazio
Digestive Disease Institute, Cleveland Clinic, Cleveland, OH, USA.

INTRODUCTION

Surgery is the most widely used modality in the treatment of rectal cancer with curative intent and has achieved rates of local recurrence in the order of 10% or less [1].

However, the results for surgery alone in locally advanced rectal cancer remain suboptimal as a significant percentage of patients are at risk of systemic failure and local recurrence albeit rare remains a devastating event. Therefore, multimodality treatment including not only surgery but also radiotherapy and chemotherapy has been gradually recognized as the most effective treatment for locally advanced rectal cancer. While multimodality treatment is widely accepted, there is a variety of different opinions regarding the timing, sequence, dosages and agents to be used.

The aim of this presentation is to illustrate some of the current issues, controversies and future directions of adjuvant treatment for rectal cancer and its influence on surgical approach with curative intent on the primary disease.

RADIATION ALONE VS. RADIATION AND CHEMOTHERAPY

Most patients with rectal cancer undergo radical surgery in the form of either low anterior resection or abdominoperineal resection. A number of studies have confirmed the role of both adjuvant chemotherapy and radiation therapy as the basis of combined modality treatment for rectal cancer. Earlier trials compared surgery alone with surgery followed by radiation with or without chemotherapy using a number of different agents.

Chemotherapeutics employed in these trials included mainly 5-fluorouracil (5-FU), biochemically modulated or not with levamisole and/or leucovorin, and other classes of drugs such as semustine and vincristine, which were subsequently abandoned based on their lack of efficacy and adverse effects based on the results of the trials. At the time when these studies were designed, these were the only chemotherapeutic agents with expected activity against rectal cancer. The method of 5-FU delivery during concurrent radiation treatment, bolus vs. continuous venous infusion, was also investigated. These studies were mainly conducted by the cooperative American groups, especially the National Surgical Adjuvant Breast and Bowel Project (NSAPB), Gastrointestinal Tumor Study Group (GTSG) and North Central Cancer Treatment Group (NCCTG) [2,3]. The results of these studies suggested that chemotherapy was an important adjunct to radiation and surgery for stage II and III carcinomas. These studies established the role of adjuvant chemoradiation using 5-FU and long-term postoperative radiation treatment and constituted the basis for the NIH recommendation for adjuvant treatment since the early 1990s in the United States for Stage II and Stage III disease [4]. While some surgeons postulate that T2N0 disease in the distal rectum should also be considered for neoadjuvant chemoradiation [5] this is not yes considered standard of care in the United States.

5-FU has continued being used as the fundamental chemotherapeutic agent during concomitant radiotherapy in studies examining preoperative vs. postoperative treatments and remains today an important drug in the treatment of locally advanced rectal carcinoma. With this respect, at least two other more recent prospective randomized studies have confirmed the value of chemotherapy in addition to radiotherapy both coming from Europe. In both the EORTC [6] and FFCD 9203 (Federation Franchophone du Chirurgie Digestif) [7] trials, the patients receiving adjuvant treatment were randomized into pre-operative radiation alone or pre-operative chemoradiation. Both trials used long-term pre-operative radiation and demonstrated significant advantage in local control associated with the use of chemotherapy in addition to radiotherapy. However, these trials did not demonstrate any significant differences in disease free or overall survival.

Current studies are assessing the value of oral fluoropyrimidines, especially capecitabine, as equivalent to 5-FU. Other chemotherapeutic agents are also being investigated as adjunct to conventional long-term radiation which is no longer recommended as standard of care for locally advanced rectal cancer without concurrent chemotherapy.

PREOPERATIVE VS. POSTOPERATIVE CHEMORADIATION

Since the introduction of adjuvant treatment for the management of rectal cancer, there has been controversy with regard to the optimal timing of adjuvant treatments with respect to surgery. Advocates of post-operative treatment have suggested that optimal decisions on treatment need to be based on the staging gold standard which is the pathologic examination of the surgical specimen. This would minimize the risk of overtreatment and optimize stratification of patients with regard to prognosis. On the other hand, advocates of preoperative chemotherapy and/or radiation therapy have suggested that delivery of treatment to fresh tissues could maximize tumoricidal effect, facilitate exclusion of small bowel and other healthy tissues from the radiation field, and reduce the size of the tumor which could facilitate the subsequent surgical procedure and possibly increase the ability to perform a sphincter-preserving procedure. In addition, the sterilizing effect derived from radiation might minimize tumor seeding at the time of surgery. This controversy has continued for several years, particularly as trials designed to address this issue in the United States met with poor patient accrual. In fact, the initial trial by the Radiation Therapy and Oncology Group (RTOG 94-01/Intergroup 0417) was prematurely closed due to poor accrual. The NSABP R-03 trial was also aimed at the evaluation of preoperative vs. postoperative 5-FU-based chemoradiation but enrolled only 267 patients out of the planned 900. A progress report indicated that treatment–related toxicity was similar in the 2 arms and a trend was described in favor of preoperative treatment in regards to tumor downstaging and sphincter preservation [8]. A more recent trial conducted in Europe has provided more solid evidence in favor of preoperative treatment. The German Rectal Cancer Study Group compared in a prospective randomized trial pre-operative vs. post-operative chemoradiotherapy for rectal cancer. The Authors randomly assigned patients with clinical Stage II or III disease to receive preoperative treatment consisting of 5040 cGy delivered in 100 cGy fractions in a schedule that is similar to the corresponding standard of care in most centers in the United States. Surgery was performed six weeks after completion of chemoradiation. One month after surgery, an additional cycle of fluorouracil was administered. Chemoradiotherapy was analogous in the post-operative treatment arm of the study whose patients also received a boost of 540 cGy. A total of 421 patients were randomly assigned to receive preoperative chemoradiotherapy vs. 402 counterparts who received post-operative treatments. The overall 5-year survival, which was the main endpoint, was comparable between the two groups with rates of 76% and 74%, respectively. The 5-year cumulative incidence of local recurrence was 6% in the preoperative chemoradiotherapy group vs. 13% in the postoperative treatment group, a difference which was statistically significant ($p = 0.006$). In this regard, it is important to note that 18% of the patients initially randomized to the postoperative treatment group ended up having Stage I disease at pathology and therefore were removed from the study. It is therefore reasonable to expect that the group undergoing preoperative radiotherapy might have been at least, in part overstaged. This is a relevant confounding variable in our interpretation on the results of the trial with respect to local recurrence. It is therefore difficult to conclude that preoperative treatment is certqinly associated with improved local control. Most importantly, there was a significant advantage in favor of preoperative treatments with regard to acute toxicity which occurred in 27% of cases vs. 40% of patients after preoperative vs. post-operative treatment, respectively. The rates of long-term toxicity were also favorable to preoperative treatment with a rate of 14% vs. 24% after postoperative treatments, respectively ($p = 0.01$) [9]. The German Rectal Cancer Study Group achieved the completion of this important trial which has contributed to reinforce an already existing trend in favor of preoperative treatments mainly by demonstrating a reduction in toxicity rates which is both statistically significant and clinically important. The results of the German trail with regard to sphincter preservation are less clear. In fact, the investigators determined at their initial evaluation whether in abdominoperineal resection would be required for all patients enrolled. Based on their own evaluations, 39% of patients initially thought to require abdominoperineal resection could actually receive a low-anterior resection as compared to 19% in the group randomized to post-operative therapy. While this difference was statistically significant (p = 0.004), the overall sphincter preservation rates were 17.1% vs 16.1%, respectively. It is therefore not possible to use the data from the German trial to support the notion that preoperative radiotherapy can achieve an increase in sphincter preservation rates.

HYPOFRACTIONATED (SHORT–TERM) RADIATION TREATMENT AS ALTERNATIVE TO CHEMORADIATION

The use of radiation treatment administered for a week followed by surgery has been mainly developed in Europe. In the last 2 decades the role of radiation treatment has been validated by prospective randomized trials, the most important of which are arguably the Swedish trial and the Dutch trial.

The Swedish trial accrued 908 patients undergoing surgery with curative intent for stages I-III rectal carcinomas situated below the promontory, as shown on a lateral projection on barium enema. It accrued patients in 70 different centers between 1987 and 1990. A total of 454 patients were randomly assigned to surgery alone vs. 454 counterparts who received preoperative radiation treatment with 25 Gy administered over 5 days followed by surgery within one week. Results from long-term follow-up at a median of 13 years have been recently published [10]. Overall survival was significantly increased after preoperative radiation treatment when compared with surgery alone (38% vs. 30%, respectively, p=0.008). Disease-specific survival (72% vs. 62%, respectively, p=0.03) and local recurrence rates (9% vs. 26%, p<0.001) also favored the preoperative radiation arm. Subgroup analyses confirmed statistically significant benefits of preoperative radiation in reducing local recurrence rates for each tumor stage and for all tumor locations except for patients with the distal edge of disease at 11 cm or higher from the anal verge. Subgroup stage-by-stage analyses for overall survival and disease-specific survival did not show significant differences except for stage I patients. There were no differences between the two groups with respect to distant metastases rates. Results from this trial confirm the widely held assumption that radiation treatment effects local control but not distant disease. As the Authors appropriately point out in the discussion of their study, this trial was conducted when total mesorectal excision was not the accepted surgical standard of care for rectal carcinoma and the pathologic evaluation of the specimen did not include evaluation of the circumferential resection margin or an accepted minimum number of lymph nodes. This might explain the relatively high local recurrence rate after surgery alone and the effect of radiation treatment on stage I carcinomas, which is generally treated with surgery alone in the United States. The long-term toxicity rates were acceptable and there was no increase in the hospital admission because of radiation toxicity after 6 months following treatment. The toxicity associated with the radiation techniques used in this trial was limited and was more than offset by the benefits in cancer outcomes [11]. While radiation treatment techniques have evolved and might allow for an even lower toxicity rate, surgical management and pathologic evaluation of the surgical specimen have also adopted new and better standards, which limit the applicability of these results to contemporary treatment of rectal cancer, particularly in the United States. A subsequent, more recent trial has been therefore designed to address these issues related to use of hypofractionated radiotherapy and surgery for rectal carcinoma and incorporated in the trial design standardization of both surgery and pathology.

HYPOFRACTIONATED RADIOTHERAPY WITH STANDARDIZATION OF SURGERY AND PATHOLOGY: THE DUTCH TRIAL

The Dutch Colorectal Cancer Group designed a prospective randomized trial comparing treatment of resectable rectal cancer with or without preoperative hypofractionated radiotherapy (CKVO 95-04). The results after a median follow-up of 6.1 years have been recently published. This is to date the only trial evaluating radiation treatment for rectal cancer which attempted to achieve standardization of surgery and pathology through the input of recognized experts, workshops and other quality-assurance metrics for the participating surgeons and pathologists. This prospective multi-center study randomized 1,861 patients with preoperative diagnosis of stage I-III rectal cancer between 1996 and 1999 after stratification according to treating center and the expected type of surgery, low anterior resection vs. abdomino-perineal resection. Eligible patients had their rectal carcinoma no farther than 15 cm from the anal verge. The primary endpoint was local recurrence, which was 5.6% at 5 years after combined treatment versus 10.9% in patients treated with surgery alone (> 0.001). In particular, patients with node-positive tumors received significant benefit from radiation treatment despite optimized surgical treatment. In fact, their 5-year local recurrence rate decreased from 20.6% after surgery alone to 10.6% after combined treatment (>0.001). While differences in local recurrence are significant, the 5-year overall survival was comparable at 64.2% after preoperative radiotherapy vs. 63.5% after surgery alone [12]. Further follow-up might reveal significant differences in survival as local recurrences of rectal cancer are usually not curable. The results from this trial are again not directly applicable to centers in the United States and wherever long-term radiation treatment is favored and concurrent chemotherapy is administered only for stages II and III. As this trial enrolled patients with stages I-III and its subgroup analyses cannot reach meaningful conclusions, it also remains uncertain to understand from the data of this trial which stages of rectal cancer really benefit from radiation treatment. One of the most important achievements of the Dutch TME trial is that it confirms the benefits of radiation treatment even in the face of optimal surgery. It is also noticeable that 31% of the local recurrence rate in patients undergoing combined treatment occurred later than 3 years following surgery versus only 10% if the patient had received no radiation treatment. In addition, there were no significant differences in outcomes among patients treated with low anterior resection vs. abdomino-perineal resection.

Adoption of hypofractionated radiotherapy could expedite care for patients and might reduce costs of treatment when compared to long-term chemoradiation. However, preoperative chemoradiation remains the accepted standard of care in stage II and III rectal carcinomas in the United States in spite of the results from the European trials. Trials comparing surgery alone with surgery and low-dose radiation treatment were conducted in the United States in the 70s and 80s and were fraught by local recurrence rates in the order of 20% and as high as 37% in one of the surgery alone arm [13,14]. At the present time the use of hypofractionated radiotherapy in the United States is uncommon. Concerns regarding hypofractionated radiotherapy include inability to achieve the same degree of tumor downsizing and downstaging, reduction of complete response rates, inability of hypofractionated radiation treatment to enhance sphincter-preservation, and concerns for possible increased rates of late toxicity [11,15-17].

SHORT-TERM RADIATION TREATMENT VS. LONG-TERM CHEMORADIATION

Direct comparisons between hypofractionated radiotherapy and long-term preoperative chemoradiation have not been conducted in the United States.

However, one randomized study from Poland has examined the oncologic results following short-term radiation treatment vs. conventional chemoradiation with 5-FU which has been the traditionally accepted chemoradiation treatment in the United States. Bujko and colleagues randomized 312 patients which were analyzed with a median follow-up of 48 months. Early radiation toxicity was higher in the chemoradiation group, but 4-year overall survival rates were comparable between the short-term radiotherapy group and the chemoradiation group at 67.2% and 66.2%, respectively. The corresponding disease-free survival rates were 58.4% vs. 55.6%, respectively and the local recurrence rates were 9.0% vs. 14.2%. These outcomes were not statistically different. Severe late toxicity was also comparable. Based on these results, the Authors concluded that neo-adjuvant chemoradiation did not result in increased survival, improved local control or late toxicity compared with short-term radiotherapy [18].

Another phase III trial examining the effect of routine short course radiation treatment is the MRC-CR07 study which has been published in an abstract form with a median follow-up of 3 years. In this trial patients with stages I-III undergoing treatment with curative intent were randomized to routine hypofractioned preoperative radiotherapy (25Gy in 5 fractions) vs. selective postoperative chemoradiation (45 Gy in 25 fraction and 5-FU) for positive radial margins and chemotherapy for involved locoregional lymph nodes at pathology. Patients were stratified by a number of factors including the operating surgeon. While overall survival was similar in the 2 arms, routine preoperative hypofractionated radiotherapy resulted in a significantly reduced local recurrence rate and increased disease-free survival when compared to select postoperative treatment (4.7% vs. 11.1% and 79.5% vs. 74.9%, respectively) [19]. When specimen were subdivided based on their histopathological assessment used as a surrogate of the quality of the surgical dissection (muscularis plane, intramesorectal plane, mesorectal plane) the benefits of routine preoperative radiation treatment remained significant for all the 3 reported planes of dissection [20]. Future studies should evaluate the relative values and indications for short-term vs. long-term radiation treatment in combination with contemporary chemotherapy.

COULD T3N0 BE TREATED WITH SURGERY ALONE?

It has been suggested that a subset of T3N0 cancers might be treated with surgery alone and achieve comparable cancer outcomes to those achieved with combined modality treatments. In fact, specialized centers have achieved a rate of local recurrence below 10% following radical surgical resection alone in stage IIa rectal carcinoma [21]. It is therefore possible to expect that at least a subset of these patients might benefit from avoiding adjuvant treatments with their inherent risks and complications and could be best served with surgery alone. A number of studies have examined the factors affecting the risk of recurrence associated with subsets of pT3N0 patients. The factor which has been most commonly evaluated is the depth of tumor penetration into the mesorectum. Various thresholds have been evaluated as markers of increased recurrence risk ranging from 2 mm [22] to 5 mm [23] or 6 mm [24]. Other studies have noted more favorable results when the penetration into the mesorectum could be detected only microscopically as opposed to grossly [25] and one study has subdivided the high-risk vs. low-risk T3 tumors on the basis of depth of penetration, tumor differentiation and presence of lymphovascular invasion [22]. In support of this, it has also been suggested based on a retrospective pooled analysis of rectal cancer adjuvant therapy trials that trimodality treatment for all patients with either T3N0 or T1-2N1 disease might be excessive when compared with other patients with stage II-III rectal carcinoma [26]. The data from these studies concur in showing that there is a subset of T3N0 tumors which present a low risk for local recurrence. However, most of these studies were based on pathologic evaluation of a non-radiated rectum and were originally intended to help in the decision-making on postoperative adjuvant treatment. As neoadjuvant treatment is increasingly preferred over postoperative chemoradiation, the data from these studies are not as pertinent to the contemporary practice of T3N0 rectal cancer diagnosed preoperatively.

With regard to the treatment of cT3N0 disease, it has been suggested that a substantial percentage of these patients is at risk of overtreatment because of inaccurate staging. However, preoperative staging also present the risk of undetected nodal disease. To clarify the role of modern neoadjuvant treatment in these patients in light of these difficulties, Guillem and colleagues reported their results on 188 cT3N0 patients with rectal carcinoma treated in six different high-volume centers. All patients were staged by endorectal ultrasound or MRI of the pelvis, and received preoperative combined modality treatment including 5-FU-based chemotherapy and a radiotherapy dose of 45 to 50.4 cGy followed by radical resection. A total of 22% of these patients had undetected mesorectal lymph node involvement demonstrated at pathologic evaluation of the specimen in spite of combined modality treatment. The Authors postulate that the rate of undetected lymph node metastases could have been even higher considering the sterilizing potential of the preoperative treatment. As 18% of patients in the German trial had preoperative stages II or III carcinomas and were assigned to postoperative treatments resulted to have pathologic stage I disease, the Authors concluded that using the currently available staging modalities cT3N0 rectal cancers should preferentially be treated with neoadjuvant chemoradiation [27]. Considering the current limitations of our ability to accurately stage rectal cancer preoperatively it is also generally accepted that cT3N0 carcinomas should be treated with neoadjuvant chemoradiation followed by surgery.

CAN NEOADJUVANT TREATMENT INFLUENCE SPHINCTER PRESERVATION?

As the effect of neoadjuvant treatment often results in the reduction of the tumor size it would be intuitive to expect that at least some patients could undergo a sphincter–saving procedure instead of an abdomino-perineal resection as a result of chemoradiotherapy. Hypofractionated radiotherapy is generally conducted over a short time and almost immediately followed by surgery. Under these circumstances the time interval between the 2 modalities is generally not sufficient to achieve significant tumor downsizing. Future trials will establish the benefit of an increased time interval between completion of hypofractionated radiotherapy and surgery.

A more controversial issue is whether conventional long-term neoadjuvant chemoradiation can results in an increased rate of low anterior resections as opposed to abdomino-perineal resections. A number of reports have suggested that downsizing of primary tumor by neoadjuvant treatments could result in an increased rate of sphincter-saving surgical procedures [28-31].

On the other hand, a number of surgeons are convinced that the treatment decision regarding sphincter preservation is determined at the time of the initial evaluation of the patient and neoadjuvant treatment does not influence the ability to perform an anterior resection. The evidence in favor of this contention is also limited. However, few carefully designed studies have been conducted to specifically examine this issue.

The GRECCAR 1 study compared high-dose radiation (45 + 18 Gy) to chemoradiotherapy in the preoperative treatment of low rectal cancers located less than 2 cm from the levator ani. Surgeons from 13 different French centers performed intersphincteric resection using a homogeneous technique. There were no significant differences in downstaging or sphincter preservation rates between the two groups and a trend was noted towards increased morbidity after high-dose radiotherapy [32]. The Polish [33] and Lyons R90-01 trials [34] also had sphincter preservation as primary end point but could not demonstrate any advantage in sphincter preservation with the adoption of preoperative treatment.

The results of the German trial suggested that the use of preoperative treatments would result in a 20% increase in the number of patients receiving sphincter sparing procedure. However, this number was calculated on the subset of patients who were deemed poor candidates for sphincter preserving surgery before receiving their treatment. When the overall number of patients enrolled in the trial is considered, the sphincter preservation rates between the two groups were comparable. The earlier NSABP R-03 trial also had sphincter preservation as a secondary end-point. In this specific trial, the authors identified benefits in the use of preoperative treatment related to sphincter preservation. Therefore, the data to assess increased sphincter-preservation as a result of preoperative treatment remains inconclusive. Several important variables affecting the ability to perform an oncologically adequate sphincter-preserving operation remain difficult to accurately evaluate. Firstly, it is accepted that there is variability among surgeons in their ability to perform coloanal anastomoses. For example, the sphincter preservation rate was 23% in the NSABP-03 trial [8] whereas it can be over 70% in specialized centers [9,35-37]. In addition, there there has been a general improvement in sphincter-sparing surgical techniques which make it difficult to compare trials performed at different times. In addition, the clinical assessment performed in the office can be different from the assessment of sphincter involvement while the patient is under general anesthesia and after a complete rectal mobilization. This assessment is subjective and self-reported by examining clinicians. For example, in the German trial 20% of patients assigned to postoperative adjuvant treatment who were deemed to require an abdomino-perineal resection could eventually undergo low anterior resection [9].

Further studies will need to be specifically focused on this issue as additional chemotherapy agents are added to the armament available to tumor response in a neo-adjuvant setting.

POSTOPERATIVE ADJUVANT CHEMOTHERAPY FOLLOWING NEOADJUVANT TREATMENT AND SURGERY

The rationale for postoperative chemotherapy after chemoradiation and surgery for locally advanced rectal cancer is that the doses of neoadjuvant chemotherapeutics administered concurrently with radiotherapy are not considered adequate to address micrometastatic disease which remains a likely event in locally advanced rectal carcinoma. While the use of postoperative chemotherapy in this situation is not supported by strong data from prospective randomized trials, there is at least some evidence supporting this practice.

The European Organization for Research and Treatment of Cancer (EORTC) 22921 trial showed an absolute increase of 6% in 5-year disease-free survival for patients who received some form of chemotherapy vs. those who did not, although this did not reach statistical significance (58.2% vs 52.2%, p=0.13) [6]. However, in a subsequent subgroup analysis, post-operative chemotherapy selectively provided benefit to patients with ypT0-2, but not for those with more advanced disease [38]. Similarly, improved oncologic outcomes from postoperative chemotherapy have been reported by Crane and colleagues only in patients who had experienced T downstaging after neoadjuvant treatment [39]. Based on these data it has been postulated that there is a subset of patients whose improved prognosis can be anticipated based on their favorable tumors response to both preoperative chemoradiotherapy and postoperative chemotherapy. On the other hand, other authors have instead noted particular advantages of postoperative chemotherapy in high-risk patients with post chemoradiation pathologic stages II and III [40] and some series have reported no benefits at all and low patients compliance [41]. There is also evidence from retrospective data suggesting that patients with ypN0 have a favorable prognosis related to their previous response to neoadjuvant treatment but this is not improved by postoperative chemotherapy. I contrast with this, patients with ypN2 disease have a poor prognosis also regardless of their use adjuvant chemotherapy [42]. In the face of such heterogeneous data, there is currently no data from prospective studies purposefully designed to evaluate the impact of postoperative adjuvant chemotherapy in these patients. The GERCOR (Groupe Cooperateur Multidisciplinaire en Oncologie) trial randomly assigned patients with locally advanced rectal cancer treated with pre-operative chemoradiation and surgery to post-operative adjuvant 5FU/leukovorin with or without irinotecan. The results of this trial are not yet available, but 340 patients have been accrued.

While most oncologist in the United States are generally in favor of postoperative chemotherapy [43], future studies are needed to clarify the benefits of postoperative chemotherapy and the subsets of patients who might benefit most from this strategy. A trial designed in Britain will formally evaluate the benefits of postoperative chemotherapy compared with observation alone following chemoradiation and R0 surgical resection (> 1 mm free radial margin) of stage II-III rectal cancer. The investigators of the British Chronicle (CHemotheRapy Or No chemotherapy In CLEar margins) trial plan to randomize 800 patients to six courses of capecitapine and oxaliplatin vs. observation following stratification by surgeon and nodal status (node positive vs. node negative vs. unknown) [44]. Other trials are also underway to examine a number of different agents used for adjuvant chemotherapy following neoadjuvant therapy and surgery (see new trials section).

VARIATIONS IN THE DELIVERY MODALITIES OF RADIATION THERAPY

A number of techniques have been used by radiation oncologists to enhance locally advanced rectal tumor response with the expectation that this would translate into improved oncologic outcomes. First of all, an increased radiation dose could be used. It is generally accepted that there is a proportional relationship between radiation dose administered and local tumor response. This hypothesis was tested in a retrospective series by Mohiuddin and coll. who showed a 67% pCR rate in 8 out of 12 patients treated with preoperative radiation doses of 55Gy or greater and continuous infusion of 5-FU which was much higher than response rates using bolus 5-FU and radiation doses lesser than 50Gy [45]. While toxicity rates were acceptable in this series, the sample size is small and most radiation oncologists still do not use the high radiation doses reported in this study. Another technique tested is referred to as hyperfractionated accelerated radiotherapy. The rationale of this approach is to deliver a high radiation dose in relatively short time to reduce toxicity and maximize radiation effect as well as convenience of treatment. In a study on 250 patients with stages II-III rectal carcinomas, preoperative radiotherapy consisted of 41.6 Gy, delivered in 2.5 weeks and followed by surgery within one week after completion of radiation treatment. This approach achieved downstaging in 38% of patients and a 5-year local recurrence rate of less than 10% [46]. Other groups have introduced hyperfractionated boost techniques or concomitant boost given during standard chemoradiation aiming at increasing both downstaging and sphincter-preservation rates [47,48]. Another possible option at least in theory is intraoperative radiation treatment, which could allow delivering radiotherapy directly onto the tumor bed at risk with minimal exposure of adjacent healthy tissue to the effects of radiation. However, it has been rarely used for stage II-III rectal disease operated with curative intent. It is available in few centers and its advantages in this area have not been demonstrated. Alternatively, in the Lyon 96-02 prospective randomized trial the addition of an endocavitary brachytherapy boost to preoperative radiotherapy was tested against standard chemoradiation and found to be associated with increased sphincter preservation rates. After a median follow-up of 35 months there were no differences between the 2 groups with respect to postoperative morbidity, local relapse and 2-year overall survival [49].

While future studies might confirm the oncologic advantages which could be associated with these modalities of radiation delivery, these studies are often reported from large centers with specific expertise in the use of various radiation techniques. It is therefore difficult to anticipate applicability of these alternative modalities of radiation treatment to the majority of patients with locally advanced rectal carcinoma treated in the United States.

Another area of interest has been the study on the effect of increasing the interval between neoadjuvant therapy and surgery. A prolonged interval time could enhance the effect of radiation treatment and potentially achieve increased tumor response. The potential value of a longer interval before surgery following preoperative radiotherapy was evaluated in the Lyon R90-01 prospective trial. In this study patients were randomized to preoperative radiation therapy followed by surgery in less than 2 weeks vs. 6-8 weeks. There were no significant differences in sphincter preservation rates at the time of surgery or in cancer outcomes after a median follow-up of 6 years [34]. Even longer intervals between radiotherapy and surgery have not shown to be associated with an increased rate of sphincter preservation in other retrospective series [50-52]. In contrast with this, another retrospective study compared patients who underwent earlier vs. later surgery for locally advanced rectal cancer following neoadjuvant chemotherapy. Patients undergoing surgery later than 7 weeks after neoadjuvant treatment experienced increased rates of pCR, near pCR, disease-free survival and decreased recurrence rates when compared to patients undergoing surgery 7 weeks or earlier following neoadjuvant treatment. The results from alternative time intervals remain inconclusive. As new chemotherapeutics are being investigated in the neoadjuvant settings, the relative impact on oncologic outcomes of different time intervals between preoperative radiotherapy and surgery vs. the specific chemotherapy regimens used will have to be further evaluated.

RELATIONSHIP BETWEEN RESPONSE TO PREOPERATIVE TREATMENT AND PROGNOSIS

A number of studies have revealed an association between response to neoadjuvant treatment and cancer outcomes [53-58], especially when patients could achieve pathologic complete response (pCR) [59-64]. While the assessment of some of these studies is complicated by the use of postoperative adjuvant chemotherapy in a significant portion of these patients, only few studies have not been able to confirm this relationship [65,66]. Other studies have introduced the classification of tumor response by histologic regression and suggested that it has prognostic value and should therefore be added as a modification of the current pathologic staging system [67-69].

Most of these studies have focused on the effects of preoperative chemoradiation. Limited data exists on the comparable evaluations after hypofractionated radiotherapy. Exceptions to this are the results from the Polish trial where responses to hypofractionated radiation were compared to responses after long- term, conventional chemoradiation. The ypN status was found to be the only independent predictor of disease-free survival. The central role of pathologic nodal status in predicting cancer outcomes confirms data from other series [70,71]. In addition, the evaluation of the Polish trial results revealed an interaction between N status and assigned treatment arm. While there was no difference between the 2 arms in disease-free survival for ypN-negative patients, ypN-positive individuals had a worse disease-free survival after long-term chemoradiation than after hypofractionated radiotherapy. These results indicate that both radiosensitive and radioresistant tumors can be node-positive after hypofractionated radiotherapy. However, radiochemoresistance of nodal metastases from rectal cancer indicate an increase potential for distant metastases [72].

To clarify the relative impact on prognosis of both treatment and tumor-related factors Quah and colleagues evaluated 342 patients with locally advance rectal cancer following preoperative chemoradiation. The degree of tumor regression was graded on each specimen using a response scale ranging from 0 to 100%. Predictive models of disease-free survival were created using information on pretherapy and postoperative staging information as well as the above-mentioned histological regression scale. The most accurate model in predicting disease-free survival was found to be the pathologic staging inclusive of both ypT and ypN. Response to preoperative treatment was again found to be a strong predictor of disease-free survival [73].

The ability to achieve pCR based on the evaluation of the specimen obtained at radical excision for rectal carcinoma suggests that some patients might not receive therapeutic benefits from radical surgery. Unfortunately, our current limitations in preoperative staging impose radical surgery as the necessary step to appropriately stage patients. Future improvements in staging [74] might achieve the identification of patients who might be spared the risks of radical resection because of their inherently favorable prognosis. In turn, these patients might be treated with either local excision or undergo no surgery at all and be treated with chemoradiation therapy alone.

LOCAL EXCISION OF RECTAL CARCINOMA AND ADJUVANT TREATMENTS

As the morbidity rate associated with radical resection remains substantial, there has been an increasing interest in the use of local excision as a sphincter-sparing, organ-preserving surgical approach. However, local excision alone has been associated with unacceptably high local recurrence rates in multiple studies and has been as reported as high as 47% for T2 carcinomas [75-77]. In spite of these suboptimal results, there is evidence that local excision for rectal cancers is increasingly used in the United States. In a study based on a patient sample from the National Cancer Database, local excision in the treatment of rectal cancer significantly increased from 1989 to 2003 for both T1 and T2 cancers. Not surprisingly, these patients had significantly lower morbidity when compared to the counterparts from the same database treated with standard radical resections. However, local excision was associated with a significantly increased five-year local recurrence rate which was 12.5% vs. 6.9% after excision of T1 tumors and 22.1% vs. 15.1% for T2 tumors following local excision vs. standard resection, respectively. The 5-year overall survival was statistically comparable for T1 tumors, but it was significantly different for T2 tumors and was mainly influenced by age and co-morbidities [78]. As local excision alone remains associated with high recurrence rates, the use of additional treatments is under investigation to determine if cancer outcomes can be improved by multimodality treatment, especially for T2 disease. In these regards, cancer cooperative groups have conducted studies to address the ability of postoperative chemoradiation to improve cancer outcomes following local excision. For example, the Cancer and Leukemia Group B (CALGB) 8984 trial included accrual of T2 patient which were treated with radiotherapy and 5-FU following transanal excision. After a median follow-up of 7.1 years the disease-free survival for T2 disease was 64 percent and the local recurrence rate was 18% [79]. In a subgroup of T2 patients from the Radiation Therapy Oncology Group (RTOG) protocol 89-02 treated similarly, local recurrence was detected alone or simultaneously with distant recurrence in 4 out of 25 cases (16%) after a minimum follow-up of 5 years. The results of these studies suggest that postoperative treatment can benefit patients when compared to surgery alone but overall cancer outcomes are still worse than after radical surgery for disease with comparable staging. Other studies have therefore focused on neoadjuvant rather than postoperative chemoradiation in addition to local excision. Single institutional series have indicated that this approach is safe and feasible and in some cases results have been encouraging and better than for local excision followed by postoperative chemoradiation. Some surgeons advocate the use of transanal endoscopic microsurgery (TEM) as a tool which could enhance completeness of tumor excision after neoadjuvant treatment of T2 and even T3 lesions [80], whose presumed advantages have not been confirmed yet on a larger scale. In a select group of patients who refused or could not tolerate an abdomino-perineal resection, neoadjuvant chemoradiation and local excision have resulted in low recurrence rates and cancer outcomes comparable to multimodality treatments including radical surgery [81-83] which was often related to a high pathologic complete response (pCR) rate. These series are from single institutions and present an often relatively small sample size with limited follow-up. Larger multicenter studies are therefore underway to asses the validity of neoadjuvant chemoradiation and local excision using a variety of agents. The American College of Surgeons Oncology Group (ACOSOG) is conducting a study to evaluate the role of neoadjuvant treatment with capecitabine and oxaliplatin followed by local excision for low T2N0 rectal cancers. Similar trials are underway in Europe [84].

While local excision for low rectal cancer remains an appropriate treatment for patients who carry prohibitive perioperative risks for major abdominal surgery, good-risk individuals should not be treated with local excision alone, particularly for T2 and T3 cancers. Results from ongoing studies will better delineate the role of neoadjuvant treatment followed by local excision.

CHEMORADIATION TREATMENT ALONE FOR RECTAL CARCINOMA

The role of chemoradiation treatment alone in the treatment of rectal cancer has been championed by Habr-Gama and colleagues from Sao Paulo, Brazil. In a sequence of reports with increasingly longer follow-up, the five-year overall survival was 93% and 5-year disease-free survival was 85% [85]. The Authors reported five cases of local recurrences which could all be salvaged. This paper has been criticized as the results pertain only to 99 out of 122 patients who were deemed to have clinical complete response [86]. It has been, therefore, assumed that the difference between these two numbers includes patients who experience local recurrence within 12 months of treatment. No other groups have been able to replicate these intriguing results [87]. On the other hand, several investigators have noted that even after complete clinical response between 40% and 75% of patients retain viable tumor detectable at pathologic examination of the surgical specimen following radical resection [65,88-90]. In addition, the salvage rates following local recurrence after local excision for rectal cancer in most reports on local recurrence of rectal cancer previously treated with local excision are in the range of 50% of cases [91]. Therefore, chemoradiation as the sole treatment for rectal cancer should be regarded with extreme caution at this time. This option at the moment may be considered for individual cases of patients with significant co-morbidities who would not be otherwise a candidate for treatment of rectal cancer with radical excision or within the confines of an investigational trial. As the results of Habr-Gama and coll. do indicate that there is a subset of patients who could be cured without surgery, future efforts are concentrated in improving the assessment of treatment response. In this regard, trials have been reported and are underway to analyze the value of MRI in the evaluation of clinical response in rectal cancer [92,93]. In addition, a number of genetic markers as possible predictor of tumor response to preoperative treatments are under investigations including apoptotic index and expression of P53, P21, P27, BCL-2, epidermal growth factor receptor, bax vascular endothelial growth factor gene, cyclo-oxygenase II and growth hormone receptor [94,95].

NEW AGENTS AND TRIALS (HTTP://WWW.CANCER.GOV/CLINICALTRIALS/SEARCH/)

A number of trials are underway to evaluate the potential of multimodality treatment combinations including alternative chemoradiotherapy schedules and techniques. Most noticeably, a number of newer chemotherapeutic agents are being tested based on their activity demonstrated in patients with metastatic colorectal carcinoma. Agents with a proven activity in the colon cancer adjuvant setting are more frequently tested in phase II trials whereas biologics and other less commonly used agents are most frequently components of earlier phase trials.

OXALIPLATIN

The role of oxaliplatin in neoadjuvant and adjuvant chemotherapy in stage II and II rectal cancer is under investigation with the expectation that it could demonstrate improved cancer outcomes similarly to what has been reported in the adjuvant treatment of colon cancer [96]. The phase III E3201 trial was designed to compare the safety of different postoperative chemotherapeutic regimens following neoadjuvant chemoradiation and surgical resection of locally advanced rectal cancer. The safety profile of FOLFOX, FOLFIRI and FU/LV were compared and it was demonstrated that the use of FOLFOX in this setting was a safe and acceptable option [97]. The Data Monitoring Committee subsequently closed E3201 and developed trial E5204 which will compare postoperative chemotherapy including FOLFOX with or without bevacizumab. The German Rectal Cancer Study Group is also planning a new study to evaluate the addition of oxaliplatin to multimodality treatment for locally advanced rectal cancer. In fact, their new study (CAO/ARO/AIO-04) will compare neoadjuvant chemoradiotherapy and adjuvant chemotherapy with 5-fluorouracil and oxaliplatin versus 5-fluorouracil alone in rectal cancer. The Authors' hypothesis is that the rate of disease-free survival will improve by 5% to 8% after 3 years of follow-up. In Italy an analogous phase III randomized trial has been conducted and the safety data presented in an abstract form. Aschele and coll. reported the results on 410 patients enrolled into the STAR (Studio Terapia Adiuvante Retto) trial. While the addition of oxaliplatin to the neoadjuvant treatment resulted in an increased frequency and severity of acute toxicity there were no major adverse events and most patients could still receive radiation treatment and undergo surgery [98]. Newer trials will attempt to assess the appropriate dosages and shedules of oxaliplatin within the context of multimodality treatments. A phase I dose-escalation study of preoperative oxaliplatin aims to establish the maximum tolerated dose on patients treated with neoadjuvant radiotherapy with oxaliplatin and 5-FU followed by surgery and adjuvant 5-FU-based chemotherapy [99]. Another trial will compare different schedules and cycle numbers of neoadjuvant FOLFOX combined with 5-FU and radiotherapy with the goal of assessing pCR rates and the impact of different treatment arms on postoperative surgical morbidity.

CAPECITABINE AND OTHER ORAL FLUOROPYRIMIDINES

The role of oral fluoropyrimidines, particularly capecitabine, which is approved in the United States, is being evaluated in the multimodality treatment of rectal cancer after clinical trials showed at least comparable effect to infusional fluorouracil in the adjuvant treatment of stage III colon carcinoma [100]. Capecitabine will therefore be evaluated as a substitute for fluorouracil during preoperative chemoradiation for locally advanced rectal cancer. The ACCORD 12 trial in France will compare capecitabine to capecitabine and oxaliplatin with radiotherapy in the treatment of T3-4 and distal T2 rectal cancer and plans to accrue 590 patients. Another trial also in France will evaluate Ftorafur (tegafur +uracil) with radiotherapy vs. radiotherapy alone in the neoadjuvant treatment of stage II and III rectal carcinomas. Other trials will examine combinations including oxaliplatin, capecitabine and biologics [101]. Another study will assess an induction chemotherapy combination of capecitabine and irinotecan followed by concomitant chemoradiotherapy again with capecitabine and then surgery.

The American NSABP R-04 trial is enrolling at the time of this writing and its investigators plan to accrue over 1600 patients within 4 years and randomize them to 4 groups who will all receive preoperative radiotherapy and either 5-FU or capecitabine with or without oxaliplatin. The trial will therefore provide data on both the use of oral fluoropyrimidines as a substitute for infusional 5-FU and the ability of oxaliplatin to be tolerated and benefit patients with rectal cancer who also receive preoperative radiotherapy. The primary endpoint will be locoregional recurrence at 3 years. Patients will be encouraged to receive postoperative adjuvant treatment. In particular, they will be eligible to participate in the above-mentioned E5204 to evaluate the impact of adjuvant FOLFOX and bevacizumab as described above.

TRIALS INCLUDING BIOLOGICS

A number of trials are also underway to evaluate the potential impact of monoclonal antibodies, especially cetuximab [102] and bevacizumab [103], on the neoadjuvant and adjuvant treatment of locally advanced rectal cancer. Several of these trials address stage II and III cancers and therefore include surgery. Bevacizumab will be tested in phase I and II trials using different neoadjuvant combinations including 5-FU, capecitabine, oxaliplatin, and radiation therapy. One trial will tests capecitabine, oxaliplatin and bevacizumab combined for induction chemotherapy followed by additional concomitant capecitabine during preoperative radiotherapy and then surgery. In another trial bevacizumab will be tested as a component of both the neoadjuvant and adjuvant treatments. The neoadjuvant therapy will also include capecitabine, oxaliplatin and radiotherapy while the adjuvant chemotherapy will be in combination with fluorouracil, leucovorin and oxaliplatin.

Cetuximab will be evaluated in phase I and II trials with a design similar to those using bevacizumab. It will therefore be included in various neoadjuvant treatment combinations including oxaliplatin, capecitabine, 5-FU, with or without radiotherapy. It will also be tested as a componenet of induction chemotherapy with capecitabine and oxaliplatin followed by concomitant chemoradiation again using the 2 latter agents and then surgery. The main endpoint in most of these early phase trials including biologics will be the rate of pathologic complete response which could prompt further phase III studies analyzing more specific cancer outcomes.

OTHER TREATMENTS

A Phase II Multicenter Study conducted by the NCCTG (North Central Cancer Treatment Gorup) will examine the addition of celecoxib to capecitabine as neoadjuvant agent in Combination With Pelvic Irradiation in Patients With Stage II or III Adenocarcinoma of the Rectum. In addition, patients will receive postoperative capecitabine.

Intensity-modulated radiotherapy, a more refined form of radiotherapy designed to enhance tumor targeting as well as sparing of surrounding healthy structures, will also be tested in a phase II trial combined with capecitabine and oxaliplatin and followed by surgery and adjuvant chemotherapy with FOLFOX.

Other less commonly used agents are also under investigations. For example, a phase II randomized study will be carried out evaluating neoadjuvant capecitabine and radiotherapy with or without adenovirus 5-Tumor Necrosis Factor Alpha (TNFerade™) followed by surgical resection in patients with either stage II, III, or locally recurrent rectal cancer. Other less commonly used agents include selenomethionine, rapamycin during short –term radiotherapy, nelfinavir and premetrexed. One phase II trial will attempt to deliver genotype-directed neoadjuvant chemotherapy based on the molecular analysis of thymidylate-synthase promoter.

REFERENCES

[1] Tzardi M. Role of total mesorectal excision and of circumferential resection margin in local recurrence and survival of patients with rectal carcinoma. *Dig Dis* 2007; 25(1):51-5.

[2] Douglass HO, Jr., Moertel CG, Mayer RJ, et al. Survival after postoperative combination treatment of rectal cancer. *N Engl J Med* 1986; 315(20):1294-5.

[3] Fisher B, Wolmark N, Rockette H, et al. Postoperative adjuvant chemotherapy or radiation therapy for rectal cancer: results from NSABP protocol R-01. *J Natl Cancer Inst* 1988; 80(1):21-9.

[4] NIH consensus conference. Adjuvant therapy for patients with colon and rectal cancer. *Jama* 1990; 264(11):1444-50.

[5] Van Cutsem E, Dicato M, Haustermans K, et al. The diagnosis and management of rectal cancer: expert discussion and recommendations derived from the 9th World Congress on Gastrointestinal Cancer, Barcelona, 2007. *Ann Oncol* 2008; 19 Suppl 6:vi1-8.

[6] Bosset JF, Collette L, Calais G, et al. Chemotherapy with preoperative radiotherapy in rectal cancer. *N Engl J Med* 2006; 355(11):1114-23.

[7] Gerard JP, Conroy T, Bonnetain F, et al. Preoperative radiotherapy with or without concurrent fluorouracil and leucovorin in T3-4 rectal cancers: results of FFCD 9203. *J Clin Oncol* 2006; 24(28):4620-5.

[8] Hyams DM, Mamounas EP, Petrelli N, et al. A clinical trial to evaluate the worth of preoperative multimodality therapy in patients with operable carcinoma of the rectum: a progress report of National Surgical Breast and Bowel Project Protocol R-03. *Dis Colon Rectum* 1997; 40(2):131-9.

[9] Sauer R, Becker H, Hohenberger W, et al. Preoperative versus postoperative chemoradiotherapy for rectal cancer. *N Engl J Med* 2004; 351(17):1731-40.

[10] Folkesson J, Birgisson H, Pahlman L, et al. Swedish Rectal Cancer Trial: long lasting benefits from radiotherapy on survival and local recurrence rate. *J Clin Oncol* 2005; 23(24):5644-50.

[11] Birgisson H, Pahlman L, Gunnarsson U, Glimelius B. Adverse effects of preoperative radiation therapy for rectal cancer: long-term follow-up of the Swedish Rectal Cancer Trial. *J Clin Oncol* 2005; 23(34):8697-705.

[12] Peeters KC, Marijnen CA, Nagtegaal ID, et al. The TME trial after a median follow-up of 6 years: increased local control but no survival benefit in irradiated patients with resectable rectal carcinoma. *Ann Surg* 2007; 246(5):693-701.

[13] Roswit B, Higgins GA, Keehn RJ. Preoperative irradiation for carcinoma of the rectum and rectosigmoid colon: reportof a National Veterans Administration randomized study. *Cancer* 1975; 35(6):1597-602.

[14] Higgins GA, Humphrey EW, Dwight RW, et al. Preoperative radiation and surgery for cancer of the rectum. Veterans Administration Surgical Oncology Group Trial II. *Cancer* 1986; 58(2):352-9.

[15] Peeters KC, van de Velde CJ, Leer JW, et al. Late side effects of short-course preoperative radiotherapy combined with total mesorectal excision for rectal cancer: increased bowel dysfunction in irradiated patients--a Dutch colorectal cancer group study. *J Clin Oncol* 2005; 23(25):6199-206.

[16] Das P, Crane CH. Preoperative and adjuvant treatment of localized rectal cancer. *Curr Oncol Rep* 2006; 8(3):167-73.

[17] Willett CG, Czito BG, Bendell JC. Radiation therapy in stage II and III rectal cancer. *Clin Cancer Res* 2007; 13(22 Pt 2):6903s-8s.

[18] Bujko K, Nowacki MP, Nasierowska-Guttmejer A, et al. Long-term results of a randomized trial comparing preoperative short-course radiotherapy with preoperative conventionally fractionated chemoradiation for rectal cancer. *Br J Surg* 2006; 93(10):1215-23.

[19] Sebag-Montefiore D SR, Quirke P, R. Grieve, S. Khanna, J. Monson, A. Holliday, L. Thompson, G. Griffiths, R. Stephens. Routine short course pre-op radiotherapy or selective post-op chemoradiotherapy for resectable rectal cancer? Preliminary results of the MRC CR07 randomised trial. *J Clin Oncol*, 2006 ASCO Annual Meeting Proceedings Part I. Vol 24, No. 18S (June 20 Supplement), 2006: 3511 2006.

[20] P. Quirke DS-M, R. Steele, S. Khanna, J. Monson, A. Holliday, L. Thompson, G. Griffiths, R. Stephens Local recurrence after rectal cancer resection is strongly related to the plane of surgical dissection and is further reduced by pre-operative short course radiotherapy. Preliminary results of the Medical Research Council (MRC) CR07 trial *J Clin Oncol*, 2006 ASCO Annual Meeting Proceedings Part I. Vol 24, No 18S (June 20 Supplement), 2006: 3512 2006.

[21] Merchant NB, Guillem JG, Paty PB, et al. T3N0 rectal cancer: results following sharp mesorectal excision and no adjuvant therapy. *J Gastrointest Surg* 1999; 3(6):642-7.

[22] Willett CG, Badizadegan K, Ancukiewicz M, Shellito PC. Prognostic factors in stage T3N0 rectal cancer: do all patients require postoperative pelvic irradiation and chemotherapy? *Dis Colon Rectum* 1999; 42(2):167-73.

[23] Merkel S, Mansmann U, Siassi M, et al. The prognostic inhomogeneity in pT3 rectal carcinomas. *Int J Colorectal Dis* 2001; 16(5):298-304.

[24] Miyoshi M, Ueno H, Hashiguchi Y, et al. Extent of mesorectal tumor invasion as a prognostic factor after curative surgery for T3 rectal cancer patients. *Ann Surg* 2006; 243(4):492-8.

[25] Steel MC, Woods R, Mackay JM, Chen F. Extent of mesorectal invasion is a prognostic indicator in T3 rectal carcinoma. *ANZ J Surg* 2002; 72(7):483-7.

[26] Gunderson LL, Sargent DJ, Tepper JE, et al. Impact of T and N stage and treatment on survival and relapse in adjuvant rectal cancer: a pooled analysis. *J Clin Oncol* 2004; 22(10):1785-96.

[27] Guillem JG, Diaz-Gonzalez JA, Minsky BD, et al. cT3N0 rectal cancer: potential overtreatment with preoperative chemoradiotherapy is warranted. *J Clin Oncol* 2008; 26(3):368-73.

[28] Allal AS, Bieri S, Pelloni A, et al. Sphincter-sparing surgery after preoperative radiotherapy for low rectal cancers: feasibility, oncologic results and quality of life outcomes. *Br J Cancer* 2000; 82(6):1131-7.

[29] Luna-Perez P, Rodriguez-Ramirez S, Rodriguez-Coria DF, et al. Preoperative chemoradiation therapy and anal sphincter preservation with locally advanced rectal adenocarcinoma. *World J Surg* 2001; 25(8):1006-11.

[30] Crane CH, Skibber JM, Birnbaum EH, et al. The addition of continuous infusion 5-FU to preoperative radiation therapy increases tumor response, leading to increased sphincter preservation in locally advanced rectal cancer. *Int J Radiat Oncol Biol Phys* 2003; 57(1):84-9.

[31] Kim DW, Lim SB, Kim DY, et al. Pre-operative chemo-radiotherapy improves the sphincter preservation rate in patients with rectal cancer located within 3 cm of the anal verge. *Eur J Surg Oncol* 2006; 32(2):162-7.

[32] Rouanet P RM, Lelong B, E. Rullier, F. Dravet, L. Mineur, L. Vanseymortier, M. Pocard, J. Faucheron, S. Gourgou, B. Saint Aubert. Sphincter preserving surgery after preoperative treatment for ultra-low rectal carcinoma. A French multicenter prospective trial: GRECCAR 1. *J Clin Oncol*, ASCO Annual Meeting Proceedings Part I. Vol 24, No. 18S (June 20 Supplement), 2006: 3527 2006.

[33] Bujko K, Nowacki MP, Nasierowska-Guttmejer A, et al. Sphincter preservation following preoperative radiotherapy for rectal cancer: report of a randomised trial comparing short-term radiotherapy vs. conventionally fractionated radiochemotherapy. *Radiother Oncol* 2004; 72(1):15-24.

[34] Glehen O, Chapet O, Adham M, et al. Long-term results of the Lyons R90-01 randomized trial of preoperative radiotherapy with delayed surgery and its effect on sphincter-saving surgery in rectal cancer. *Br J Surg* 2003; 90(8):996-8.

[35] Heald RJ, Moran BJ, Ryall RD, et al. Rectal cancer: the Basingstoke experience of total mesorectal excision, 1978-1997. *Arch Surg* 1998; 133(8):894-9.

[36] Rengan R, Paty PB, Wong WD, et al. Ten-year results of preoperative radiation followed by sphincter preservation for rectal cancer: increased local failure rate in nonresponders. *Clin Colorectal Cancer* 2006; 5(6):413-21.

[37] Wu XJ, Wang JP, Wang L, et al. Increased rate change over time of a sphincter-saving procedure for lower rectal cancer. *Chin Med J (Engl)* 2008; 121(7):636-9.

[38] Collette L, Bosset JF, den Dulk M, et al. Patients with curative resection of cT3-4 rectal cancer after preoperative radiotherapy or radiochemotherapy: does anybody benefit from adjuvant fluorouracil-based chemotherapy? A trial of the European Organisation for Research and Treatment of Cancer Radiation Oncology Group. *J Clin Oncol* 2007; 25(28):4379-86.

[39] Crane C, Thames, H, Skibber, J, et al. . 5-FU based aduvant chemotherapy given after neoadjuvant chemoradiation improves survival only among responders (abstract). *Eur J Cancer* 2001; 37(6 suppl): 271s.

[40] Chan A, Wong, A, Jenken, D, et al. . Is postoperative adjuvant chemotherapy necessary in locally advanced rectal cancers after preoperative chemoradiation (abstract). *Int J Radiat oncol Biol Phys* 2004; 60:S297.

[41] Cionini L, Manfredi, B, Sainato, A, et al. . Randomized study of postoperative chemotherapy (CT) after preoperative chemoradiotherapy (CRT) in locally advanced rectal cancer (LARC). Preliminary results (abstract). *Eur J Cancer* 2001, 37 (6 suppl):S300

[42] Fietkau R, Barten M, Klautke G, et al. Postoperative chemotherapy may not be necessary for patients with ypN0-category after neoadjuvant chemoradiotherapy of rectal cancer. *Dis Colon Rectum* 2006; 49(9):1284-92.

[43] O'Neil BH, Tepper JE. Current options for the management of rectal cancer. *Curr Treat Options Oncol* 2007; 8(5):331-8.

[44] Glynne-Jones R, Meadows H, Wood W. Chemotherapy or no chemotherapy in clear margins after neoadjuvant chemoradiation in locally advanced rectal cancer: CHRONICLE. A randomised phase III trial of control vs. capecitabine plus oxaliplatin. *Clin Oncol (R Coll Radiol)* 2007; 19(5):327-9.

[45] Mohiuddin M, Regine WF, John WJ, et al. Preoperative chemoradiation in fixed distal rectal cancer: dose time factors for pathological complete response. *Int J Radiat Oncol Biol Phys* 2000; 46(4):883-8.

[46] Coucke PA, Notter M, Stamm B, et al. Preoperative hyper-fractionated accelerated radiotherapy (HART) in locally advanced rectal cancer (LARC) immediately followed by surgery. A prospective phase II trial. *Radiother Oncol* 2006; 79(1):52-8.

[47] Movsas B, Diratzouian H, Hanlon A, et al. Phase II trial of preoperative chemoradiation with a hyperfractionated radiation boost in locally advanced rectal cancer. *Am J Clin Oncol* 2006; 29(5):435-41.

[48] Janjan NA, Crane CN, Feig BW, et al. Prospective trial of preoperative concomitant boost radiotherapy with continuous infusion 5-fluorouracil for locally advanced rectal cancer. *Int J Radiat Oncol Biol Phys* 2000; 47(3):713-8.

[49] Gerard JP, Chapet O, Nemoz C, et al. Improved sphincter preservation in low rectal cancer with high-dose preoperative radiotherapy: the lyon R96-02 randomized trial. *J Clin Oncol* 2004; 22(12):2404-9.

[50] Stein DE, Mahmoud NN, Anne PR, et al. Longer time interval between completion of neoadjuvant chemoradiation and surgical resection does not improve downstaging of rectal carcinoma. *Dis Colon Rectum* 2003; 46(4):448-53.

[51] Dolinsky CM, Mahmoud NN, Mick R, et al. Effect of time interval between surgery and preoperative chemoradiotherapy with 5-fluorouracil or 5-fluorouracil and oxaliplatin on outcomes in rectal cancer. *J Surg Oncol* 2007; 96(3):207-12.

[52] Habr-Gama A, Perez RO, Proscurshim I, et al. Interval Between Surgery and Neoadjuvant Chemoradiation Therapy for Distal Rectal Cancer: Does Delayed Surgery Have an Impact on Outcome? *Int J Radiat Oncol Biol Phys* 2008.

[53] Mohiuddin M, Hayne M, Regine WF, et al. Prognostic significance of postchemoradiation stage following preoperative chemotherapy and radiation for advanced/recurrent rectal cancers. *Int J Radiat Oncol Biol Phys* 2000; 48(4):1075-80.

[54] Janjan NA, Crane C, Feig BW, et al. Improved overall survival among responders to preoperative chemoradiation for locally advanced rectal cancer. *Am J Clin Oncol* 2001; 24(2):107-12.

[55] Valentini V, Coco C, Picciocchi A, et al. Does downstaging predict improved outcome after preoperative chemoradiation for extraperitoneal locally advanced rectal cancer? A long-term analysis of 165 patients. *Int J Radiat Oncol Biol Phys* 2002; 53(3):664-74.

[56] Kim NK, Baik SH, Seong JS, et al. Oncologic outcomes after neoadjuvant chemoradiation followed by curative resection with tumor-specific mesorectal excision for fixed locally advanced rectal cancer: Impact of postirradiated pathologic downstaging on local recurrence and survival. *Ann Surg* 2006; 244(6):1024-30.

[57] Kuo LJ, Liu MC, Jian JJ, et al. Is final TNM staging a predictor for survival in locally advanced rectal cancer after preoperative chemoradiation therapy? *Ann Surg Oncol* 2007; 14(10):2766-72.

[58] Gavioli M, Luppi G, Losi L, et al. Incidence and clinical impact of sterilized disease and minimal residual disease after preoperative radiochemotherapy for rectal cancer. *Dis Colon Rectum* 2005; 48(10):1851-7.

[59] Willett CG, Warland G, Hagan MP, et al. Tumor proliferation in rectal cancer following preoperative irradiation. *J Clin Oncol* 1995; 13(6):1417-24.

[60] Bozzetti F, Baratti D, Andreola S, et al. Preoperative radiation therapy for patients with T2-T3 carcinoma of the middle-to-lower rectum. *Cancer* 1999; 86(3):398-404.

[61] Rodel C, Martus P, Papadoupolos T, et al. Prognostic significance of tumor regression after preoperative chemoradiotherapy for rectal cancer. *J Clin Oncol* 2005; 23(34):8688-96.

[62] Stipa F, Chessin DB, Shia J, et al. A pathologic complete response of rectal cancer to preoperative combined-modality therapy results in improved oncological outcome compared with those who achieve no downstaging on the basis of preoperative endorectal ultrasonography. *Ann Surg Oncol* 2006; 13(8):1047-53.

[63] Wiig JN, Larsen SG, Dueland S, Giercksky KE. Clinical outcome in patients with complete pathologic response (pT0) to preoperative irradiation/chemo-irradiation operated for locally advanced or locally recurrent rectal cancer. *J Surg Oncol* 2005; 92(1):70-5.

[64] Capirci C, Valentini V, Cionini L, et al. Prognostic Value of Pathologic Complete Response After Neoadjuvant Therapy in Locally Advanced Rectal Cancer: Long-term Analysis of 566 ypCR Patients. *Int J Radiat Oncol Biol Phys* 2008.

[65] Onaitis MW, Noone RB, Fields R, et al. Complete response to neoadjuvant chemoradiation for rectal cancer does not influence survival. *Ann Surg Oncol* 2001; 8(10):801-6.

[66] Pucciarelli S, Toppan P, Friso ML, et al. Complete pathologic response following preoperative chemoradiation therapy for middle to lower rectal cancer is not a prognostic factor for a better outcome. *Dis Colon Rectum* 2004; 47(11):1798-807.

[67] Dworak O, Keilholz L, Hoffmann A. Pathological features of rectal cancer after preoperative radiochemotherapy. *Int J Colorectal Dis* 1997; 12(1):19-23.

[68] Wheeler JM, Warren BF, Mortensen NJ, et al. Quantification of histologic regression of rectal cancer after irradiation: a proposal for a modified staging system. *Dis Colon Rectum* 2002; 45(8):1051-6.

[69] Vecchio FM, Valentini V, Minsky BD, et al. The relationship of pathologic tumor regression grade (TRG) and outcomes after preoperative therapy in rectal cancer. *Int J Radiat Oncol Biol Phys* 2005; 62(3):752-60.

[70] Onaitis MW, Noone RB, Hartwig M, et al. Neoadjuvant chemoradiation for rectal cancer: analysis of clinical outcomes from a 13-year institutional experience. *Ann Surg* 2001; 233(6):778-85.

[71] Shivnani AT, Small W, Jr., Stryker SJ, et al. Preoperative chemoradiation for rectal cancer: results of multimodality management and analysis of prognostic factors. *Am J Surg* 2007; 193(3):389-93; discussion 393-4.

[72] Bujko K, Michalski W, Kepka L, et al. Association between pathologic response in metastatic lymph nodes after preoperative chemoradiotherapy and risk of distant metastases in rectal cancer: An analysis of outcomes in a randomized trial. *Int J Radiat Oncol Biol Phys* 2007; 67(2):369-77.

[73] Quah HM, Chou JF, Gonen M, et al. Pathologic stage is most prognostic of disease-free survival in locally advanced rectal cancer patients after preoperative chemoradiation. *Cancer* 2008; 113(1):57-64.

[74] Diagnostic accuracy of preoperative magnetic resonance imaging in predicting curative resection of rectal cancer: prospective observational study. *Bmj* 2006; 333(7572):779.

[75] Mellgren A, Sirivongs P, Rothenberger DA, et al. Is local excision adequate therapy for early rectal cancer? *Dis Colon Rectum* 2000; 43(8):1064-71; discussion 1071-4.

[76] Paty PB, Nash GM, Baron P, et al. Long-term results of local excision for rectal cancer. *Ann Surg* 2002; 236(4):522-29; discussion 529-30.

[77] Madbouly KM, Remzi FH, Erkek BA, et al. Recurrence after transanal excision of T1 rectal cancer: should we be concerned? *Dis Colon Rectum* 2005; 48(4):711-9; discussion 719-21.

[78] You YN, Baxter NN, Stewart A, Nelson H. Is the increasing rate of local excision for stage I rectal cancer in the United States justified?: a nationwide cohort study from the National Cancer Database. *Ann Surg* 2007; 245(5):726-33.

[79] Greenberg JA, Shibata D, Herndon JE, 2nd, et al. Local Excision of Distal Rectal Cancer: An Update of Cancer and Leukemia Group B 8984. *Dis Colon Rectum* 2008.

[80] Guerrieri M, Baldarelli M, Organetti L, et al. Transanal endoscopic microsurgery for the treatment of selected patients with distal rectal cancer: 15 years experience. *Surg Endosc* 2008.

[81] Kim CJ, Yeatman TJ, Coppola D, et al. Local excision of T2 and T3 rectal cancers after downstaging chemoradiation. *Ann Surg* 2001; 234(3):352-8; discussion 358-9.

[82] Ruo L, Guillem JG, Minsky BD, et al. Preoperative radiation with or without chemotherapy and full-thickness transanal excision for selected T2 and T3 distal rectal cancers. *Int J Colorectal Dis* 2002; 17(1):54-8.

[83] Bonnen M, Crane C, Vauthey JN, et al. Long-term results using local excision after preoperative chemoradiation among selected T3 rectal cancer patients. *Int J Radiat Oncol Biol Phys* 2004; 60(4):1098-105.

[84] Ortholan C, Gerard JP, Benezery K, Francois E. State of the art and recent advance in the treatment of resectable nonmetastatic rectal cancer. *Surg Oncol* 2007; 16 Suppl 1:S125-8.

[85] Habr-Gama A, Perez RO, Proscurshim I, et al. Patterns of failure and survival for nonoperative treatment of stage c0 distal rectal cancer following neoadjuvant chemoradiation therapy. *J Gastrointest Surg* 2006; 10(10):1319-28; discussion 1328-9.

[86] Bujko K, Kepka L, Nowacki MP. Chemoradiotherapy alone for rectal cancer: a word of caution. *Lancet Oncol* 2007; 8(10):860-2; author reply 862-3.

[87] Nakagawa WT, Rossi BM, de OFF, et al. Chemoradiation instead of surgery to treat mid and low rectal tumors: is it safe? *Ann Surg Oncol* 2002; 9(6):568-73.

[88] Chari RS, Tyler DS, Anscher MS, et al. Preoperative radiation and chemotherapy in the treatment of adenocarcinoma of the rectum. *Ann Surg* 1995; 221(6):778-86; discussion 786-7.

[89] Zmora O, Dasilva GM, Gurland B, et al. Does rectal wall tumor eradication with preoperative chemoradiation permit a change in the operative strategy? *Dis Colon Rectum* 2004; 47(10):1607-12.

[90] Hiotis SP, Weber SM, Cohen AM, et al. Assessing the predictive value of clinical complete response to neoadjuvant therapy for rectal cancer: an analysis of 488 patients. *J Am Coll Surg* 2002; 194(2):131-5; discussion 135-6.

[91] Weiser MR, Landmann RG, Wong WD, et al. Surgical salvage of recurrent rectal cancer after transanal excision. *Dis Colon Rectum* 2005; 48(6):1169-75.

[92] O'Neill BD, Brown G, Heald RJ, et al. Non-operative treatment after neoadjuvant chemoradiotherapy for rectal cancer. *Lancet Oncol* 2007; 8(7):625-33.

[93] Maretto I, Pomerri F, Pucciarelli S, et al. The potential of restaging in the prediction of pathologic response after preoperative chemoradiotherapy for rectal cancer. *Ann Surg Oncol* 2007; 14(2):455-61.

[94] Ghadimi BM, Grade M, Difilippantonio MJ, et al. Effectiveness of gene expression profiling for response prediction of rectal adenocarcinomas to preoperative chemoradiotherapy. *J Clin Oncol* 2005; 23(9):1826-38.

[95] Chang HJ, Jung KH, Kim DY, et al. Bax, a predictive marker for therapeutic response to preoperative chemoradiotherapy in patients with rectal carcinoma. *Hum Pathol* 2005; 36(4):364-71.

[96] Andre T, Boni C, Mounedji-Boudiaf L, et al. Oxaliplatin, fluorouracil, and leucovorin as adjuvant treatment for colon cancer. *N Engl J Med* 2004; 350(23):2343-51.

[97] Benson AB CP, Meropol NJ, B. J. Giantonio, E. R. Sigurdson, J. A. Martenson, R. P. Whitehead, F. Sinicrope, R. J. Mayer, P. J. O'Dwyer. ECOG E3201: Intergroup randomized phase III study of postoperative irinotecan, 5- fluorouracil (FU), leucovorin (LV) (FOLFIRI) vs oxaliplatin, FU/LV (FOLFOX) vs FU/LV for patients (pts) with stage II/ III rectal cancer receiving either pre or postoperative radiation (RT)/ FU. *J Clin Oncol*, ASCO Annual Meeting Proceedings Part I. Vol 24, No. 18S (June 20 Supplement), 2006: 3526 2006.

[98] C. Aschele CP, S. Cordio, G. Rosati, A. Bonetti, O. Alabiso, S. Siena, S. Pucciarelli, L. Boni, L. Cionini,. Preoperative FU-based chemoradiation with or without weekly oxaliplatin in locally advanced rectal cancer: Preliminary safety findings of the STAR

(Studio Terapia Adiuvante Retto)-01 randomized trial. *Journal of Clinical Oncology*, 2007 ASCO Annual Meeting Proceedings Part I. Vol 25, No. 18S (June 20 Supplement), 2007: 4040 2007.

[99] D. I. Rosenthal PC, D. G. Haller, J. C. Landry, E. R. Sigurdson, F. R. Spitz, A. B. Benson. ECOG 1297: A phase I study of preoperative radiaton therapy (RT) with concurrent protracted continuous infusion 5-FU and dose escalating oxaliplatin followed by surgery, adjuvant 5-FU, and leucovorin for locally advanced (T3/4) rectal adenocarcinoma *Proc Am Soc Clin Oncol 22* (abstr 1094) 2003.

[100] Twelves C, Wong A, Nowacki MP, et al. Capecitabine as adjuvant treatment for stage III colon cancer. *N Engl J Med* 2005; 352(26):2696-704.

[101] Machiels JP, Duck L, Honhon B, et al. Phase II study of preoperative oxaliplatin, capecitabine and external beam radiotherapy in patients with rectal cancer: the RadiOxCape study. *Ann Oncol* 2005; 16(12):1898-905.

[102] Machiels JP, Sempoux C, Scalliet P, et al. Phase I/II study of preoperative cetuximab, capecitabine, and external beam radiotherapy in patients with rectal cancer. *Ann Oncol* 2007; 18(4):738-44.

[103] Czito BG, Bendell JC, Willett CG, et al. Bevacizumab, oxaliplatin, and capecitabine with radiation therapy in rectal cancer: Phase I trial results. *Int J Radiat Oncol Biol Phys* 2007; 68(2):472-8.

In: Rectal Cancer: Etiology, Pathogenesis and Treatment
Editors: Paula Wells and Regina Halstead

ISBN 978-1-60692-563-8
© 2009 Nova Science Publishers, Inc.

Chapter III

THREE-DIMENSIONAL ENDORECTAL ULTRASONOGRAPHY IN RECTAL CANCER STAGING

G.A. Santoro[1], S. Magrini[2] and L. Cancian[1]

[1]Regional Hospital, Treviso, Italy;
[2]Veneto Hospital, Vittorio Veneto, Italy.

ABSTRACT

Management of rectal cancer is influenced by local factors such as depth of rectal wall invasion, presence of mesorectal lymph node metastases and status of circumferential resection margin (CRM). Accurate preoperative staging plays a decisive role in selecting patients suitable to local resection, radical surgery with total mesorectal excision or neoadjuvant chemoradiotherapy (CRT). Imaging modalities used for local staging include computed tomography, two-dimensional endorectal ultrasonography (2D-ERUS) and magnetic resonance.

The new technique of high-resolution three-dimensional ERUS, constructed from a synthesis of standard 2D cross-sectional images, promises to further improve the accuracy in rectal cancer staging. This tool seems to offer best information on early tumoral invasion into the rectal wall, presence of mesorectal lymph node metastases, prediction of surgical CRMs, restaging rectal carcinomas after neoadjuvant CRT and detection of local recurrence after primary treatment. It has also the advantage of being an office-based procedure, well tolerated, with fast acquisition times and relatively low cost.

INTRODUCTION

Rectal cancer will affect approximately 40000 people in the United States in 2008 [1]. Cure is achieved in approximately 45% of all patients and poor prognosis is associated with advanced disease, local recurrences and distant metastases [1]. The optimal treatment for rectal cancer is still matter of debate. Several improvements have been made in the last 25 years, transforming a surgically managed disease into a multidisciplinary treatment model. Refined surgical techniques (transanal endoscopic microsurgery, laparoscopic resection with total mesorectal excision, sphincter-saving procedures) and neoadjuvant or adjuvant chemoradiotherapy (CRT) have been demonstrated to both improve the quality of life and the local control of the disease [2-17].

Accurate preoperative staging plays a fundamental role in therapeutic decision-making. Imaging modalities used for local staging include conventional two-dimensional endorectal ultrasound (2D-ERUS), magnetic resonance imaging (MRI) and computed tomography (CT) [18-24]. The recent advent of high-resolution three-dimensional (3D) ERUS, constructed from a synthesis of standard 2D cross-sectional images, and of "Volume Render Mode" (VRM), a technique to analyze information inside a three-dimensional volume by digitally enhancing individual voxels, promises to further improve the accuracy in rectal cancer staging [25,26]. This new technique seems to offer best information on early tumoral invasion into the rectal wall, presence of mesorectal lymph node metastases, prediction of surgical circumferential resection margin (CRM), restaging rectal carcinomas after neoadjuvant CRT and detection of local recurrence after primary treatment [26-28].

This chapter is devoted to discussing the method for generating and using 3D-ERUS, particularly with regard to the advantages of this application in the preoperative staging of rectal tumors.

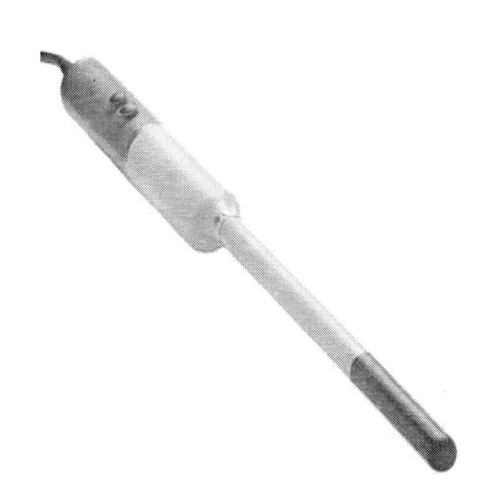

Figure I. B-K Medical anorectal probe type 2050.

EQUIPMENT AND TECHNIQUE

The most widely used ERUS system is the B-K Medical scanner (ProFocus 2202, B-K Medical A/S, Mileparken 34, DK-2730 Herlev, Denmark) with a hand-held rotating endoprobe type 2050, which gives a 360-degree axial view of the rectal wall, and a built-in 3D automatic acquisition system (Figure I) [25]. The radial probe has a 270 mm metal shaft with a double crystal at its tip, frequency range from 6.0 to 16.0 MHz and 90 degree scanning plane. It is rotated at 4-6 cycles per second to get radial scan of the rectum and surrounding structures. The probe is covered with a latex balloon that is filled with degassed water to maintain acoustic coupling between the transducer and the tissue (Figure II) [25]. It is important to eliminate all bubbles within the balloon to avoid artifacts that limit the overall utility of the study. The rectum can be of varying diameters and therefore the volume of water in the balloon may have to be adjusted intermittently.

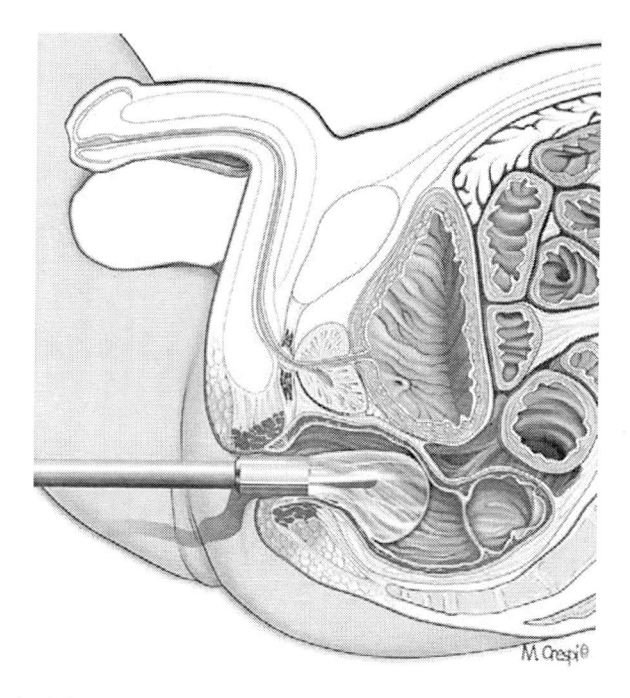

Figure II. Contact method for endorectal ultrasound. To maintain acoustic coupling between the transducer and the tissue, the probe is covered with a latex balloon that is filled with degassed water (with permission from: Santoro GA, Di Falco G. Atlas of endoanal and endorectal ultrasonography. Springer-Verlag 2004).

The acquisition of a 3D data volume and the underlying techniques are different from application to application. With the conventional 2D ultrasound, the screen resolution is measured in number of pixels (the display matrix), with each pixel having X- and Y-plane only. A 3D model may be constructed from a synthesis of a high number of parallel transaxial 2D images (Figure III) [26]. Such reconstruction is possible by combining the ultrasound apparatus and the integrated computer technology with 3D software (BK3Di, B-K Medical, Herlev, Denmark). Adding the third dimension means that the pixel is transformed in a small 3D picture element called a voxel. Ideally, a voxel should be a cubic structure, however the dimension in the Z-plane is often slightly larger than that in the X- and Y-planes. The depth of the voxel is critical to the resolution of the 3D image, and this depth is directly related to the spacing between two adjacent images. High resolution 3D ultrasound acquires four to five transaxial images sampled per 1mm of acquisition length in the Z-plane. This means that an acquisition based upon a sampling of transaxial images over a distance of 60 mm in the human body will result in a data volume block consisting of between 240 and 300 transaxial images. High-resolution data volumes will consist of typical voxel sizes around 0.15 x 0.15 x 0.2 mm. Because of this resolution in the longitudinal plane, which is close to the axial and transverse resolution of the 2D image, this technique ensures true dimensions of the 3D data cube also in the reconstructed Z-plane and provides accurate distance, area, angle and volume measurements [26]. The 2050 probe is designed so that no moving parts come in contact with human tissue. The transducer's 360° rotating head, the proximal-distal actuation mechanism and the electronic mover are fully enclosed within the housing of the probe.

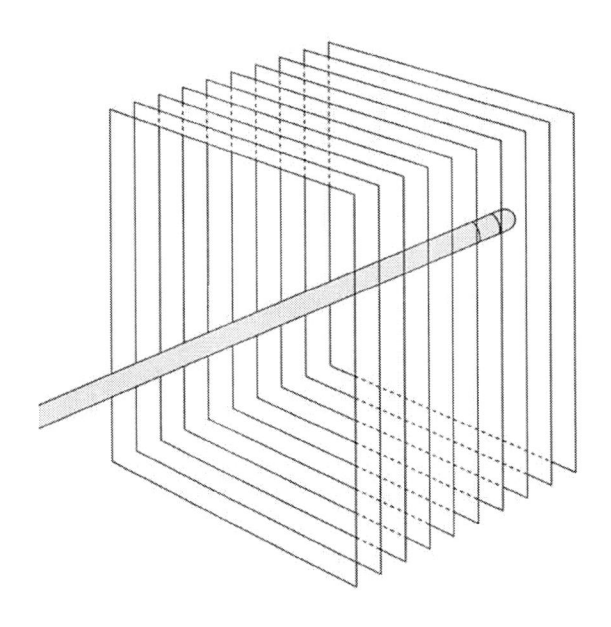

Figure III. Schematic model for acquisition of 3-D anorectal endo image as a synthesis of a high number of parallel transaxial 2D images.

The ability to visualize information in the 3D image depends critically on the rendering technique [26]. Three basic types of technique are used: 1) *Surface Render Mode* (SRM). An operator or algorithm identifies the boundaries of the structures to create a wire-rame representation. It is the most commonly known version of *Render Mode* and it is extensively used by some medical centers in producing perhaps the very first images of an unborn baby's facial contours. Surface rendering techniques only give good results when a surface is available to render. These technique fail when a strong surface cannot be found such as in the subtly layered structures within the anal canal and the rectal wall; 2) *Multiplane viewing techniques*. Three perpendicular planes (axial, tranverse and longitudinal) are displayed simultaneously and can be moved, rotated, tilted and sliced to allow the operator to infinitely vary the different section parameters and visualize the lesion at different angles and to get the most information out of the data. After a data is acquired it is immediately possible to select coronal anterior-posterior or posterior-anterior as well as sagittal right-left views. The multiview function allows to see up to six different and specialized views at once with real-time reconstruction (Figure IV); 3) *Volume Render Mode*. It is a special feature that can be applied to high-resolution 3D data volume so information inside the cube is reconstructed to some extent. This technique uses a ray tracing model as its basic operation. A ray or beam is projected from each point on the viewing screen (the display) back into and through the volume data. As the ray passes through the volume data it reaches the different elements (voxels) in the data set. Depending on the various render mode settings, the data from each voxel may be discarded, it may be used to modify the existing value of the ray, or it may be stored for reference to the next voxel and used in a filtering calculation. All of these calculations result in the current color or intensity of the ray being modified in some way. In normal VRM the following four different post-processing display parameters can be used: 1) *Opacity*. Sets the relative transparency of the volume. The higher the value, the further into the volume the ray can travel before being terminated. Because of accumulated brightness as the ray traverses the volume, the net effect is to make the volume appear brighter as this control value is increased; 2) *Luminance*. Sets the inverse of the self luminance value for the pixels, and should be used in conjunction with the opacity control for displaying certain voxel values for optimal visualization. The final image impression should be adjusted to the readers requirements by setting the normal brightness and contrast controls; 3) *Thickness*. Sets an upper limit to the penetration of the rays into the volume. This value is used in conjunction with the opacity parameter to determine when the ray traversal is terminated. Increasing the thickness setting allows deeper penetration and the result is often a slightly smother presentation together with a significant increase in the visual depth impression of a lesion; 4) *Filter*. Sets the lower threshold value for pixel intensities. Pixel values less than the filter value are not included in determining the intensity of the ray final value. In normal VRM, the rendering mode stops each ray when the value found reaches a specified value of opacity. This is affected by the setting of some of the controls (opacity, thickness and to some extent luminance). Some rendering modes apply global operations to the ray calculations: "Maximum Intensity Projection" (MIP) tries to find the brightest or most significant color or intensity along a ray path and "Transparent Mode" allows the separation of color and intensity data and selective control of the transparency of the two components. Using this method, it is possible to reduce the intensity of the grey scale voxels so that they appear as a light fog over the color information. Both of these methods require the ray to pass through the entire volume and, in the case of transparent display methods, to pass through the entire volume twice. In the MIP mode, none of the controls are present and they have no effect on the final image, and the pixel brightness shown on the screen is the maximum intensity value found along the path. Such processes, however, decrease the information. This may be desirable if an image is cluttered with noise and the observer's visual perception is overloaded. The loss of information can reduce the geometric accuracy and consequently many details may be missed. For this reason, it is always essential to display unprocessed images together with processed images, so that misinterpretations do not occur as a result of image processing [26].

    Endoluminal ultrasound is usually performed with the patient in the left lateral decubitus position. An enema is administered 2 hours before the examination to clean the rectum. Initially a digital rectal examination should identify the size, fixation, morphology and location of the tumor, if it is low enough. Proctoscopy with a dedicated rectosigmoidoscope (A.4522, Sapimed, Alessandria, Italy) is then performed (Sapimed, Alessandria, Italy) (Figure V) [29]. Proctoscopy serves several purposes: 1) it allows visual examination of the rectal tumor with exact determination of its location both with respect to circumferential involvement of the rectal wall and the distance from the anal verge; 2) it allows suctioning of any residual stool or enema fluid that might interfere with the acoustic pathways of the ultrasound wavers which may alter the image; 3) it allows easy passage of the probe above the tumor. The presence of a double-graduated scale to measure the distance of the tip of the proctoscope and the tip of the probe from the anal verge, respectively, allows ascertainment of the correct positioning of both devices. The entire rectum from the upper third to the anal sphincter is evaluated while progressively withdrawing conjoined the probe and the rectoscope. This is of extreme importance as the lower border of a rectal cancer can differ significantly in the depth of invasion than the center or upper portions of the cancer and lymph nodes in the perirectal region are often just above the level of the tumor and will be missed if complete imaging is not obtained [29].

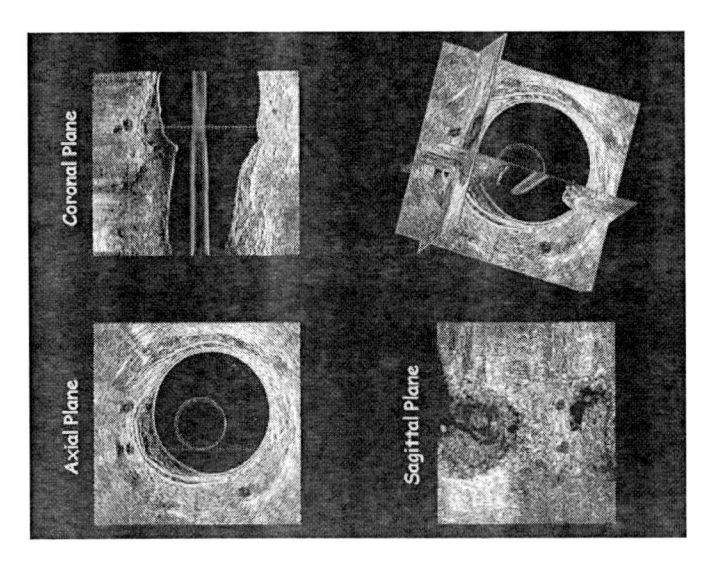

Figure IV. Multiplanes viewing technique. This function allows to see four different and specialized views at once.

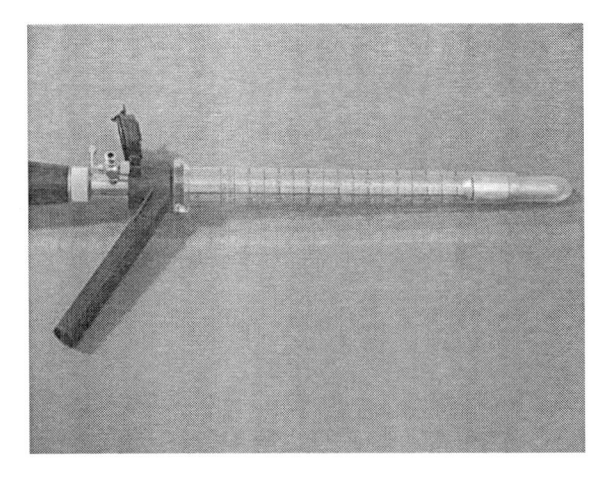

Figure V. Dedicated proctoscope rectosigmoidoscope (A.4522, Sapimed, Alessandria, Italy) for assembled with ultrasonographic probe.

On the screen the anterior aspect of the rectum will be superior (12 o'clock), right lateral will be left (9 o'clock), left lateral will be right (3 o'clock) and posterior will be inferior (6 o'clock) (just like the image on axial CT scan). The tip of the ultrasound probe should be maintained in the center of the rectal lumen to gain optimal imaging of the rectal wall and perirectal structures.

ULTRASOUND ANATOMY

On ultrasound the normal rectal wall is 2-3 mm thick and is composed of a five-layer structure [30]. The first hyperechoic layer corresponds to the interface of the balloon with the rectal mucosal surface, the second hypoechoic layer to the mucosa and muscularis mucosa, the third hyperechoic layer to the submucosa, the fourth hypoechoic layer to the muscularis propria and the fifth hyperechoic layer to the serosa or to the interface with the fibrofatty tissue surrounding the rectum (mesorectum) (Figure VI). The mesorectum contains blood vessels, nerves and lymphatics and has an inhomogeneous echo pattern. Very small, round to oval, hypoechoic lymph nodes should be distinguished from blood vessels which also appear as circular hypoechoic structures. Two-dimensional ERUS is limited by the inability to distinguish the mesorectal fascia.

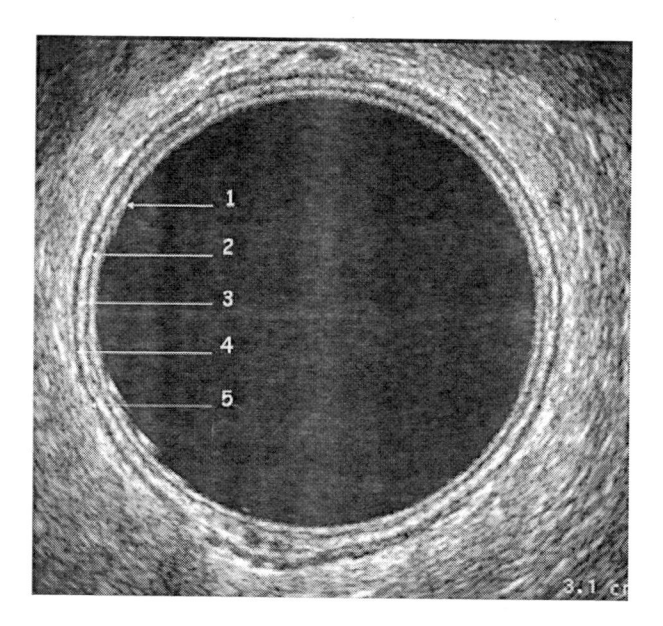

Figure VI. Two-dimensional ultrasonographic five layer structure of the normal rectal wall. The first hyperechoic layer (1) corresponds to the interface of the balloon with the rectal mucosal surface, the second hypoechoic layer (2) to the mucosa and muscularis mucosa, the third hyperechoic layer (3) to the submucosa, the fourth hypoechoic layer (4) to the muscularis propria and the fifth hyperechoic layer (5) to the serosa or to the interface with the mesorectum.

Three-dimensional ERUS offers a valuable supplement to conventional 2D-ERUS (30). The five layers of the rectal wall are clearly illustrated in the coronal plane as well as in the transaxial and sagittal planes (Figure VII). Blood vessels can be followed longitudinally and distinguished from lymph nodes (Figure VIII). It is also possible, by using the rendering technique, to accurately image the outer limit of the mesorectum where the mesorectal fascia is located (Figure IX). Moreover, 3D reconstruction allows an accurate depiction of pelvic organs (Figures X-XI).

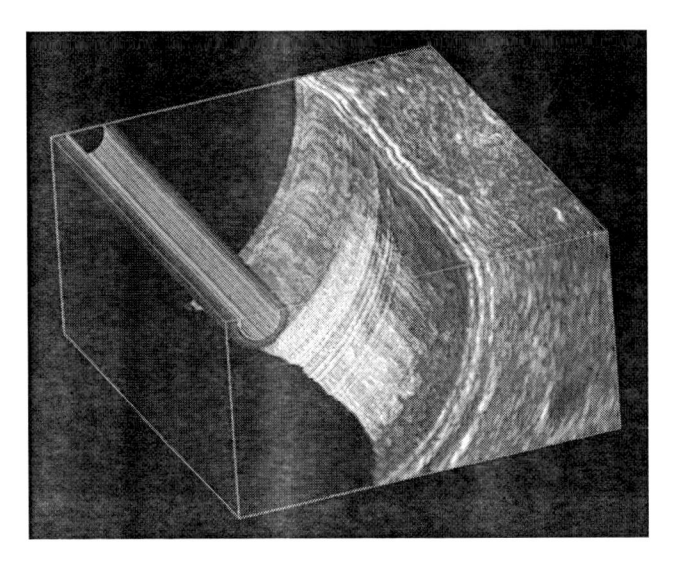

Figure VII. Three-dimensional ultrasonographic five layer structure of the normal rectal wall.

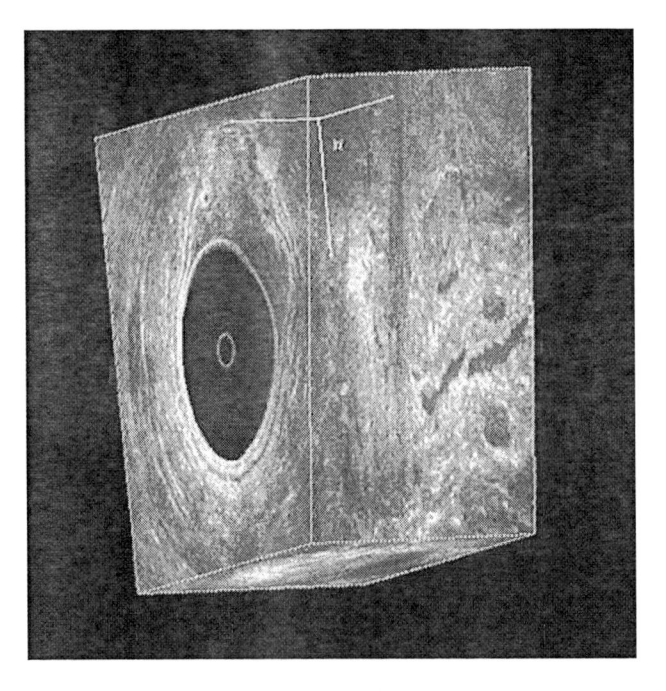

Figure VIII. Blood vessels can be followed longitudinally and distinguished from lymph nodes on reconstructed sagittal plane.

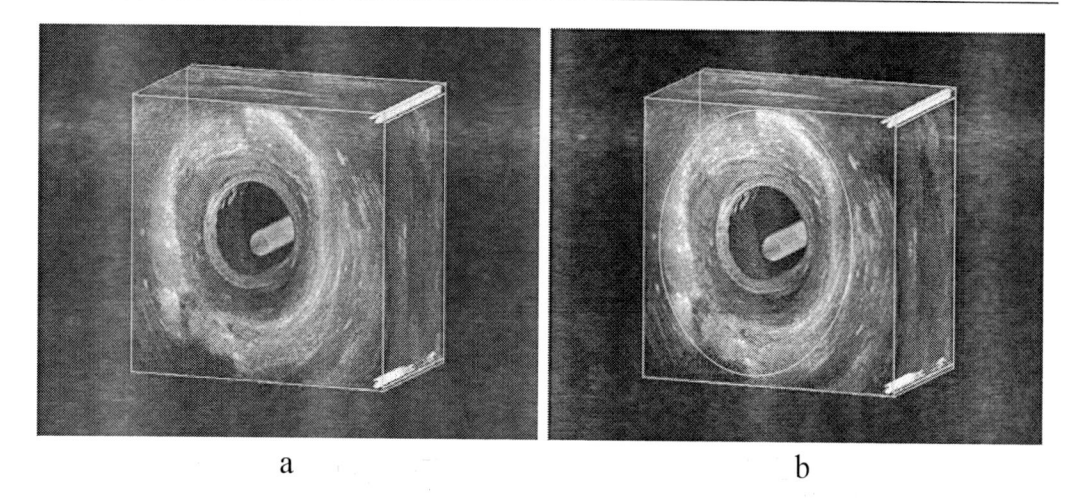

Figure IX. By using the rendering technique it is possible to accurately image the outer limit of the mesorectum (a). This interface should be considered as the mesorectal fascia (b).

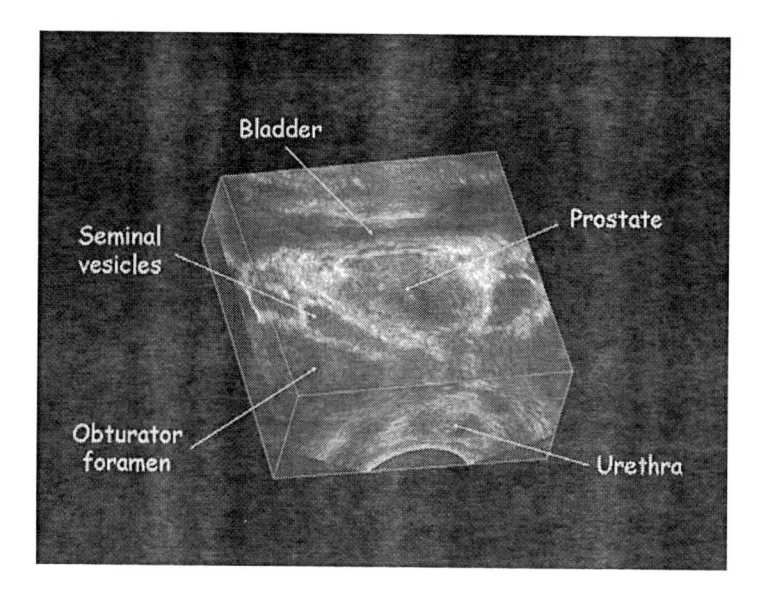

Figure X. Pelvic organs in male visualized on the reconstructed coronal plane.

ULTRASONOGRAPHIC STAGING OF RECTAL CANCER

Ultrasonographic criteria to determine the depth of tumor invasion, based on the classification proposed by Hildebrandt and Feifel [18], are as follows: a) uT0 lesion: the mucosal layer is expanded but the third hyperechoic submucosal layer remains intact around the entire breadth of the tumor (Figure XII); b) uT1 lesion: the hyperechoic submucosal layer is irregular or interrupted consistent with tumor invasion. The fourth hypoechoic layer of the muscularis propria is intact (Figure XIII); c) uT2 lesion: a distinct break is seen in the submucosal layer and the muscularis propria is thickened. The surrounding hyperechoic layer corresponding to the serosa or perirectal fat remains intact (Figure XIV); d) uT3 lesion: disruption of the hyperechoic layer corresponding to the submucosa, thickening of the hypoechoic layer representing the muscolaris propria and presence of irregularities of the outer hyperechoic layer which corresponds to the serosa or perirectal fat interface (Figure XV) and e) uT4 lesion: extensive local invasion with loss of the normal hyperechoic interface between tumor and the adjacent organs or invasion of the serosa in tumors above the peritoneal reflection (Figure XVI). Undetectable or benign lymph nodes are classified as uN-. Pathologic lymph nodes (uN+) appear as circular or slightly oval-shaped structures, often with an irregular border, with an echogenicity similar to the tumor and most commonly found adjacent or in the mesorectum proximal to the primary tumor (Figure XVII) [19].

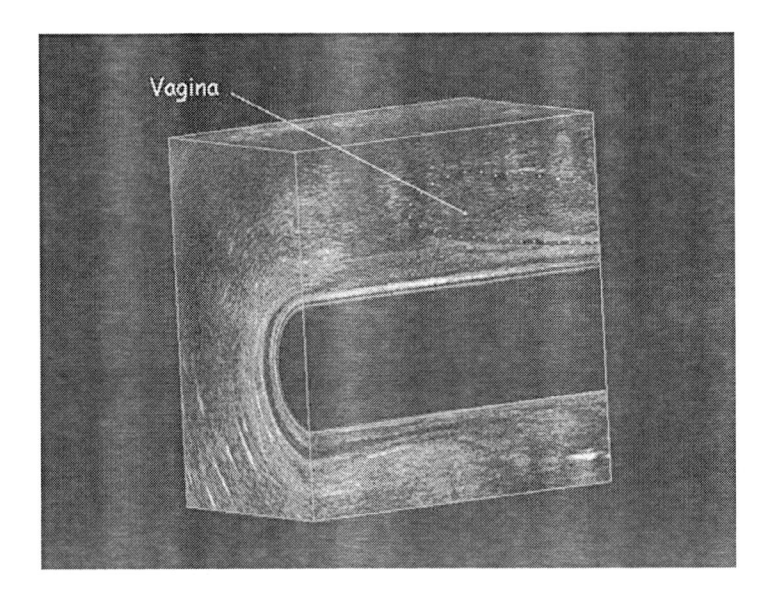

Figure XI. Vagina visualized on the reconstructed longitudinal plane.

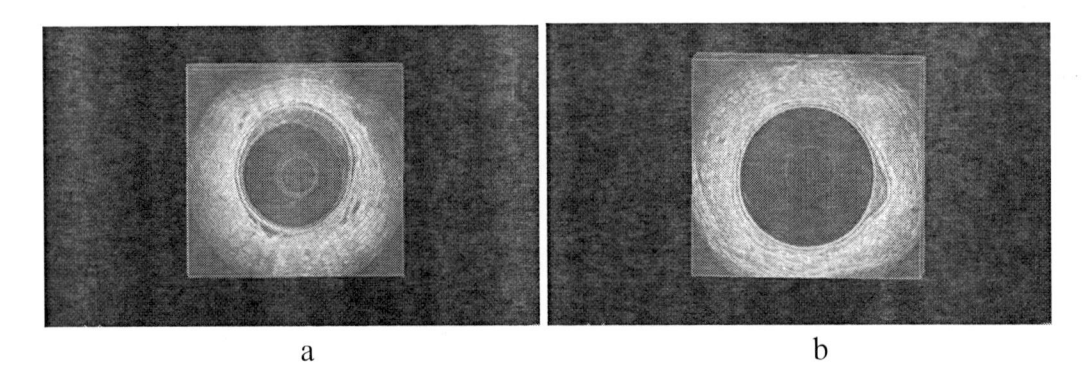

Figure XII. uT0 lesions (a,b). The mucosal layer is expanded but the third hyperechoic submucosal layer remains intact around the entire breadth of the tumor.

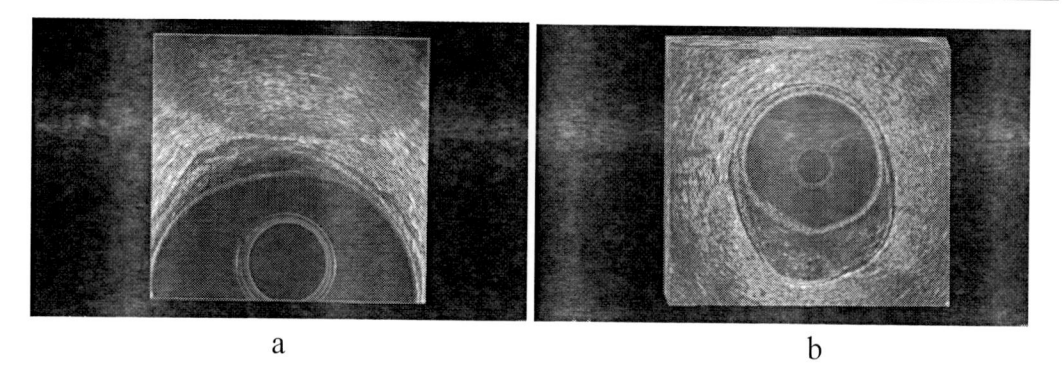

Figure XIII. uT1 lesions (a,b). The hyperechoic submucosal layer is irregular or interrupted consistent with tumor invasion. The fourth hypoechoic layer of the muscolaris propria is intact.

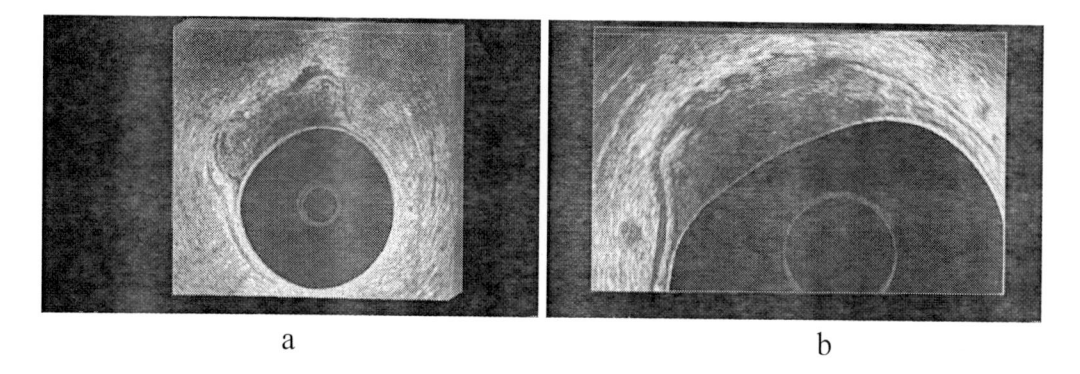

Figure XIV. uT2 lesions (a,b). A distinct break is seen in the submucosal layer and the muscolaris propria is thickened. The surrounding hyperechoic layer corresponding to the serosa or perirectal fat remains intact.

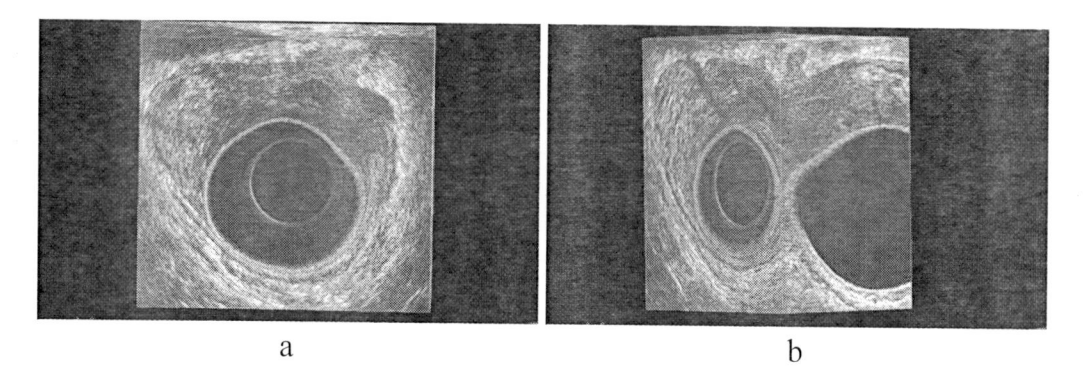

Figure XV. uT3 lesions (a,b). Disruption of the hyperechoic layer corresponding to the submucosa, thickening of the hypoechoic layer representing the muscolaris propria and presence of irregularities of the outer hyperechoic layer which corresponds to the serosa or perirectal fat interface.

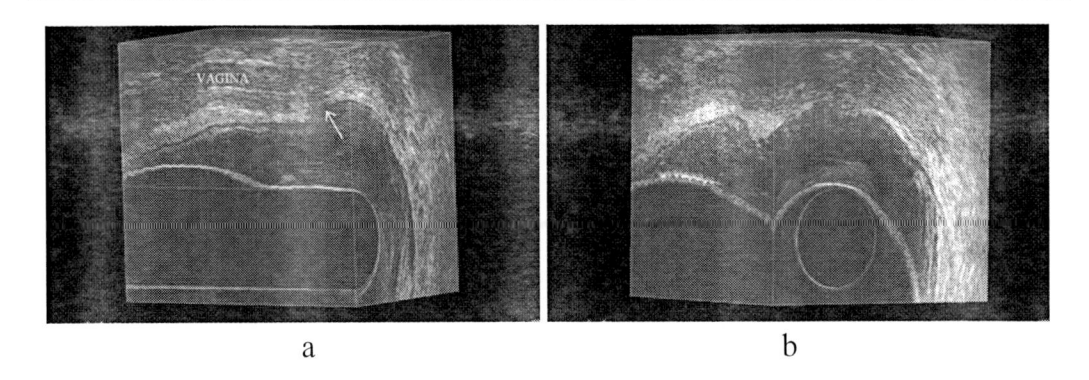

Figure XVI. uT4 lesions (a,b). Extensive local invasion with loss of the normal hyperechoic interface between tumor and the adjacent organ.

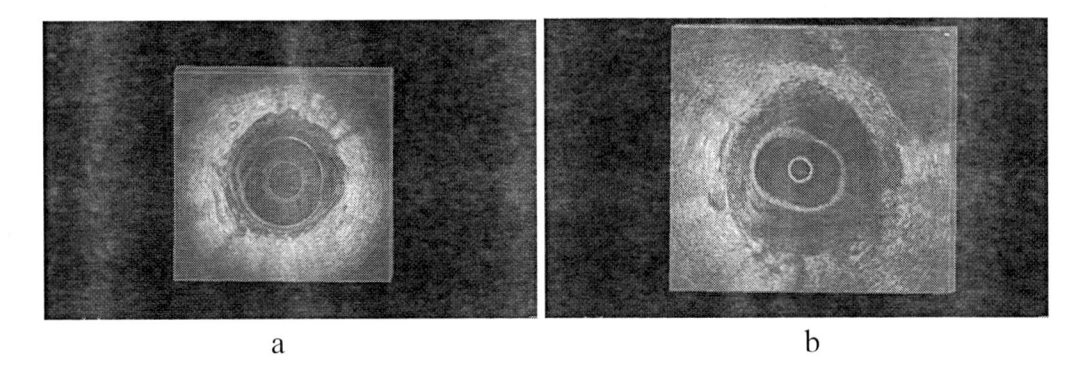

Figure XVII. Sonogram of enlarged, hypoechoic, malignant appearing lymph nodes (a,b) of the mesorectum.

Stage uT0: Benign Lesion

Sonographic evaluation of a villous rectal lesion is helpful in determining the presence of tumor invasion. The presence of an intact hyperechoic submucosal interface indicates lack of tumor invasion into the submucosa (Figure XVIII). Heintz et al. [31] believe that ERUS cannot differentiate between villous adenoma and invasive cancer because of neither the muscolaris mucosae nor the submucosa is sonographically definable and that the first hypoechoic layer corresponds anatomically with the mucosa and the submucosa. They suggest that uT0 and uT1 tumors, that manifest as a broadening of the first hypoechoic layer, should be classified together. Instead Adams and Wong [32] disagree with this interpretation and consider the first hypoechoic layer as the mucosa and muscolaris mucosae and the middle hyperechoic layer as the submucosa. Consequently for such authors lesions that expand the inner hypoechoic layer and are surrounded by a uniform middle hyperechoic layer are considered villous adenoma and lesions that expand the inner hypoechoic layer and have distinct echo defects of the middle hyperechoic layer are considered uT1 tumors. Doornebosch et al. [33] recently reported that ERUS is very reliable in diagnosing tubolovillous adenoma (sensitivity: 89% and specificity: 86%), and therapeutic decision-making regarding local excision vs. radical surgery based on ERUS is valid. By adding ERUS to preoperative biopsies the rate of missed carcinomas could be reduced from 21 to 3% ($P<0.001$).

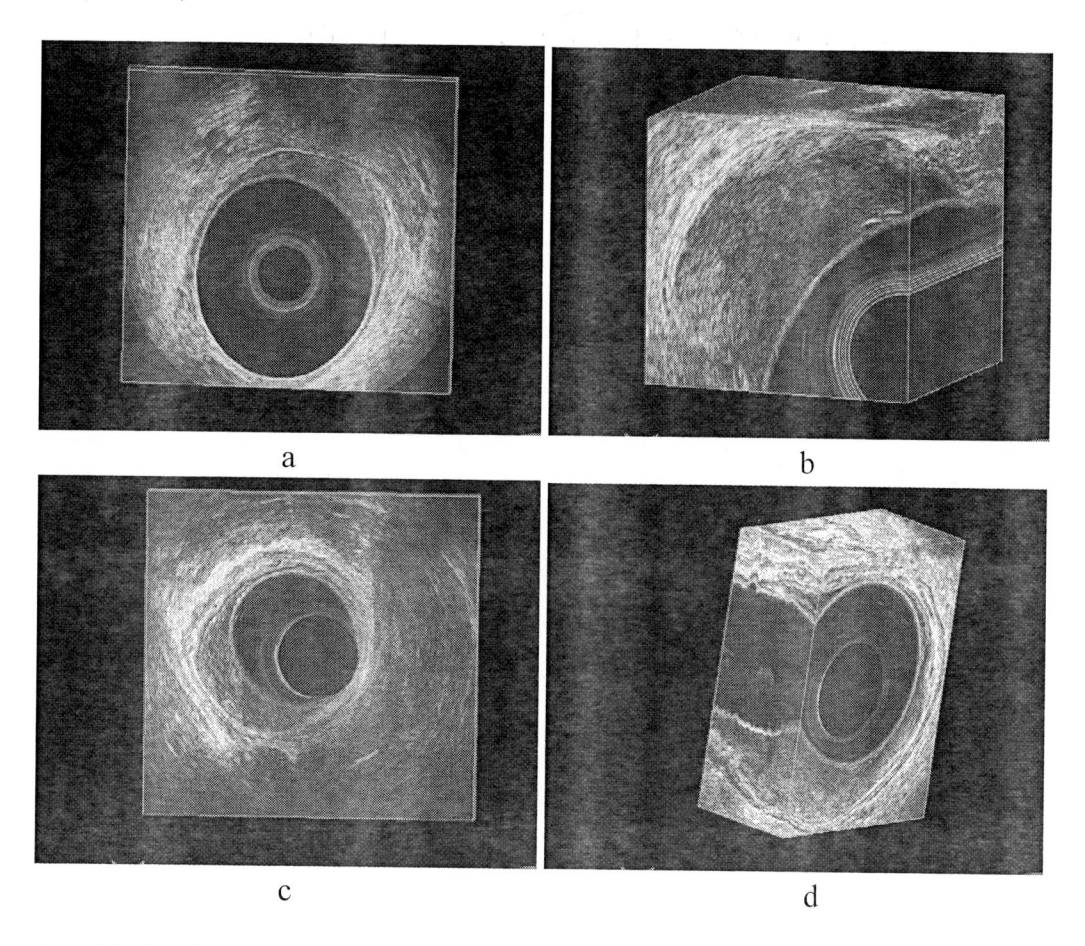

Figure XVIII. uT0 lesions (a-d). The presence of an intact hyperechoic submucosal interface indicates lack of tumor invasion into the submucosa.

Technical difficulties associated with scanning villous adenoma can be due to very large exophytic lesions that tend to attenuate rectal layers or to produce fixed artefacts over one part of the rectal wall, obscuring the image [34]. In large carpeting lesions, careful evaluation of the entire tumor is necessary to determine that a small area of invasion has not be overlooked. Snare biopsy of lesions before referral to ERUS produces a burn artefact, which can also lead to overstaging [34].

Stage uT1: Submucosal Invasion

If a tumor arises in a polyp it is important to determine whether the stalk is invaded. Differences in classification are reported between Western and Japanese pathologists. In 1985 Haggitt et al. [35] divided the depth of invasion into four levels: Level 0: carcinoma in situ or intramucosal carcinoma; Level 1: carcinoma invading through the muscolaris mucosa into the submucosa but limited to the head of the polyp; Level 2: carcinoma invading the level of the neck of the adenoma; Level 3: carcinoma invading any part of the stalk; Level 4: carcinoma invading into the submucosa of the bowel wall below the stalk of the polyp. By definition all sessile polyps with invasive adenocarcinoma are in level 4. They studied 129 patients with pTis to pT1 colorectal tumors and found that level 4 invasion was a statistically significant factor ($P<0.001$) predicting positive nodes. Similar results were reported by Nivatvongs et al. [36] on 151 patients with pT1 colorectal tumors undergoing bowel resection in which invasion into the submucosa of the bowel wall at the base of the stalk (level 4) was the single most significant risk factor for positive nodes. For sessile polyps the risk was 10% and for peduncolated polyps 27%. Suzuki et al. [37] determined the risk of lymph node metastases in 65 patients having Haggitt's level 4 invasion into the submucosa. Lymph node metastasis was noted in 11 (16.9%) of the 65 patients, however the width of submucosal invasion was significantly greater in node-positive than in node-negative patients ($P=0.001$). When 5-mm-wide submucosal invasion was used as an indicator for intestinal resection, 37 patients were found to have indications for bowel resection and 11 (29.7%) of the 37 had lymph node metastases. The positive predictive value increased from 17 to 30% when the width of submucosal invasion was added to Haggitt's level 4 as an indicator for bowel resection. Seitz et al. [38] suggested that Haggitt's classification applies well for pedunculated polyps however it should not be used for malignant sessile polyps. Kudo et al. [39] were the first to differentiate three different types of early invasive cancers: 1) SM-1 tumor, invading the superior third of the submucosa, 2) SM-2 tumor, invading the superficial two/third of the submucosa and 3) SM-3 tumor, invading the deep third of the submucosa. Within the group type SM-1, there are three subtypes: type SM-1a (indicates that invasion is <1/4 of the submucosa), type SM-1b (indicates that invasion is <1/2 of the submucosa) and type SM-1c (indicates that invasion is >1/2 of the submucosa). Kikuchi et al [40] found that the risk of lymph node metastasis was 0% for SM-1 lesions, 10% for SM-2 lesions and 25% for SM-3 lesions ($P<0.001$). In their study tumoral invasion of the deep third of the submucosa (SM-3) was the only independent risk factor of lymph node metastasis. Akasu et al. [41] proposed a classification of the depth of submucosal cancer in two groups: 1) SM-slight (SM-s): extent limited to the upper third of the submucosa and 2) SM-massive (SM-m): tumor invasion extended to the middle or lower third of the submucosa (Figure XIX). In their series incidences of lymph node metastasis in pT1-slight and pT1-massive were 0% and 22%, respectively. They suggested that patients with massive submucosal invasion should be best treated by radical surgery. Another study from the Mayo Clinic confirmed these data [42]. Among patients with T1 carcinoma in the middle or lower third of the rectum the multivariate risk factors for long-term cancer-free survival was invasion into the lower third of the submucosa. For lesions with SM3 invasion, the oncologic resection group had lower rates of distant metastases and better survival compared with patients who underwent local excision. Therefore a decision whether to perform radical surgery or local excision or polypectomy should be based principally on assessment of invasion depth.

At preoperative ERUS, we propose to classify the depth of submucosal cancer invasion in two subtypes: 1) slight (SM-s): extent limited to the upper third of the third layer. The fourth hypoechoic layer of the muscolaris propria appears intact (Figure XX) and 2) massive

(SM-m): tumor invasion extended to the middle or lower third of the third layer. The fourth hypoechoic layer is thickened consistent with peritumoral inflammation and desmoplastic reaction (Figure XXI) [43].

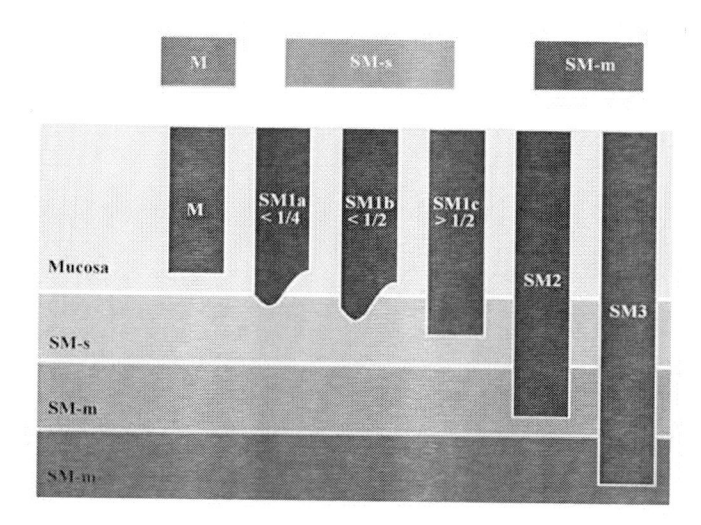

Figure XIX. Level of submucosal invasion according to the Japanese classification (40).

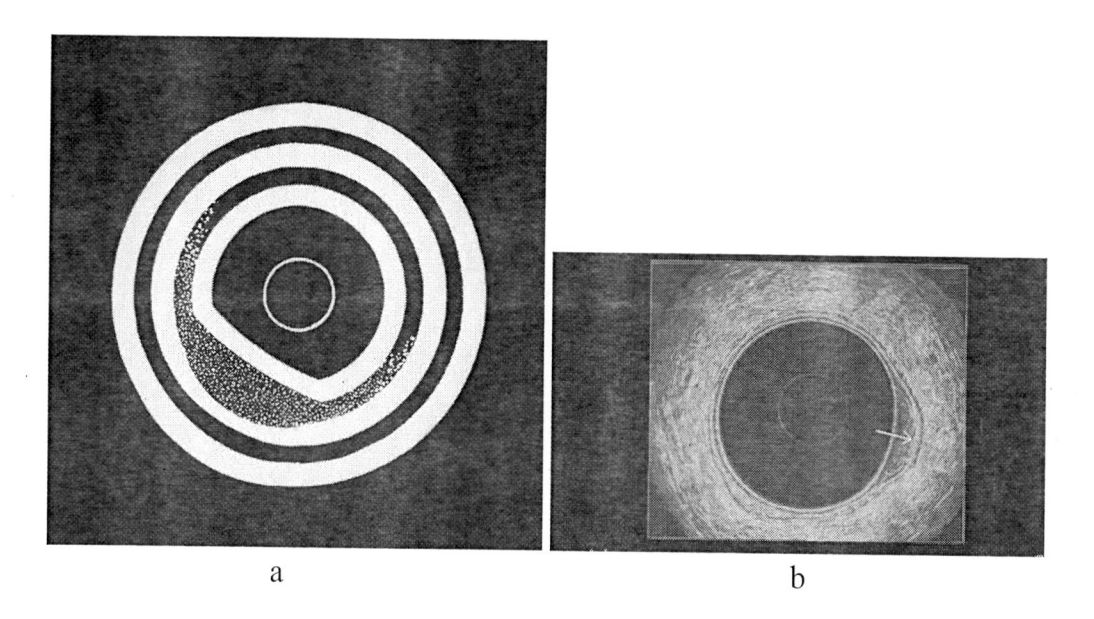

a   b

Figure XX. uT1 rectal tumor with slight submucosal invasion (SM-s: extent limited to the upper third of the third layer. The fourth hypoechoic layer of the muscolaris propria is intact).

Stage uT2: Invasion of the Muscular Layer

Sonographic diagnosis of uT2 tumor is based on a distinct break in the hyperechoic submucosal layer with thickening of the hypoechoic layer representing the muscolaris propria

(Figure XXII). Since the tumor is also hypoechoic, early muscolar invasion is difficult to detect. The surrounding hyperechoic layer corresponding to the perirectal fat interface remains intact. Lymph node metastases occur in approximately 15% to 20% of patients with T2 tumors.

Interpretative errors can occur in distinguishing uT1 from uT2 tumors. Overstaging of pT1 lesions can be due to severe inflammatory infiltrate underlying a tumor, which is sonographically indistinguishable from malignant tissue. Understaging of pT2 tumors, on the other hand, may be caused by a failure to detect microscopic cancer infiltration owing to the limits of resolution of the equipment [19].

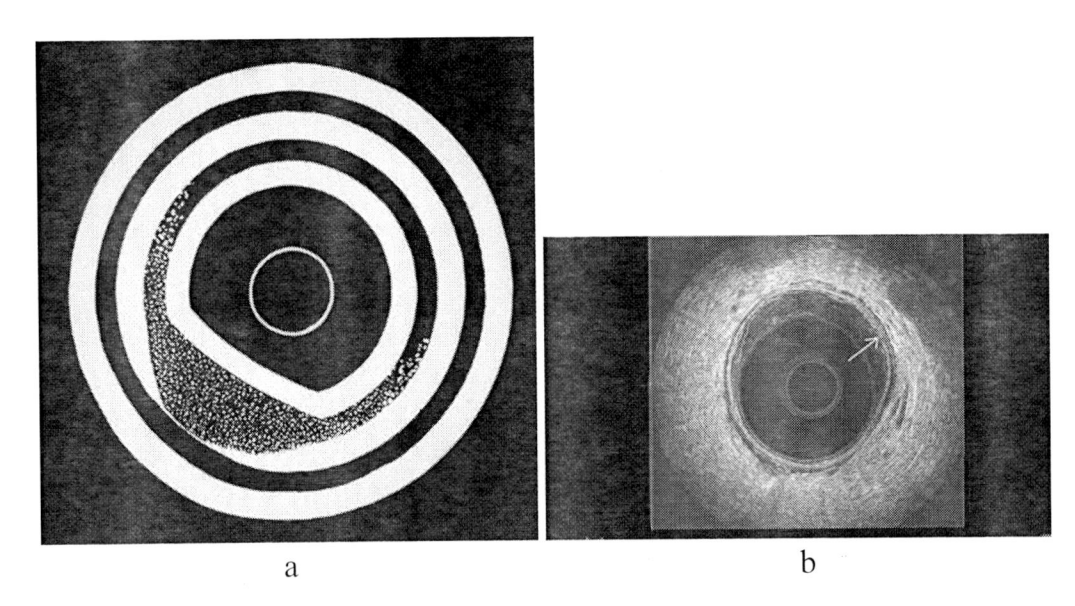

Figure XXI. uT1 rectal tumor with massive submucosal invasion (SM-m: tumor invasion extended to the middle or lower third of the third layer. The fourth hypoechoic layer is thickened consistent with peritumoral inflammation and desmoplastic reaction).

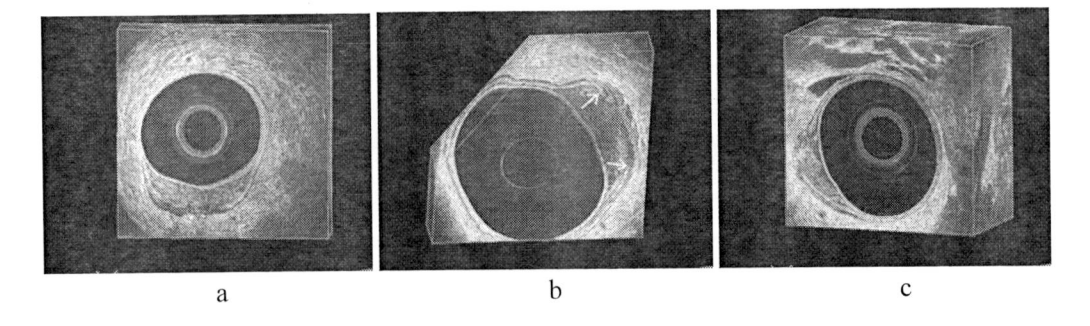

Figure XXII. uT2 rectal tumors (a-c).

Stage uT3: Perirectal Fat Invasion

Perirectal fat invasion is diagnosed sonographically by the presence of irregularity of the outer hyperechoic layer which corresponds to the perirectal fat interface. These findings should be associated with disruption of the hyperechoic layer corresponding to the submucosa and thickening of the hypoechoic layer representing the muscolaris propria (Figure XXIII). Contiguous organs are not involved. About 10% of such tumors are accompanied by a narrowing of the lumen and angulation and it may be difficult or impossible to advance the probe proximal to the lesion. Under these circumstances the study may be incomplete and the presence of enlarged lymph nodes may not be ascertained with accuracy since nodes are often located proximal to the tumor. The incidence of regional lymph node metastases in uT3 tumors is approximately 30% to 50%.

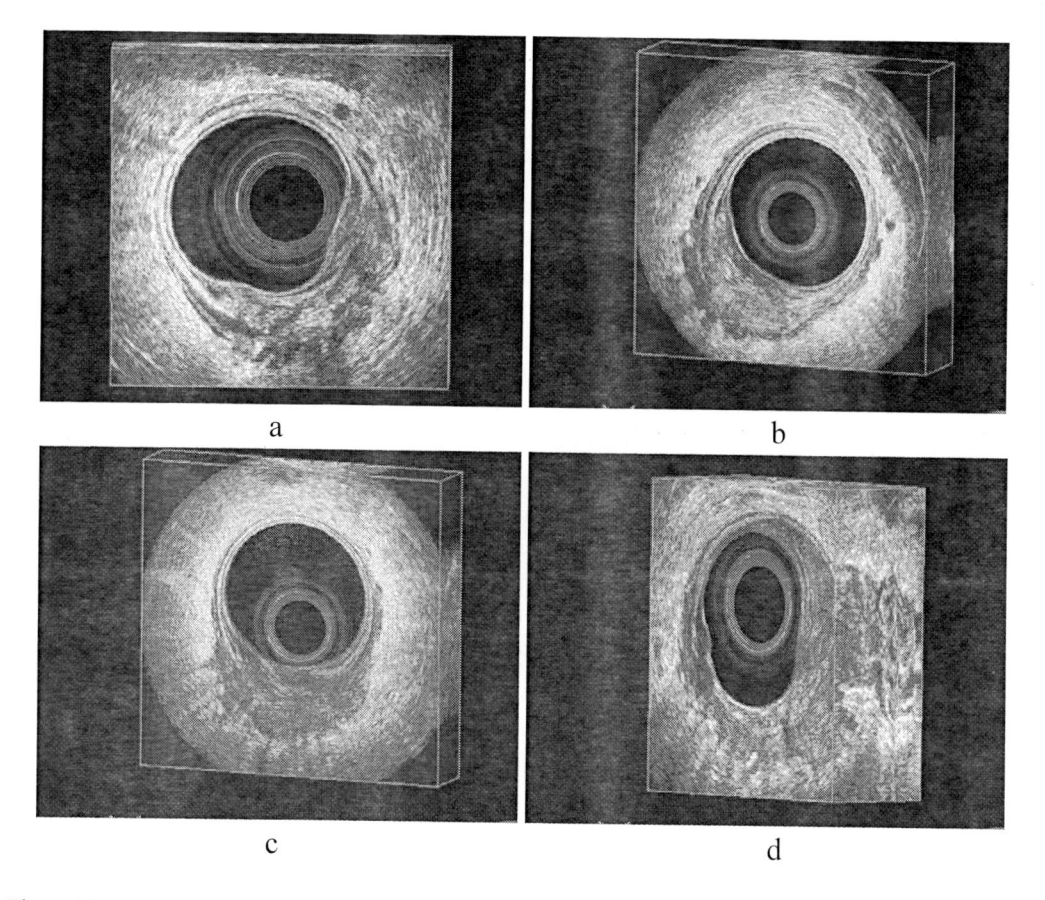

Figure XXIII. uT2 rectal tumors (a-d).

The recognition of perirectal fat invasion is an important determination to select appropriate patients for preoperative combined CRT. One of the most important drawbacks in the staging of tumor with extramural infiltration is in providing information regarding the mesorectal fascia and the relation of the tumor to it (CRMs) [23] (Figure XXIV). Currently MRI is considered the most accurate technique for determining CRMs, while ERUS is limited by the inability to distinguish the mesorectal fascia [44]. The recent advance in ultrasonographic technique with 3D reconstruction and rendering allows the outer interface of the mesorectum, where the mesorectal fascia is located, to be clearly visualized and the depth of extramural penetration (CRM) to be measured (Figure XXV, Figure XXVI).

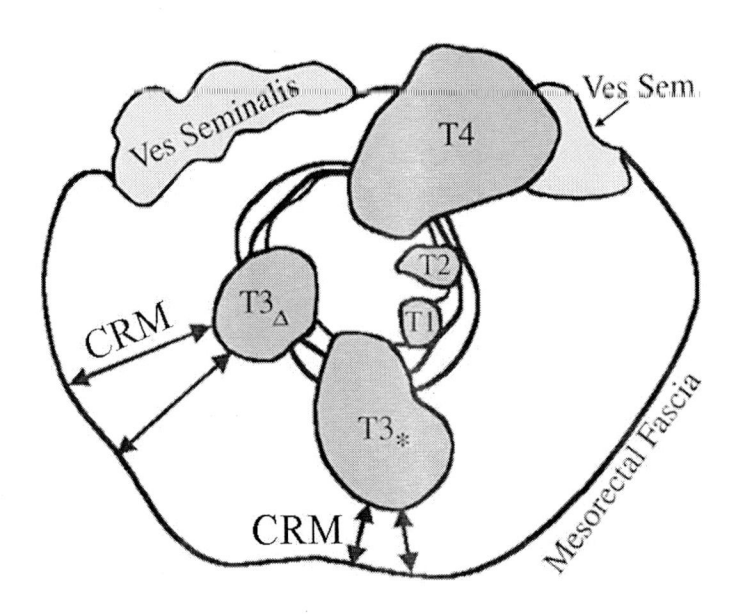

Figure XXIV. Schematic representation of mesorectal fascia and circumferential resection margins.

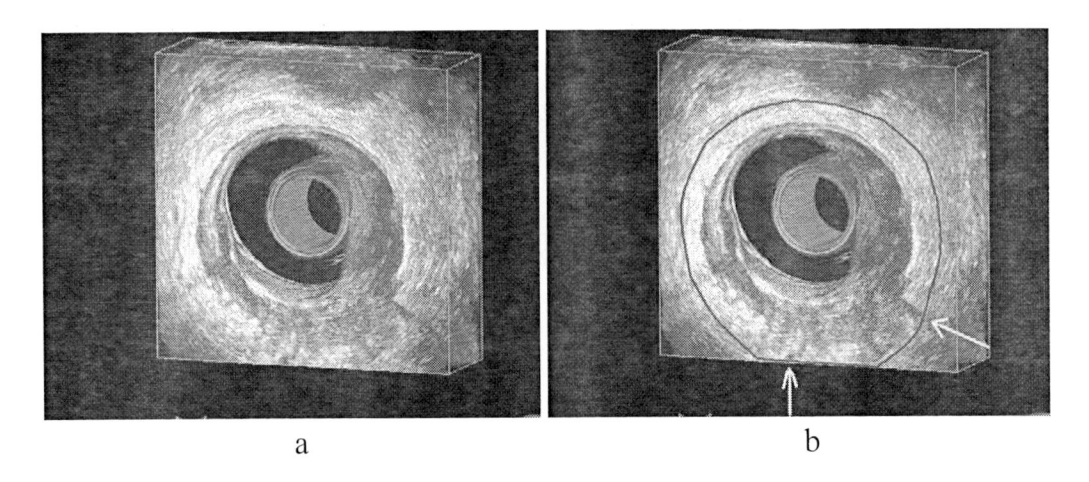

Figure XXV. uT3 rectal tumor. By using the rendering technique it is possible to accurately depict the mesorectal fascia and to measure the circumferential resection margins.

A recent report from the Memorial Sloan-Kettering Cancer Center [45] showed that ERUS can also identify T3 rectal cancer patients unlikely to respond well to combined modality therapy. On multivariate analysis, deep radial extension on ERUS (>2.5mm) was associated with limited or lack of tumor downstaging. Moreover, five-year recurrence free-survival was related with tumor downstaging on ERUS after preoperative treatment: 89% in the cohort that obtained tumor downstaging compared with 45% in the cohort that obtained no tumor downstaging.

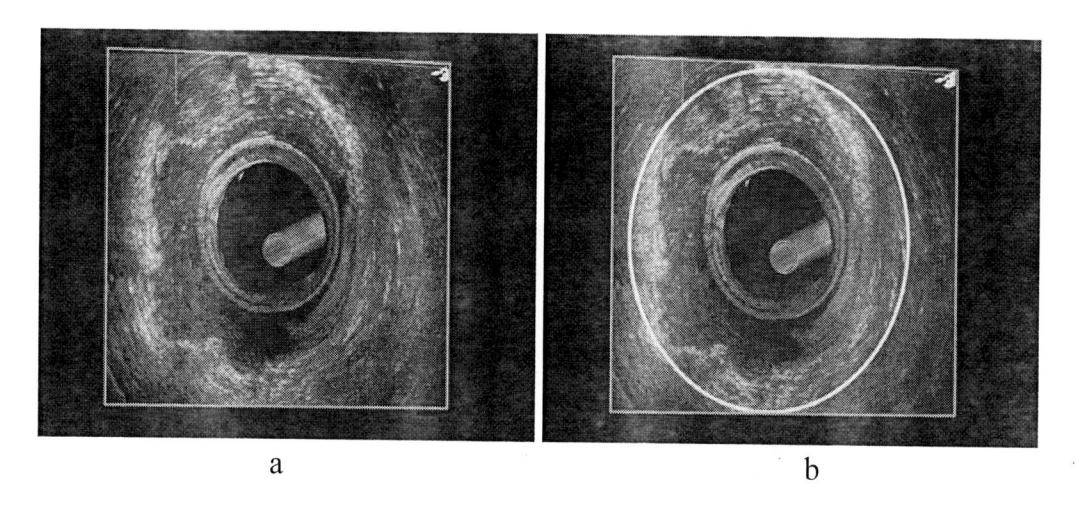

Figure XXVI. uT3 rectal tumor. By using the rendering technique it is possible to accurately depict the mesorectal fascia and to measure the circumferential resection margins.

Stage uT4: Extensive Local Invasion

Advanced lesions are clinically fixed or tethered and may locally invade into contiguous organs such as bladder, uterus, cervix, vagina, prostate and seminal vesicles. Sonographically there is a loss of the normal hyperechoic interface between tumor and the adjacent organ (Figure XXVII). The inability of ERUS to distinguish between malignant infiltration or peritumoral inflammation results in a somewhat lower staging accuracy with regard to T4 cancer. Stenotic lesions represent a limit to accurate endosonographic staging by precluding the passage of the probe or by causing angulation of the probe to the tumor axis.

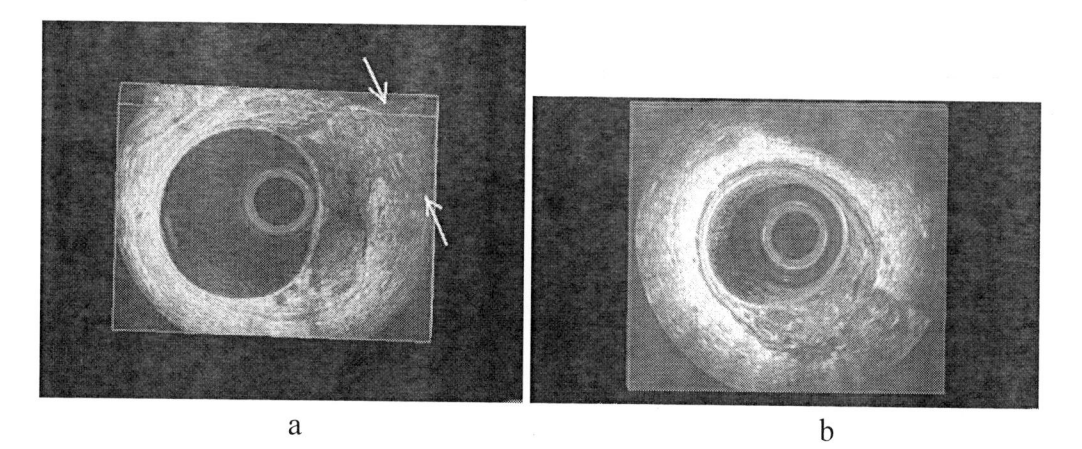

Figure XXVII. uT4 rectal tumors (a-b).

Stage uN-/N+: Lymph Node Metastases

Metastatic involvement of the mesorectal lymph node is a major independent prognostic factor. It has been observed that the presence of >3 nodes is associated with a poor prognosis. Moreover, identification of a metastatic perirectal lymph node is important as these patients may benefit from preoperative CRT [14-17] and some of the early T1 or T2 lesions with mesorectal node involvement are not suitable for local excision.

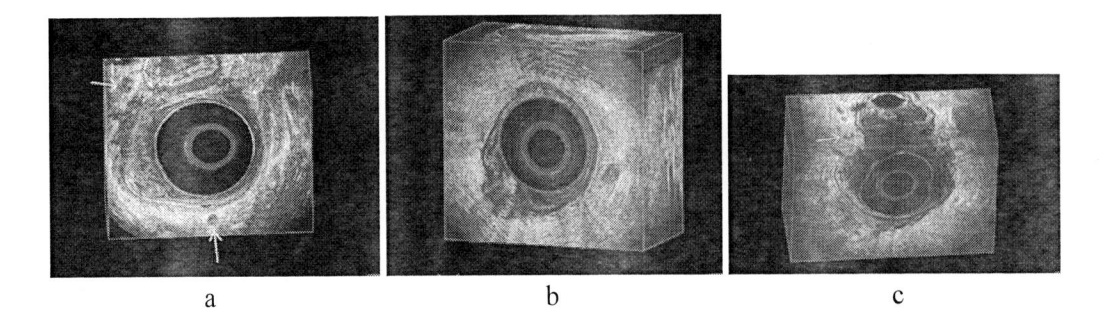

Figure XXVIII. Three-dimensional endorectal ultrasound showing malignant lymph nodes.

Sonographic evaluation of lymph node metastases is somewhat less accurate than depth of wall invasion [19]. Undetectable or benign appearing lymph nodes are classified as uN-. Malignant appearing lymph nodes are classified as uN+. The criteria used to identify metastatic lymph nodes in most of the studies are echogenicity, border demarcation and node diameter. Normal, nonenlarged perirectal nodes are not usually seen on ERUS. Inflamed, enlarged lymph nodes appear hyperechoic, with ill-defined borders. Much of the sound energy is reflected because of the lymphatic tissue architecture is intact. In contrast, metastatic lymph nodes that have been replaced with tumor appear hypoechoic with an echogenicity similar to the primary lesion (Figure XXVIII). Malignant lymph nodes tend to be circular rather than oval, have discrete borders and are most commonly found adjacent to the primary tumor or in the mesorectum proximal to the tumor (Figure XXIX). The sonographic features of lymph nodes generally can be distributed into four groups [19]: 1) if lymph nodes are not visible by ultrasound, the probability of lymph node metastases is low; 2) hyperechoic lymph nodes are often benign and result from nonspecific inflammatory changes; 3) hypoechoic lymph nodes larger than 5 mm are highly suggestive for lymph node metastases; 4) lymph nodes larger than 5 mm that are visible with mixed echogenic patterns should be considered metastatic. On size characteristics alone, sonographically detected nodes in the mesorectum greater than 5 mm in diameter have 50-70% chance of being involved, whereas those smaller than 4 mm have less than 20% chance. However up to 20% of patients have involved nodes of less than 3 mm, limiting the accuracy of the technique. Hulsmans et al. [46] studied several features by correlating pathologic and sonographic findings in the lymph nodes of specimens obtained from a series of 21 consecutive patients with resected rectal cancer. These features included ratio of long axis to short axis diameter, referred to as roundness index; lobulations (multiple notches); echogenicity; inhomogeneity (not uniform); border delineation; echo-poor rim (the outer rim being more hypoechoic than the rest of the node); peripheral halo and hilar reflection. The authors showed that the contemporary presence of sonographic short axis diameter, inhomogeneity and absence of hilar reflection were significantly related to histopathologic malignant findings.

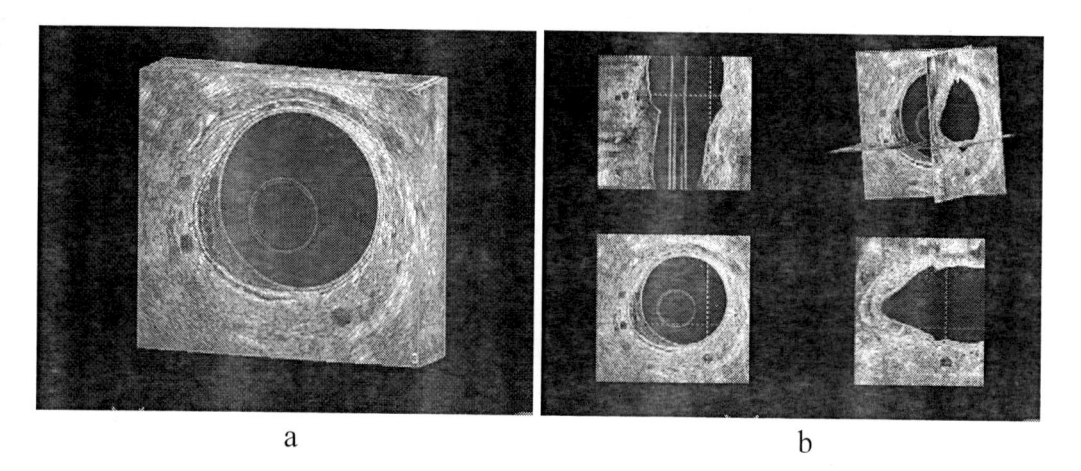

Figure XXIX. Multiplanes viewing technique showing malignant lymph nodes.

Overstaging and understaging can occur during assessment of lymph node involvement (19). At conventional 2D-ERUS the cross-sectional appearance of blood vessels in the perirectal fat may be confused with positive lymph nodes. Three-dimensional reconstruction allows to differentiate vessels from lymph nodes by following their branching pattern (Figure VIII). However, even with an improved understanding of the ultrasonographic characteristics of malignant lymph node, micrometastases and granulomatous inflammation are impossible to be detected. In these cases ERUS-guided needle biopsy or ERUS-guided fine-needle aspiration biopsy may improve diagnostic accuracy. Malignant lymph nodes located distant from the primary tumor remain undetected if they exceed the depth of penetration of the transducer. This is particularly true for nodes in the proximal mesorectum above the reach of the rigid probe.

ACCURACY

Accurate staging of rectal carcinoma is of major importance for the surgical strategy and the indications of neoadjuvant CRT. The tumor is categorized according to the degree of penetration into the rectal wall (T stage), the presence of mesorectal lymph nodes (N stage) and distant metastases (M stage). At present, pre-treatment assessment also includes the evaluation of CRM and mesorectal fascia, that has become an essential anatomic landmark for the definition of prognosis and the planning of a correct multidisciplinary management.

Conventional 2D-ERUS has become the most common imaging modality for loco-regional staging of rectal cancer and several studies have reported good accuracy rates (range: 63-96%) for T stage [18,47-52]. Garcia-Aguilar et al. [53] demonstrated that 2D-ERUS was reliable in assessing depth of tumor infiltration into the rectal wall. The overall accuracy was 69%, with 18% of tumors overstaged and 13% understaged. More recently,

Ptok et al. [54] found that the overall accuracy of 2D-ERUS was higher for pT1 and pT3 lesions (76.4% and 71.2%, respectively) comparing to pT2 and pT4 tumors (56% and 48.6%, respectively). Overstaging was more frequent than understaging. Discrepancies in 2D-ERUS accuracy between studies could be accounted by several factors. Most series are limited in size and represent the initial institutional experience with this technique. Moreover the examination is often performed with not dedicated, low frequency probes. Moreover ERUS is highly operator-dependant and a learning curve is present [53,55-58]. Nesbakken et al. [59] reported poor sensitivities (<40%) in 71 cancers staged by two examiners with no prior ultrasonographic experience. Carmody and Otchy [60] showed that the accuracy of a single operator improved from 58% to 92% after 24 examinations. The Minneapolis group had similar improvements from 59.3% to 95% over 3 years [61]. Marusch et al. [62] showed considerably lower accuracies in a multicenter study involving 75 hospitals. They stressed the need for highly trained surgeons with large case loads, possibly achieved thanks to the centralization of ERUS service. In a recent review on ERUS, Harewood et al. [63] underlined the issue of potential publication bias since the reported ERUS accuracies appeared inversely proportional to study sizes.

Interpretative errors may occur for stenotic lesions due to the incapacity of the probe to achieve sufficient contact with angulated tumors [34,64]. Bulky lesions may lied outside the focal length of the transducer and be inadequately imaged [64]. ERUS can be inaccurate for tumors located in the proximal rectum or low at the level of the anal canal. However, the distance of the tumor from the anal verge and its location did not influence accuracy when the ERUS probe was inserted through a specially designed 22 cm rigid rectosigmoidoscope, as we already reported in a series of 173 patients [29]. Transvaginally inserted probe may also help to define the local extent of tumor infiltration [65].

According to the literature, 2D-ERUS is the most accurate technique for determining the depth of tumor invasion in early stage rectal cancer. In a systematic literature review, Worrell et al. [66] reported that ERUS correctly established a cancer diagnosis in 81% of 62 biopsy-negative rectal adenomas, which had focal carcinoma on histopathology. In another study from the Cleveland Clinic Florida [67] the final pathology results confirmed the preoperative ERUS diagnosis of non-invasive villous rectal tumors in 26 out of 27 patients. Akasu et al. [41] reported the results of a study on 154 patients with early stage rectal cancer, evaluated preoperatively by ERUS. Sensitivity, specificity and overall accuracy rates for detection of slight and massive submucosal invasion were 99%/74%/96% and 98%/88%/97%, respectively. Konishi et al. [68] reported that the overall accuracy of ERUS based evaluation of tumor invasion depth was 60% in villous lesions and 91% in non villous lesions. In differentiating mucosal neoplasias from submucosal cancers the accuracy of ERUS in villous and nonvillous lesions were 66% and 96%, respectively. Akahoshi et al. [69] improved the accuracy of ERUS by using a high frequency (12 MHz) ultrasound catheter probe. The depth of invasion was correctly assessed in 87% (46/53) of pT1 tumors. Starck et al. [70] reported their experience on the adoption of high multifrequency probes. Their conclusion was that endosonography reliably distinguished benign from early invasive rectal lesions.

ERUS assessment of lymph nodes is more difficult and accuracy is inferior to T stage [19,71]. Overall accuracy has been reported to range from 63% to 86% [41,72,73]. Discrepancies could be partly due to the variable criteria used as markers of nodal involvement. The use of multiple criteria has been suggested to improve accuracy [74]. As already mentioned in the chapter sonographic criteria for involved nodes include hypoechogenicity, size greater than 3 mm, circular rather than oval shape, irregular margins and the absence of hilar reflection. In rectal cancer, over half of the metastatic nodes measure less than 5 mm and are located within 3 cm from the primary tumor [75,76]. A node measuring > 8 mm in the short axis is probably malignant [77]. Enlarged nodes, however, may be benign and reactive whereas small nodes, that are difficult to identify, may be infiltrated. The size of nodal metastasis is proportional to pT stage. This explains the relationship between nodal staging accuracy and T stage: < 50% accuracy for pT1 lesions and > 80% for pT3 lesions [78].

A number of comparative studies have been performed to assess the efficacy of ERUS, CT and MRI in the preoperative staging of rectal cancer [21,22]. Some studies have shown a clear superiority for ERUS whereas other studies have shown little difference [79,80]. CT is regarded as inferior to the other staging modalities for prediction of tumor invasiveness and lymph node status [21,81]. Overall accuracy of this procedure for the staging of rectal tumors is approximately 50% to 75% [21,82]. However it still has the advantage over ERUS that can combine local, regional and distal evaluation. Compared to ERUS, MRI with phased-array coil also resulted in images that reliably differentiate the rectal wall layers [83]. At MRI, such as at ERUS, errors in T staging mainly occur at limits of T2-T3 and T3-T4 tumors due to the difficulties in distinguishing between peripheral reactive fibrous and inflammatory change and neoplastic growth in the mesorectum. The prediction of nodal involvement by MRI is more accurate than T stage, particularly when the morphological features, such as spiculated or indistinct borders and a mottled heterogeneous appearance were used rather than size alone [83]. Guillem et al. [84] reported that the accuracy of preoperative ERUS/MRI for staging T3N0 rectal cancer was limited because 22% of their patients had undetected mesorectal lymph nodes involvement.

New software technology has allowed a series of 2D images to be assembled, giving a three-dimensional representation of the rectum and mesorectum [26]. After a 3D dataset has been acquired, it is immediately possible to select coronal anterior-posterior or posterior-anterior as well as sagittal right-left views, together with any oblique image plane. The 3D image can be rotated, tilted, and sliced to allow the operator to infinitely vary the different section parameters, visualize the lesion at different angles, and measure accurately distance, area, angle and volume. By using a combination of the different postprocessing display parameters, the 3D image can be rendered to provide better visualization performance when there are not large differences in the signal levels of pathologic structures compared with surrounding tissues [26]. Several studies have been shown an important benefits of 3D high-resolution ERUS in terms of better parietal staging [26-29]. In a recent comparative study on 86 patients examined with 3D-ERUS, 2D-ERUS and CT, Kim et al. [85] demonstrated that 3D-ERUS was greatly superior to the other modalities in both T staging and N staging. In this series, the accuracy of 3D-ERUS for T and N staging was 78% and 65%, respectively, but by eliminating examiner errors, the most frequent cause being misinterpretation, accuracy increased to 91% for T and 90% for N staging. In a study from Memorial Sloan-Kettering Cancer Center [86] the use of the new implemented 3D-ERUS appeared to facilitate the understanding of the spatial relations between different structures, compared to 2D-ERUS and MRI. However, no definitive conclusions over the new diagnostic tool were drawn. Vyslouzil et al. [87] reported an accuracy of 100% in the pT1 stage using 3D-ERUS and concluded that preoperative 3D ultrasonographic staging plays a decisive role in selecting patients suitable for local resection. Giovannini et al. (28) reported that the mesorectal margins are better defined by using 3D-ERUS than 2D-ERUS. In six of 15 patients classified as having T3N0 lesions, 3D-ERUS revealed malignant lymph nodes, a finding that was confirmed surgically in five of the six cases. Moreover 3D-ERUS correctly assessed the degree of infiltration of the mesorectum in all cases, demonstrating complete invasion of the mesorectum in eigth cases. Two-dimensional ERUS correctly assessed 71.4% of rectal tumors and 3D-ERUS increased this figure to 88.6%. In a preliminary study [43] we reported that the accuracy of 3D-ERUS was significantly superior to 2D-ERUS in determining the presence of submucosal invasion in 89 patients with rectal villous lesions (85 *vs.* 62.5%, respectively; $P=0.022$). Moreover 3D-ERUS with render mode provided better delineation of the superficial invasion of submucosa (SM-s lesions) compared to 2D-ERUS (83.3 *vs.* 54.1%, respectively; $P=0.029$). To provide a higher resolution image of the different layers of the rectal wall, render mode was used with high opacity, high thickness, normal filter and luminance setting, adjusted with high contrast and brightness. Compared with normal mode, VRM with this setting offered a clear view of the submucosal layer and helped to differentiate slight from massive submucosal invasion. Three-dimensional ERUS with VRM can also be useful in measuring CRMs. Even if, compared to MRI [83], the mesorectal fascia cannot be delineated, it is possible to visualize the outer interface of the mesorectal fat, where the mesorectal fascia is located. By using this criteria we are conducting a prospective study to compare the accuracy of 3D-ERUS to MRI in determining CRMs. Preliminary results are so far extremely encouraging with good agreement between the two techniques.

Conclusion

The great transformation in the management of rectal cancer has increased the importance of accurate preoperative staging on therapeutic decision-making. Among the different imaging modalities, 3D-ERUS has evolving as the best procedure, due to enhanced spatial resolution, providing detailed information on early tumoral invasion into the rectal wall, presence of mesorectal lymph node metastases and prediction of surgical circumferential resection margins. It has also the advantage of being an office-based procedure, well tolerated, with fast acquisition times and relatively low cost.

References

[1] American Cancer Society. *Cancer facts & figures* 2008. Atlanta: American Cancer Society; 2008

[2] Heintz A, Morschel M, Junginger T. Comparison of results after transanal endoscopic microsurgery and radical resection for T1 carcinoma of the rectum. *Surg Endosc* 1998;12:1145-8

[3] Hemingway D, Flett M, McKee RF, Finlay IG. Sphincter function after transanal endoscopic microsurgical excision of rectal tumours. *Br J Surg* 1996;83:51-2

[4] Heald RJ, Husband EM, Ryall RD. The mesorectum in rectal cancer surgery – the clue to pelvic recurrence? *Br J Surg* 1982;69:613-6

[5] Heald RJ. The holy plane of rectal surgery. *J R Soc Med* 1988;81:503-8

[6] Hainsworth PJ, Egan MJ, Cunliffe WJ. Evaluation of the policy of total mesorectal excision for rectal and rectosigmoid cancers. *Br J Surg* 1997;84:652-6

[7] Cavaliere F, Pemberton JH, Cosimelli M, Fazio VW, Beart RW. Coloanal anastomosis for rectal cancer. Long-term results at the Mayo and Cleveland Clinics. *Dis Col Rectum* 1995;38:807-12

[8] Williams NS, Price R, Johnston D. The long-term effect of sphincter preserving operations for rectal carcinoma on function of the anal sphincter in man. *Br J Surg* 1980;67:203-8

[9] Parc R, Tiret E, Frileux P, Moszkowoski E, Loygue J. Resection and coloanal anastomosis with colonic reservoir for rectal carcinoma. *Br J Surg* 1986;73:138-41

[10] Santoro GA, Makhdoomi KR, Eitan BZ, Bartolo DCC. Functional outcome after coloanal anastomosis with J-colonic pouch for rectal cancer. *Ann Ital Chir* 1998;LXIX,4:485-9

[11] Scheidbach H, Scneider C, Hugel O, et al. Oncological quality and preliminary long-term results in laparoscopic colorectal surgery. *Surg Endosc* 2003;17: 903-10

[12] Hazebroek EJ. COLOR. A randomised clinical trial comparing laparoscopic and open resection for colon cancer. *Surg Endosc* 2002;16:949-53

[13] Morino M, Parini U, Giraudo G, et al. Laparoscopic total mesorectal excision. A consecutive series of 100 patients. *Ann Surg* 2003;237:335-42

[14] Kapiteijn E, Corrie M, Nagtegaal ID, et al. Preoperative radiotherapy combined with total mesorectal excision for resectable rectal cancer. *N Engl J Med* 2001;34:638-46

[15] Cionini L, Cartei F, Manfredi B, et al. Randomized study of preoperative chemoradiation (CTRT) in locally advanced rectal cancer. Preliminary results. *Int J Radiat Oncol Biol Phys* 1999;45:S178

[16] Valentini V, Coco C, Cellini N, et al. Preoperative chemoradiation for extraperitoneal T3 rectal cancer: acute toxicity, tumor response and sphincter preservation. *Int J Radiat Oncol Biol Phys* 1998; 40:1067-75

[17] Valentini V, Coco C, Cellini N, et al. Ten years of preoperative chemoradiation for extraperitoneal T3 rectal cancer: acute toxicity, tumor response and sphincter preservation in three years consecutive studies. *Int J Radiat Oncol Biol Phis* 2001; 51:371-83

[18] Hildebrandt U, Feifel G. Preoperative staging of rectal cancer by intrarectal ultrasound. *Dis Colon Rectum* 1985; 28:42-6

[19] Santoro GA, Di Falco G. Endorectal ultrasound in the preoperative staging of rectal cancer. In: Santoro GA, Di Falco G. *Atlas of endoanal and endorectal ultrasonography*. Springer-Verlag 2004;11-21

[20] Glaser F, Schlag P, Herfarth CH. Endorectal ultrasonography for the assessment of invasion of rectal tumors and lymph node involvement. *Br J Surg* 1990;77:883-7

[21] Holdsworth PJ, Johnston D, Chalmers AG, et al. Endoluminal ultrasound and computed tomography in the staging of rectal cancer. *Br J Surg* 1988;75:1019-22

[22] Joosten FB, Jansen JB, Joosten HJ, Rosenbusch G. Staging of rectal carcinoma using MR doudle surface coil, MR endorectal coil and intrarectal ultrasound: correlation with histopathologic findings. *J Comput Assist Tomogr* 1995;19:752-8

[23] Brown G, Richards CJ, Newcombe RG, et al. Rectal carcinoma: thin section MR imaging for staging in 28 patients. *Radiology* 1999; 211:215-22

[24] Beets-Tan RG, Lettinga T, Beets GL. Pre-operative imaging of rectal cancer and its impact on surgical performance and treatment outcome. *Eur J Surg Oncol* 2005;31:681-8

[25] Santoro GA, Di Falco G. Endoanal and endorectal ultrasonographic techniques. In: Santoro GA, Di Falco G. *Atlas of endoanal and endorectal ultrasonography*. Springer-Verlag 2004;11-21

[26] Santoro GA, Fortling B. The advantages of volume rendering in three-dimensional endosonography of the anorectum. *Dis Colon Rectum* 2007;50:359-68

[27] Kim JC, Cho YK, Kim SY, Park SK, Lee MG. Comparative study of three-dimensional and conventional endorectal ultrasonography used in rectal cancer staging. *Surg Endosc* 2002;16:1280-5

[28] Giovannini M, Bories E, Pesenti C, et al. Three-dimensional endorectal ultrasound using a new freehand software program: results in 35 patients with rectal cancer. *Endoscopy* 2006; 38:339-43

[29] Santoro GA, D'Elia A, Battistella G, Di Falco G. The use of dedicated rectosigmoidoscope for ultrasound staging of tumors of the upper and middle third of the rectum. *Colorectal Dis* 2007; 9: 61-6

[30] Santoro GA, Di Falco G. Surgical and endosonographic anatomy of the rectum. In: Santoro GA, Di Falco G. *Atlas of endoanal and endorectal ultrasonography*. Springer-Verlag 2004;37-41

[31] Heintz A, Buess G, Frank K, et al. Endoluminal ultrasonic examination of sessile polyps and early carcinomas of the rectum. *Surg Endosc* 1989;3:92-5

[32] Adams WJ, Wong WD. Endorectal ultrasonic detection of malignancy within rectal villous lesions. *Dis Colon Rectum* 1995;38:1093-6

[33] Doornebosch PG, Bronkhorst PJB, Hop WCJ, et al. The role of endorectal ultrasound in therapeutic decision-making for local vs. transabdominal resection of rectal tumors. *Dis Colon Rectum* 2008;51:38-42

[34] Kim J, Yu CS, Jung HY, et al. Source of errors in the evaluation of early rectal cancer by endoluminal ultrasonography. *Dis Colon Rectum* 2001;44:1302-9

[35] Haggitt RC, Glotzbach RE, Soffer EE, Wruble LD. Prognostic factors in colorectal carcinomas arising in adenomas: implications for lesions removed by endoscopic polypectomy. *Gastroenterology* 1985;89:328-36

[36] Nivatvongs S, Rojanasakul A, Reiman HM, et al. The risk of lymph node metastasis in colorectal polyps with invasive adenocarcinoma. *Dis Colon Rectum* 1991;34:323-8

[37] Suzuki T, Sadahiro S, Mukoyama S, et al. Risk of lymph node and distant metastases in patients with early invasive colorectal cancer classified as Haggitt's level 4

invasion:image analysis of submucosal layer invasion. *Dis Colon Rectum* 2003;46:203-8

[38] Seitz U, Bohnacker S, Seewald S, et al. Is endoscopic polypectomy an adequate therapy for malignant colorectal adenomas? Presentation of 114 patients and review of the literature. *Dis Colon Rectum* 2004;47:1789-97

[39] Kudo S. Endoscopic mucosal resection of flat and depressed types of early colorectal cancer. *Endoscopy* 1993;25:455-61

[40] Kikuchi R, Takano M, Takagi K, et al. Management of early invasive colorectal cancer: risk of recurrence and clinical guidelines. *Dis Colon Rectum* 1995; 38: 710-7

[41] Akasu T, Kondo H, Moriya Y, et al. Endorectal ultrasonography and treatment of early stage rectal cancer. *World J Surg* 2000;24:1061-8

[42] Nascimbeni R, Nivatvongs S, Larson DR, Burgart LJ. Long-term survival after local excision for T1 carcinoma of the rectum. *Dis Colon Rectum* 2004;47:1773-9

[43] Santoro GA, Bara Egan D, Di Falco G. Three-dimensional endorectal ultrasonography in the evaluation of early invasive rectal cancer. *Colorectal Dis* 2004; 6 (Suppl 2): O-20

[44] LeBlanc JK. Imaging and management of rectal cancer. *Nat Clin Pract Gastroenterol Hepatol* 2007;4:665-76

[45] Lin AY, Wong WD, Shia J, et al. Predictive clinicopathologic factors for limited response of T3 rectal cancer to combined modality therapy. *Int J Colorectal Dis* 2008;23:243-9

[46] Hulsmans FJ, Bösma A, Mulder PJ, Reeders JW, Tytgat GN. Perirectal lymph nodes in rectal cancer: in vitro correlation of sonographic parameters and histologic findings. *Radiology* 1992;184:553

[47] Beynon J, Foy DM, Roe AM, et al. Preoperative staging of local invasion in rectal cancer using endoluminal ultrasound. *J R Soc Med* 1987;80:23-4

[48] Sailer M, Leppert R, Kraemer M, Fuchs KH, Thiede A. The value of endorectal ultrasound in the assessment of adenomas, T1- and T2-carcinomas. *Int J Colorectal Dis* 1997;12:214-9

[49] Katsura Y, Yamada K, Ishizawa T, Yoshinaka H, Shimazu H. Endorectal ultrasonography for the assessment of wall invasion and lymph node metastasis in rectal cancer. *Dis Colon Rectum* 1992;35:362-8

[50] Sentovich S, Blatchford G, Falk P, Thorson A, Christensen M. Transrectal ultrasound of rectal tumors. *Am J Surg* 1993;166:638-41

[51] Senesse P, Khemissa F, Lemanski C, et al. Contribution of endorectal ultrasonography in preoperative evaluation for very low rectal cancer. *Gastroenterol Clin Biol* 2001;25:24-8

[52] Herzog U, von Flue M, Tondelli P, Schuppisser JP. How accurate is endorectal ultrasound in the preoperative staging of rectal cancer? *Dis Colon Rectum* 1993;36:127-34

[53] Garcia-Aguilar J, Pollack J, Lee S-K, et al. Accuracy of endorectal ultrasonography in preoperative staging of rectal tumors. *Dis Colon Rectum* 2002;45:10-15

[54] Ptok H, Marusch F, Meyer F, et al. Feasibility and accuracy of TRUS in the pretreatment staging for rectal carcinoma in general practice. *Eur J Surg Oncol* 2006;32:420-5

[55] Steele SR, Martin MJ, Place RJ. Flexible endorectal ultrasound for predicting pathologic stage of rectal cancers. *Am J Surg* 2002;184:126-30

[56] Solomon MJ, McLeod RS. Endoluminal transrectal ultrasonography: accuracy, reliability, and validity. *Dis Colon Rectum* 1993;36:200-5

[57] Massari M, De Simone M, Cioffi U, Rosso L, Chiarelli M, Gabrielli F. Value and limits of endorectal ultrasonography for preoperative staging of rectal carcinoma. *Surg Laparosc Endosc* 1998;8:438-44

[58] Kim HJ, Wong WD. Role of endorectal ultrasound in the conservative management of rectal cancers. *Semin Surg Oncol* 2000;19:358-66

[59] Nesbakken A, Løvig T, Lunde OC, Nygaard K. Staging of rectal carcinoma with transrectal ultrasonography. *Scand J Surg* 2003;92:125-9

[60] Carmody BJ, Otchy DP. Learning curve of transrectal ultrasound. *Dis Colon Rectum* 2000; 43:193-7

[61] Orrom WJ, Wong WD, Rothenberger DA, Jensen LL, Goldberg SM. Endorectal ultrasound in the preoperative staging of rectal tumors. A learning experience. *Dis Colon Rectum* 1990;33:654-9

[62] Marusch F, Koch A, Schmidt U, et al. Routine use of transrectal ultrasound in rectal carcinoma: results of a prospective multicenter study. *Endoscopy* 2002;34:385-90

[63] Harewood GC. Assessment of publication bias in the reporting of EUS performance in staging rectal cancer. *Am J Gastroenterol* 2005;100:808-16

[64] Kumar A, Scholefield JH. Endosonography of the anal canal and rectum. *World J Surg* 2000;24:208-15

[65] Dhamanaskar KP, Thurston W, Wilson SR. Transvaginal sonography as an adjunct to endorectal sonography in the staging of rectal cancer in women. *Am J Radiol* 2006;187:90-8

[66] Worrell S, Horvath K, Blakemore T, Flum D. Endorectal ultrasound detection of focal carcinoma within rectal adenomas. *Am J Surg* 2004;187:625-9

[67] Pikarsky A, Wexner S, Lebensart P, et al. The use of rectal ultrasound for the correct diagnosis and treatment of rectal villous tumors. *Am J Surg* 2000;179:261-5

[68] Konishi K, Akita Y, Kaneko K, et al. Evaluation of endoscopic ultrasonography in colorectal villous lesions. *Int J Colorectal Dis* 2003;18:19-24

[69] Akahoshi K, Yoshinaga S, Soejima A, et al. Transit endoscopic ultrasound of colorectal cancer using 12MHz catheter probe. *Br J Rad* 2001;74:1017-22

[70] Starck M, Bohe M, Simanaitis M, Valentin L. Rectal endosonography can distinguish benign rectal lesions and invasive early rectal cancers. *Colorectal Dis* 2003;5:246-50

[71] Bipat S, Glas AS, Slors FJ, Zwinderman AH, Bossuyt PM, Stoker J. Rectal cancer: local staging and assessment of lymph node involvement with endoluminal US, CT, and MR imaging-a meta-analysis. *Radiology* 2004;232:773-83

[72] Beynon J. An evaluation of the role of rectal endosonography in rectal cancer. *Ann R Coll Surg Engl* 1989;71:131-9

[73] Rifkin MD, Wechsler RJ. A comparison of computed tomography and endorecatl ultrasound in staging rectal cancer. *Int J Colorectal Dis* 1986;1:219-23

[74] Kim J, Han MS, Lee HK, et al. Distribution of carcinoembryonic antigen and biologic behavior in colorectal carcinoma. *Dis Colon Rectum* 1999;42:640-8

[75] Dworak O. Number and size of lymph nodes and node metastases in rectal carcinomas. *Surg Endosc* 1989;3:96-9

[76] Monig SP, Baldus SE, Zirbes TK, et al. Lymph node size and metastatic infiltration in colon cancer. *Ann Surg Oncol* 1999;6:579-81

[77] Kim JH, Beets GL, Kim MJ, Kessels AG, Beets-Tan RG. High-resolution MR imaging for nodal staging in rectal cancer: are there any criteria in addition to the size? *Eur J Radiol* 2004;52:78-83

[78] Landmann RG, Wong WD, Hoepfl J, et al. Limitations of early rectal cancer nodal staging may explain failure after local excision. *Dis Colon Rectum*. 2007;50:1520-5

[79] Goldman S, Arvidson H, Normig U, et al. Transrectal ultrasound and computed tomography in preoperative staging of lower rectal adenocarcinoma. *Gastrointestinal Radiol* 1991;16:259-63

[80] Meyenberger C, Huch Boni RA, Bertschinger P, et al. Endoscopic ultrasound and endorectal magnetic resonance imaging: a prospective, comparative study for preoperative staging and follow-up of rectal cancer. *Endoscopy* 1995;27:469-79

[81] Civelli EM, Gallino G, Mariani L, et al. Double-contrast barium enema and computerised tomography in the pre-operative evaluation of rectal carcinoma: are they still useful diagnostic procedures? *Tumori* 2000;86:389-92

[82] Brown G, Daniels IR. Preoperative staging of rectal cancer: the MERCURY research project. *Recent Results Cancer Res* 2005;165:58-74

[83] Brown G, Richards CJ, Bourne MW, et al. Morphologic predictors of lymph node status in rectal cancer with use of high-spatial-resolution MR imaging with histopathologic comparison. *Radiology* 2003;227:371-7

[84] Guillem JG, Diaz-Gonzalez JA, Minsky BD, et al. cT3N0 rectal cancer: potential overtreatment with preoperative chemoradiotherapy is warranted. *J Clin Oncol* 2008;26:368-73

[85] Kim JC, Kim HC, Yu CS. Efficacy of 3-dimensional endorectal ultrasonography compared with conventional ultrasonography and computed tomography in preoperative rectal cancer staging. *Am J Surg* 2006;192:89-97

[86] Schaffzin DM, Wong WD. Endorectal ultrasound in the preoperative evaluation of rectal cancer. *Clin Colorectal Cancer* 2004;4:124-32

[87] Vyslouzil K, Cwiertka K, Zboril P, et al. Endorectal ultrasonography in rectal cancer staging and indication for local surgery. *Hepatogastroenterolgy* 2007;54:1102-6

In: Rectal Cancer: Etiology, Pathogenesis and Treatment
Editors: Paula Wells and Regina Halstead

ISBN 978-1-60692-563-8
© 2009 Nova Science Publishers, Inc.

Chapter IV

TRANSANAL ENDOSCOPIC MICSROSURGERY (TEM) IN EARLY RECTAL CANCER

A. Suppiah and J. R. T. Monson
Castle Hill Hospital, East Yorkshire, United Kingdom.

ABSTRACT

Radical resection with total mesorectal excision is the mainstay of rectal cancer treatment. However, it is associated with significant surgical morbidity/mortality, possible stoma surgery/complications and long-term gastrointestinal dysfunction with deterioration in quality of life. Re-assessment of surgical treatment is required in view of new cancer trends. There is an observable stage migration towards early stage cancer due to cancer screening and increased patient awareness, especially in the West. Simultaneously, better health care provision leads to an increasingly elderly population. The result is an elderly population group with significant co-morbidity and the probability of non-cancer related death which have early stage cancers with low recurrence rates. Radical resection risks over-treatment in these patients by attempting to achieve lowest recurrence rates but at the risk of non-cancer related death or deterioration in quality of life.

Transanal endoscopic microsurgery (TEM) is relatively new method of local excision without the morbidity associated with radical resection. It is superior to other local excision techniques. Published long-term outcomes in selected cancers appear to be comparable to radical resection although this is unproven in the context of randomised control trial. TEM may be an acceptable surgical alternative with minimal morbidity and gastrointestinal dysfunction but with acceptable compromise in recurrence rates. This chapter discusses the role of TEM in modern oncological surgery where the aim of oncological surgery should not just emphasise lowest recurrence rates but rather a balance of surgical risk, an acceptable post-operative quality of life and the possibility of non-cancer related death. TEM appears to balance all this areas and in selected cancers groups, TEM may well prove to be the treatment of choice in the future.

INTRODUCTION

Radical resection (RR), which includes Anterior resection (AR) and Abdomino-perineal Resection (APR) is the current mainstay of treatment for colorectal cancer. In the United Kingdom, colorectal cancer is the third most common cancer in men and the second most common cancer in women and a third of these are rectal cancers [1]. As such, it has enormous cost and health implications. Although radical resection is the mainstay of treatment, it comes at significant morbidity and mortality. There is immediate risk of post-operative death (1-12.5%) and morbidity such anastomatic leakage (5%) and wound complications. Long-term morbidity includes genitourinary and gastrointestinal dysfunction and deterioration in quality of life. In addition, perineal wound complications and long-term stoma lead to significant impact on body image, depression and psychological morbidity [2,3]. Finally, despite the risks associated with surgery, a third eventually die of disease.

The "gold standard" of cancer treatment emphasises recurrence rates as the primary outcomes measure. However, the aim of oncological surgery should be to balance disease control whilst maintaining quality of life. This is especially true of colorectal cancer where significant proportions of patients are elderly and at risk of non-cancer related death. Furthermore, a large proportion of these patients have early stage cancer which have a low risk of recurrence. In such cases, radical resection risks over-treatment. Radical resection may well lead to lowest recurrence rates, but to the detriment of the patient, causing excess morbidity/mortality with decreased quality of life, and yet the possibility (*and the likely probability*) that the patient will eventually die of non-cancer related causes. In view of this, various local excision methods such as a transanal excision (Parks), transcoccygeal (Kraske), trans-sphincteric (York-Mason), endoscopic posterior mesorectal excision (EPMR), fulguration and endocavitary radiation have been tried but with limited success [4,5,6,7,8,9].

Buess et al introduced Transanal Endospcic Microsurgery in the 1980s [10]. This involves passage of a 40mm rectoscope which forms an airtight seal within the rectum. Gas insufflation leads to pneumorectum thus creating a large field view with optical-enhancement up to six times magnification. Simultaneous instrumentation is performed via air-tight ports of the rectoscope. Access up to 20 cm from the anal verge is possible. During surgery, the patient is positioned such that the lesion is accessible and in a dependant position. Markers for the resection margins are scored with diathermy at various points 1 cm away from the lesion. Adrenaline is occasionally injected into the submucosal layer. Excision is performed by joining the pre-marked resection margin markers. Excision should be full thickness to incorporate the mesorectum. This results in a conical/pyramid tissue specimen where the lesion forms the narrow apex of the specimen and the submucosa/mesorectal tissue forms the wider base. The resulting defect in the rectum can either be closed transanally or left open depending on surgeon choice. The concern is defects sutured close could lead to rectal stenosis whereas defects left open could result in bleeding or intraperitoneal leaks. Although some studies conclude there is no difference, the general consensus is large high intraperitoneal defects should be closed whereas small low extraperitoneal defects can be left open [11,12].

Outcomes of TEM are superior to other local transanal procedures [13]. Recurrence rates are lower primarily due to the better view and instrumentation which allows the ability to obtain complete resection margins. The TEM-resected specimen also allows more accurate pathological assessment. In addition, morbidity is less than transacral/ transphincteric approaches. Hence, TEM should be the local excision method of choice for treating in selected early rectal cancer. This chapter aims to evaluate the role of TEM in rectal cancer.

Transanal Endoscopic Microsurgery vs. Radical Resection

The ongoing discussion of TEM compared to Radical Resection (RR) is largely based on 4 trials. The most commonly quoted is the study by Winde et al which is also the only randomised trial to date [14]. The remaining 3 studies are retrospective case comparisons [15,16,17]. To facilitate discussion, the results of these 4 pivotal studies are divided by the 2 important treatment outcomes measures – cancer outcome/recurrence, and procedure safety. Individual trials results are summarised in Table 1 (Cancer Outcomes) and Table 2 (Procedure safety). Finally, and most recently, a second randomised trial of TEM has been published where TEM was compared to Laproscopic resection [18]. These results are discussed later.

Table 1. Comparative studies in TEM vs. Radical Resection (RR) – Cancer related Outcomes

Reference	Tumour	Procedure (n)	FU	Outcome Measures (TEM vs. RR)
Winde (1996) [14]	50 T1 (G1/2)	TEM (24) RR (26)	TEM 40.9 AR 45.8	Local Recurrence: 4.1% (1/24) vs. 3.8% (1/26) Metastases: 0% vs. 3.8% (1/26) 5 year survival: 96% vs. 96%
Heintz (1998) [15]	80 low risk T1 23 high risk T1	TEM (56) Parks (2) RR (45)	52$^\infty$ (+/-23) 43 (+/-22)	Low risk: Local Recurrence: 4.3% (2/46) vs. 29% (1/34) 5 year survival: 79% vs. 81% High-risk: Local recurrence: 33% (4/12) vs. 0% (0/11) 5 year survival: 62% vs. 69%
Langer (2003) [16]	118 Ad 59 T1 (G1/2) 5 other	TEM-ES(45) TEM-UC(34) TP(76) RR(27)	TEM 21.6 RR 33.7	Local recurrence for carcinoma: TEM 10% vs. RR 4% vs. TP 15% TEM-UC 4% vs. TEM-ES 15.4% 2 year survival: TEM 100% vs. RR 96%
Lee (2003) [17]	52 T1 22 T2 100 T1/2N0	TEM (74) RR (100)	TEM 31 RR 35	Local recurrence at 5 years - T1: 4% vs. 0% - T2: 20% vs. 9% (p = 0.04) Disease free survival at 5 years - T1: 96% vs. 94% - T2: 81% vs. 83%

All results are *not statistically significant* unless stated otherwise. Follow up in Median unless Mean(∞); (G1/2) well/ moderately differentiated; (LR) Local recurrence; (Mets) Metastatic disease; (DFS) Disease Free Survival; (RR) radical resection; (AR) anterior resection; (TEM-ES) electrosurgery; (TEM-UC) Ultracision; (y) years;

Cancer-related Outcomes Measures

The results of cancer-related outcomes are summarised in Table 1.

Winde et al represents the strongest single study level of evidence on TEM and radical resection despite being published more than 20 years ago [14]. The mean follow up was sufficiently long in both groups (40-45 months) and there was no difference in survival (96%). However, the study does not mention methods of pre-operative staging and excludes 2 patients who were understaged pre-TEM and who were later excluded from analysis. This study, as with all other published studies, has only a small population and is not powered to detect difference in survival.

Heintz et al also demonstrated no difference in 5 year survival in patients treated with TEM or RR in a retrospective case-comparison study [15]. More interestingly, 5-year survival was similar (62% vs. 69%) in patients with high-risk T1 treated with TEM despite the fact that these patients were significantly older than those treated with RR (mean 74y vs. 63y p=0.048). Although this is likely due to selection bias, it also suggests that elderly patients may benefit from less invasive treatment, even those with unfavourable early stage cancers. At the very least, outcomes are not worse as a result of TEM, which is also far less traumatic than RR.

It is further possible that the overall survival benefit of all T1 cancers treated with TEM may be under-reported in this study due to change in trial protocol. T1 tumours were stratified into low- and high-risk tumours only midway through the trial. After 1988, only low-risk tumours were treated with TEM. Thus, the high-risk T1 cancers prior to 1988 were inappropriately treated with TEM which most likely leads to a falsely lower survival rates. However, strong conclusions on cancer outcomes cannot be made due to the retrospective nature of this trial, the non-randomised case controls and insufficient power. All recurrences after local excision in this study occurred with resection margin tumour involvement which is one of the most important predictors of recurrence.

Heintz et al also demonstrate another problem with obtaining long-term cancer outcomes in trials of TEM vs. Radical resection - patient selection/ patient refusal leading to protocol deviation. TEM is often offered with curative intent but most likely in highly selected patients with especially significant co-morbidity who would not tolerate radical resection. Even at present, many surgeons consider patients for TEM only when the patient is deemed unfit for RR. In unfit patients, if the tumour is early stage and deemed resectable, TEM will be labelled "curative" although the reality remains that it is offered as a compromise between curative and palliation. This inadvertently selects out an unfit population, who due to their co-morbidity, refuse salvage RR if TEM is deemed inadequate (e.g. due to incomplete resection margins, or upstaged on pathological assessment). This is demonstrated in this study by Heintz et al where 23 patients were pre-operatively staged low-risk but subsequently deemed high-risk following pathological examination of the cancer. More than half of these patients (n=12) refused salvage surgery as recommended by trial protocol. Thus although TEM is often labelled as offered with "curative" intent, published results are often that of TEM used as a compromise between curative and palliative treatment.

Langer et al again demonstrated comparable outcomes of TEM with RR but with less morbidity [16]. This study also reported lowest complication rates when using a Parks retractor for transanal excision. This method was associated with the shortest operation time and least blood loss. This apparent benefit was offset by Park's transanal excision having the highest recurrence rate (27%). High recurrence rates using other local excision methods have also been documented in other studies [19,20]. A systematic review reported 25% recurrence following transanal excision compared to 10% following TEM [13].

None of the above studies are sufficiently powered to detect differences in cancer survival outcomes. A randomised control trial comparing TEM *vs.* RR using survival as primary outcome can be logistically challenging due to the good outcomes with total mesorectal excision (TME). The Dutch TME trial reported 5 year local recurrence rates of 0.7% in T1 cancer treated with neo-adjuvant short course radiotherapy and TME [21]. Other centres report slightly higher recurrence rates but still <5%. Assuming current neo-adjuvant short course radiotherapy and TME has a 3-year local recurrence rate of 5%, a two-tailed randomised trial powered to detect a 2.5% difference in survival will require 500 patients per trial arm i.e. 1000 trial patients with highly-selected T1. Furthermore, this assumes 100% accurate pre-operative staging, no patient drop out, no treatment side effects and 100% compliance with trial protocol. Hence, in reality the number of patients required to conduct a trial with survival as the end-point and may prove logistically unfeasible. Surrogate outcome measures such as morbidity/mortality scores and measurements of gastrointestinal functional and quality of life could be used in future. These outcome measures would be more appropriate when attempting to establish the role of TEM in treating early rectal cancer. A trial using these multifactorial outcomes measures may even demonstrate TEM to be gold-standard treatment (in selected cancer) from a patient perspective but not necessarily for recurrence rates.

In summary, there are several problems with the published evidence. Firstly, tumour selection criteria are often not stipulated and pre-operative staging methods are not mentioned. There is lack of prospective case controls and the change of intent of surgery as dictated by patient selection affects long-term outcomes. None of the studies are powered to detect survival difference. Regardless, bearing these limitations, all published comparative studies favour TEM over RR in selected early rectal cancer.

Safety and Outcome Measures in Comparative Trials

The key advantage of TEM compared to RR is safety. Results of 4 trials comparing morbidity and mortality between TEM and RR are summarised in Table 2. The only published randomised control trial by Winde et al demonstrates TEM superiority in terms of operative parameters [14]. In addition, there was also less post-operative analgesic requirement in the TEM group. Similarly, TEM was associated with far less morbidity than RR in the three remaining studies [15,16,17]. A recent review of TEM showed a median 19% morbidity from published studies [13]. Furthermore, not only is the frequency of complications less, but the severity is also less disastrous than complications following RR as seen in study by Lee et al. (Table 2) [17]. Finally, these studies under-report long-term complications of RR. The current evidence does not take into account complications which are more likely following RR such as repeat hospital attendances (e.g. for adhesive obstruction), care in the community, stoma problems and psychological burden. Such problems should intuitively, be even less with TEM. Hence, complications following TEM are less frequent, less severe when they do occur, and its long-term safety advantage over RR is likely to be under-reported.

Table 2. Comparative Studies in TEM vs. Radical Resection (RR): Operative and Safety Outcomes

Reference	Procedure (n)	Outcome Measures (TEM vs. RR)
Winde (1996) [14]	TEM (24) AR (26)	Complications: Early: 20.8% (5/24) vs. 34.5% (9/26) Late: 8.3% (2/24) vs. 23.3 (6/26) Mean Operating time: 103 min vs. 149 min Blood loss: 143 ml vs. 745 ml Length of stay: 5.7 d vs. 15.4 d
Heintz (1998) [15]	TEM (56) Parks (2) RR (45)	Complications: Low-risk T1: 2% (1/46) vs.15% (5/34) High risk T1: 8% (1/12) vs.27% (3/11) (NS) Mortality: Low-risk T1: 0% vs.6% (2/34) (NS) High-risk T1: 0% both groups (NS)
Langer (2003) [16]	TEM-ES(45) TEM-UC(34) TP(76) RR(27)	Complications: 8% vs. 56% Mortality 0% vs. 3.7% Mean operating time: 100 min vs.152 min Transfusion requirement: 9% vs. 43% Length of stay: 8.2 d vs. 14.5 d
Lee (2003) [17]		Complications (4.1% vs. 48%) All TEM complications (n=3) were minor and treated conservatively (bleeding, urinary difficulty, faecal incontinence) RR: Early complications n=20; 2 anastomatic leak, 1 bleeding, 1 rectovaginal fistula requiring surgery. Late complications n=30

All differences shown are *statistically significant* unless stated otherwise; (NS) not significant; (RR) radical resection; (AR) anterior resection; (TEM-ES) electro-surgery; (TEM-UC) Ultracision; (min) minutes; (ml) mililitres; (d) days.

Transanal Endoscopic Microsurgery and Laparoscopic Colorectal Resection

Laparoscopic resection has extended to colorectal surgery in an attempt to minimise the trauma caused by major abdominal surgery. TME is possible with laproscopic resection thus avoiding major laparotomy whilst providing lowest recurrence rates and an adequate specimen for lymph node assessment. Lezoche et al performed the only study comparing TEM with laproscopic resection [18]. A highly selected group of 40 T2 tumours with G1/2 and diameter <3cm within 6 cm of the anal verge were subjected to neo-adjuvant chemoradiotherapy (CRT) followed by TEM or laparoscopic resection. TEM was associated with better operative parameters – decreased operative time (95 *vs.* 170 minutes), blood loss (50 *vs.* 200ml) and hospital stay (4.5 *vs.* 7.5 days) although complication rates were similar between the 2 procedures. There was a prolonged follow-up (median 56 months). 2 patients in each group developed recurrence/metastases. Both patients with recurrence following LapR died at 31 and 51 months. In the 2 patients with recurrence following TEM, 1 died at 39 months and another is disease free at 21 moths following salvage LapR. The numbers are too small to determine statistical significance. However, it would appear that TEM *and* neoadjuvant CRT can offer similar survival in long-term for highly selected T2 tumours but TEM is safer.

Table 3. TEM Individual Case Series

Reference	N	Morbidity	FU	Local Recurrence % (n)
Serra-Aracil 2008 [41]	Ad 122 Tis 22 T1 16 T2 11	Morbidity 9% Mortality 0%	52, >24 months Median 59 months	Tis/T1 5.3% (2/38) Tis 4.5% (1/22) T1 6.25% (1/16) T2 2/11 (22.2%) Kaplan Meir probability of non recurrence Tis 94.4% T1 92.3% T2 77.8%
Bretagnol F 2007 [42]	Ad 148 T1 31 T2 17 T3 4	Morbidity 14% (28 / 200) Mortlaity 0.5% (1 / 200)	33 (2 – 133)	Ad 7.6% (11 / 148) T1 3/31 T2 2/17 T3 3/4 5y DFS 65%
Guerrieri M 2006 [43]	ad 530 T1 58	Minor 8% (48) Major 1.2% (7) Mortality 0	ad 44 (15-74) T1 35 (27-48)	Ad: 4.3% (23) T1: 0%; 96% survival at 120m 5.3% (31) died non-cancer cause
Floyd ND 2006 [44]	T1 37	Minor 20% (10) Major 0 Mortality 0	34 ∞	11% (4) 5y DFS 100%
Jotautas V 2005 [45]	ad 23 T1≠ 22 T2 3	Morbidity 4.2% (2) Mortality 0	3-17 (n=26)	ad 2% (1) T1/2 0%
Duek SD 2005 [46]	ad 74 T1 25 T2 14 T3 3	Morbidity 7% (5) Mortality 0	-	T1 0% T2 9% (1)
Suzuki H 2005 [47]	ad 7 Tis 5 T1≠ 9	Morbidity 0 Mortality 0	27.2 (2-52)	ad 0% Tis/1 17% (1)
Palma P 2004 [48]	ad 71 T1 21	Morbidity 7% (7) Mortality 0	30 (6-54)	ad 7% (5) T1 5% (1)
Stipa F 2004 [49]	Tis 9 T1 39 T2 23 T3 12	Morbidity 18% (15) Mortality 0	37 (18-118)	LR 5y Survival Tis 0% 100% T1 13% 92% T2 17% 75% T3 50% 69%
Meng WC 2004 [50]	31 ad/Tis	Morbidity 16% (5) Mortality 0	23 (2-92)	0%
Dafnis G 2004 [51]	ad 46 T1 10 T2 2	Morbidity 19% (11) Mortality 0	8 (3-40)	ad 11% (5) T1/2 14% (2)

Table 3. (Continued)

Neary P 2003 [52]	ad 21 T0/is 5 T1 5 T2 8 T3 1	Minor 10% (4) Major 2.5% (1) Mortality 0	20 (1-47)	0%
Lloyd GM 2002 [53]	T1 6 T2 10	Major 4.4% Mortality 0	32.2	0%
Lezoche E 2002 [54]	T2# 35	Minor 14% (5) Major 0% Mortality 0%	38 (24-96)	LR 3% (1), SR 11.4% (4) Survival probability 83% at 96m. 17.2% (6) died non cancer cause.
de Graaf EJ 2002 [55]	Tis 32 T1 21 T2 18 T3 5	Minor 17% (14) Major 3% (2) Mortality 1.3% (1)	10 (1-52)	18% at 3 y 1 death in T3 day 4
Farmer C 2002 [40]	ad 36 T1 10 T2 3 T3 1	Early 10% (5) Late 6% (3) Mortality 2% (1)	33	ad 5% T1/2/3 0%
Demartines N 2001 [56]	ad 35 T1# 9 T2 3	Minor 8% (4) Major 2% (1) Mortality 0	31 (11-54)	ad 2% (1) T1 8.3%
Benoist S 2001 [57]	ad 30 ca 13	Morbidity 18% Mortality 0	26∞	ad 3% (1) T1 0 T2 75%
Azimuddin 2000 [58]	ad 8 ca 23	Major 3.2% (1) Mortality 0	15	6.5% (2)
Arribas D 2000 [59]	ad 29 ca 13	Morbidity 5% (2) Mortality 0	11∞ (1-36)	ad 7% (2) ca 8%(1)
Lev-Chelouche D 2000 [60]	ad 46 T1 10 T2 10 T3 9	Minor 21% (16) Major 11% (8) Mortality 1.3% (1)	ad 36∞ (5-76) ca 34∞ (4-72)	T1 0% (0/8) T2 25% (2/8) T3 33% (2/6) 1 non cancer related death
Saclarides T 1998 [61]	ad 28 Tis 14 T1 16 T2 13	Morbidity 25% (18) Mortality 0		ad 14% (4) Tis 15% T1 13% (2) T2 80% (8)
Mentges B 1997 [62]	T1 64 T2 33 T3 16	Major 7% (8) Mortality 0	29 (3-65)	T1 3% (2) T2 0% T3 40% (2)
Said S 1997 [63]	ad 260 T1 19	Major 2.8% Morality 0.5% (2)	ad 60 T1 12	ad 6.5% (17) T1 10.5% (2) Low risk T1: 91% 3y survival
Steele RJ 1996 [64]	ad 77 T1 7 T2 14 T3 2	Major 6% (6) Mortality 1% (1)	ad 7.4 ca 6.7	ad 5% (4) T1 0
Smith LE 1996 [65]	ad 82 T1 30 T2 15 T3 6	Early 15% (20) Late 5% (7)		ad 11% (9) T1 10% (3) T2 40% (6) T3 66% (4)

Neary P 2003 [52]	ad 21 T0/is 5 T1 5 T2 8 T3 1	Minor 10% (4) Major 2.5% (1) Mortality 0	20 (1-47)	0%
Lloyd GM 2002 [53]	T1 6 T2 10	Major 4.4% Mortality 0	32.2	0%
Lezoche E 2002 [54]	T2# 35	Minor 14% (5) Major 0% Mortality 0%	38 (24-96)	LR 3% (1), SR 11.4% (4) Survival probability 83% at 96m. 17.2% (6) died non cancer cause.
de Graaf EJ 2002 [55]	Tis 32 T1 21 T2 18 T3 5	Minor 17% (14) Major 3% (2) Mortality 1.3% (1)	10 (1-52)	18% at 3 y 1 death in T3 day 4
Farmer C 2002 [40]	ad 36 T1 10 T2 3 T3 1	Early 10% (5) Late 6% (3) Mortality 2% (1)	33	ad 5% T1/2/3 0%
Demartines N 2001 [56]	ad 35 T1# 9 T2 3	Minor 8% (4) Major 2% (1) Mortality 0	31 (11-54)	ad 2% (1) T1 8.3%
Benoist S 2001 [57]	ad 30 ca 13	Morbidity 18% Mortality 0	26∞	ad 3% (1) T1 0 T2 75%
Azimuddin 2000 [58]	ad 8 ca 23	Major 3.2% (1) Mortality 0	15	6.5% (2)
Arribas D 2000 [59]	ad 29 ca 13	Morbidity 5% (2) Mortality 0	11∞ (1-36)	ad 7% (2) ca 8% (1)
Lev-Chelouche D 2000 [60]	ad 46 T1 10 T2 10 T3 9	Minor 21% (16) Major 11% (8) Mortality 1.3% (1)	ad 36∞ (5-76) ca 34∞ (4-72)	T1 0% (0/8) T2 25% (2/8) T3 33% (2/6) 1 non cancer related death
Saclarides T 1998 [61]	ad 28 Tis 14 T1 16 T2 13	Morbidity 25% (18) Mortality 0		ad 14% (4) Tis 15% T1 13% (2) T2 80% (8)
Mentges B 1997 [62]	T1 64 T2 33 T3 16	Major 7% (8) Mortality 0	29 (3-65)	T1 3% (2) T2 0% T3 40% (2)
Said S 1997 [63]	ad 260 T1 19	Major 2.8% Morality 0.5% (2)	ad 60 T1 12	ad 6.5% (17) T1 10.5% (2) Low risk T1: 91% 3y survival
Steele RJ 1996 [64]	ad 77 T1 7 T2 14 T3 2	Major 6% (6) Mortality 1% (1)	ad 7.4 ca 6.7	ad 5% (4) T1 0
Lirici MM 1994 [66]	ad 58 T1 21 T2 21	Minor 29% (16) Major 0% Mortality 0%	7-16	ad 10.5% (6) T1 4.7% (1) 19% (4)

Table 3. (Continued)

Buess G 1993 [67]	ad 191 T1 29 T2 16	Major 9% (21) Mortality 0.5% (1)	12	ad 3.5% (6) T1 3.5% (1) T2 6% (1)
Buess G 1988 [68]	ad 110 T1 12	Morbidity 4.5% Mortality 0%	12.3	0%

*Salm is questionnaire study from 57 surgical departments in Germany. (Ad) adenoma; ($\dagger$) well/moderately differentiated carcinoma; (ca) carcinoma; (FU) Median follow-up in months unless; (∞) mean; (m) months; (LR) Local Recurrence; (SR) Systemic Recurrence; (DFS) Disease Free Survival.

This study suggests highly selected T2 tumours can be treated with CRT and TEM. However, several problems arise with this blanket approach mainly due to the lack accurate pre-operative staging methods. T1/2 staging inaccuracies can vary between 5-20%. As many as 1 in 5 patients with T1 cancers overstaged as T2 would be receiving unnecessarily toxic CRT. Conversely, patients with T3/4 or node positive tumours understaged as T2 N0 may miss out on early TME which may impact on their survival. The decision to proceed with TEM or RR following CRT is also not possible due to further decrease in staging accuracy caused by CRT-induced changes. Finally, the long-term function of an irradiated rectum left in-situ is not known as current practice of mesorectal excision removes the irradiated segment. This is among the limitation of TEM treatment and is discussed later (*Limitations of Transanal Endoscopic Microsurgery*).

Non-comparative case series' of Transanal Endoscopic Microsurgery

The results of other case series' of TEM are summarised in Table 3. Results are variable due to different population, case selection, use of adjuvant therapy, protocol deviation and change in practice.

Gastrointestinal Function and Quality of Life Following Transanal Endoscopic Microsurgery

Radical resection of colorectal cancer can cause significant functional problems and the carry the risk of stoma requirement. This is especially true in patients suitable for TEM or RR. These patients will have rectal tumours with greater continence issues and higher rates of stoma formation than more proximal colonic surgery. Table 4 summarises the results of studies reporting either gastrointestinal function scores, anorectal manometry/ physiology measurements or quality of life scores.

TEM can cause transient gastrointestinal dysfunction which usually recovers fully within 6 weeks [22]. This is probably due to anal dilatation caused by the 40mm rectsoscope. Most patients return to pre-TEM continence levels within 6 weeks although some reports require up to a year for full recovery [23,24]. Risk factors for anorectal dysfunction include >50%

circumferential excision, prolonged operation time (>2 hours), pre-operative low sphincter pressures or anorectal dysfunction [25,26]. Anorectal physiology and manometry measurements show a deterioration post-procedure compared to clinical continence scores. These measurements also takes longer to recover and some persist > 6 weeks [26,27] However, these usually do not impact on clinical continence. This is consistent with other reports showing poor correlation between anorectal measurements and clinical continence. All patients receiving TEM should be counselled with regards to this risk of this transient dysfunction. These results are still superior to continence following RR.

Table 4. Gastrointestinal function and Quality of Life following TEM

Author	N	Assessment	Method	Result
Doornebosch 2008 [29]	47	Pre- and 6m	FISI; FIQL	Improvement in functional continence (FISI), especially in tumours within 7cm of dentate line. Improvement in quality of life
Cataldo 2005 [22]	37	Pre- and 6 w	FISI; FIQL	No change in function 6 w post TEM
Dafnis 2004 [51]	48	Median 22m	Questionnaire Wexner / Kamm	37% (18/48) decreased continence.
Wang 2003 [69]	22	Pre-, 2 and 6w, 3m, 1y	AR manometry Questionnaire	Transient lower squeeze pressures at 2, 6w but recovered at 1 year. Mean continence better at 3m vs. pre-TEM (NS)
Kennedy 2002 [26]	13	Pre-, 3 and 6w	AR manometry PNTML Electrosensitivity Interview	Decrease sphincter tone at 6w correlates with duration of procedure >2h. No change in continence
Herman 2001 [25]	33	Pre-, 3w, 6m	AR manometry ISS	Decrease ISS at 3w. Risk factors for anorectal dysfunction post-TEM was post-operative internal anal sphincter defects, low pre-operative resting anal pressure, disturbed anorectal co-ordination, >50% circumferential excision and full thickness excision in this study
Kreis 1996 [24]	42	Pre-, 3m, 1y	AR manometry Interview	Decreased squeeze pressure and continence at 3m with full recovery at 1y
Banerjee 1996 [27]	36	Pre- and 12m	AR manometry Questionnaire	Decreased resting pressures but not continence
Hemmingway 1996 [23]	6	Pre-, 48hours, 6 weeks	AR manometry Interview	Decreased resting and squeeze pressure to 75% and 653% pre-op levels at 48 hours. All pressures normal at 6 weeks. No incontinence

Quality of Life (QOL) is more complex and multi-factorial than simple clinical continence. Many QOL assessment tools are generic e.g. Hospital Anxiety and Depression scale. The Rockwood FIQOL is amongst the only validated questionnaires which combine QOL scores with measurements of continence [28]. The Rockwood FIQOL is used in the only 2 studies reporting QOL as an outcome [22,29]. Both studies report no change in QOL scores before and after TEM. None of the above studies compare QOL in TEM *vs.* RR. The only comparative study of QOL following TEM and RR is a small retrosepective case comparison. There was no difference in QOL between the 2 groups but patients with TEM had less defecation disorders than those with RR [30]. This would play an important part in the decision making for treatment of early rectal cancer.

Limitations of Transanal Endoscopic Microsurgery

Despite the promising role of TEM, it is subject to several limitations. These are
1. Pre-operative staging
2. Tumour favourability
3. Tumour location
4. Cost-effectiveness

1. Pre-operative Staging

Accurate pre-operative staging is required to select patients suitable for TEM as patients with T3 cancer or nodal involvement are not suitable for TEM. Similarly patients with T1 disease should be differentiated form T2 disease as T1 can be treated with TEM only whereas T2 patients may require neo-adjuvant treatment. Magnetic Resonance Imaging or Endorectal/anal Ultrasound (ERUS) have higher accuracy rates (up to 95%) compared to CT (52-75%) although the latter is still used due to lower cost [31,32]. Despite advances in radiological technology, current staging modalities are still considered too inaccurate to select patients who will benefit from TEM. This remains one of the biggest hurdles to patient selection. Furthermore, accuracy further decreases if neo-adjuvant CRT is used. This is because imaging modalities are not able to differentiate between scar tissue or viable tumour depth (T-stage). Scarring and reactive changes secondary to CRT-induced inflammation also reduce accuracy of nodal staging. Hence, MRI cannot be used to decide if patients should undergo RR or TEM [33].

2. Tumour Favourability

Radical resection excises the tumour en-block with the mesorectal fat/fascia and the vascular/lymphatic chain thus allowing accurate nodal staging. Nodal assessment is not possible with TEM excision. It is estimated that nodal involvement occurs in 0-12% T1, 12-28% T2 and 30-60% T3. [34,35] Hence 1 in 10 (10%) T1 patients are nodal status understaged and miss out on beneficial chemotherapy leading to shorter survival. Other predictive factors on pathological assessment of the TEM specimen are used to increase the accuracy of nodal prediction. One such example is tumour differentiation. Well differentiated tumours have 0-3% nodal involvement compared to poorly differentiated tumours which have up to 12% nodal involvement [35,36]. The current favourable pathological features for TEM only treatment are T1 tumours < 3cm with < 40% wall circumference, well/moderate differentiation, no lymphovascular invasion or tumour budding and Kikuchi Sm1 level [37,38]. These are extremely important pathological criteria as patients with poor predictive factors cannot be treated for curative purposes with TEM only. Additional adjuvant treatment or salvage radical resection is required!

3. Tumour Location

In addition to the stipulated "favourable" pathological and staging criteria, the tumour has to be in a suitable location. High rectal tumours may be treated with mesorectal excision with acceptable minor disturbance in gastrointestinal function. Tumours in the low rectum are occasionally too low to be accessible by TEM. A Parks transanal excision is favoured which is cheaper and associated with less operative time and bleeding [16]. The combination of these factors make TEM suitable for only a select group of tumours, which in addition to being T1, also have to display the favourable prognostic factors, and finally located within a suitable region in the rectum. This highly select criteria restricts its utility and cost-effectiveness.

4. Cost-effectiveness

The initial capital expenditure for TEM equipment is costly, estimated at £40,000. This outlay can be offset by savings using TEM provided sufficient cases are performed. In one study, the cost of RR is estimated at £4000-£6000 whereas TEM costs £560 [39]. The main reason for high expense of RR is longer operating time and prolonged hospital stay, especially high dependency units. Patients who have a temporary defunctioning stoma also require re-admission and re-operation. An Australian study reported similar findings [40]. In a recent systematic review, the cost of RR *vs.* TEM for adenoma was US$2081 *vs.* US$3309 and carcinoma US$2542 *vs.* US$5679. Hence substantial savings can be made provided sufficient cases are performed. Our own retrospective case comparison study suggested 11.5 cases were required to offset capital cost [39]. As only small numbers of highly selected tumours are suitable for TEM, it is probably cost-effective only in larger hospitals. Alternatively, smaller hospitals could set up referral pathways to one nominated tertiary centre to make up the case volume required.

CONCLUSION

TEM appears to be a viable alternative and possibly the treatment of choice in selected early rectal cancer. It is safe with minimal complications and almost no mortality. Surgical complications, if present, (e.g. perforation/ suture line dehiscence) are less disastrous than those of radical resection (e.g. abdominal wound dehiscence/ anastomatic leakage). Furthermore, the current published complication rates are from initial experiences. The complications rates should decrease further with time, consistent with a steep learning curve. Reported recurrence and disease-free rates are variable between studies due to case selection and pre-operative staging, technical surgical aspects (e.g. resection margin involvement), treatment intent (curative or palliative), patient refusal for salvage procedures and use of (neo)adjuvant treatment. Even so, the recurrence rates appear to be comparable to RR in selected tumours but with less morbidity/mortality and better function. Hence, TEM appears to have a promising role in the future of rectal cancer treatment, possibly even treatment of choice in selected tumours, but further controlled trials are required.

REFERENCES

[1] Registrations of Cancers Diagnosed in 2002. In: *Registration CS*, editor. London: National Statistics; 2005.

[2] Nastro P, Beral D, Hartley J, Monson JR. Local excision of rectal cancer: review of literature. *Dig Surg* 2005; 22(1-2): 6-15.

[3] Williams NS, Johnston D. The quality of life after rectal excision for low rectal cancer. *Br J Surg* 1983; 70(8): 460-462

[4] Parks AG, Stuart AE. The management of villous tu ours of the large bowel. *Br J Surg* 1973; 60(9): 688-95

[5] Chirstiansen J. Excision of mid-rectal lesions by the Kraske sacral approach. *Br J Surg*. 1980 Sep;67(9):651-2.

[6] Thompson BW, Tucker WE. Transsphincteric approach to lesions of the rectum. *South Med J.* 80(1): 41-3

[7] Schilberg FW, Wenk H. [Sphincter-preserving interventions in rectal tumors. The posterior approach to the rectum] *Chirurg.* 1986 Dec;57(12):779-91

[8] Mason AY. Trans-sphincteric exposure of the rectum. *Ann R Coll Surg Engl.* 1972 Nov;51(5):320-31

[9] Tarantino I. Hetzer FH, Warschkow R, Zund M, Stein HJ, Zerz A. Local excision and endoscopic posterior mesorectal resection versus low anterior resection in T1 rectal cancer. *Br J Surg.* 2008 Mar;95(3):375-80

[10] Buess G, Kipfmuller K, Hack D, Grussner R, Heintz A, Junginger T. Technique of transanal endoscopic microsurgery. *Surg Endosc.* 1988;2(2):71-5

[11] Gavagan JA, Whiteford MH, Swanstrom LL. Full-thickness intraperitoneal excision by transanal endoscopic microsurgery does not increase short-term complications. *Am J Surg.* 2004; 187(5): 630-4

[12] Ramirez JM, Aguilella V, Arribas D, Martinez M. Transanal full-thickness excision of rectal tumours: should the defect be sutured? a randomized controlled trial. *Colorectal Dis.* 2002 Jan;4(1):51-55.

[13] Middleton PF, Sutherland LM, Maddern GJ. Transanal endoscopic microsurgery: a systematic review. *Dis Colon Rectum* 2005; 48(2): 270-284

[14] Winde G, Nottberg H, Keller R, Schmid KW, Bunte H. Surgical cure for early rectal carcinomas (T1). Transanal endoscopic microsurgery vs. anterior resection. *Dis Colon Rectum* 1996; 39(9): 969-976

[15] Heintz A, Morschel M, Junginger T. Comparison of results after transanal endoscopic microsurgery and radical resection for T1 carcinoma of the rectum. *Surg Endosc* 1998; 12(9): 1145-1148.

[16] Langer C, Liersch T, Suss M, Siemer A, Markus P, Ghadimi BM, Fuzesi L, Becker H. Surgical cure for early rectal carcinoma and large adenoma: transanal endoscopic microsurgery (using ultrasound or electrosurgery) compared to conventional local and radical resection. *Int J Colorectal Dis* 2003; 18(3): 222-229.

[17] Lee W, Lee D, Choi S, Chun H. Transanal endoscopic microsurgery and radical surgery for T1 and T2 rectal cancer. *Surg Endosc* 2003; 17(8): 1283-1287.

[18] Lezoche E, Guerrieri M, Paganini AM, D'Ambrosio G, Baldarelli M, Lezoche G, Feliciotti F, De Sanctis A. Transanal endoscopic versus total mesorectal laparoscopic resections of T2-N0 low rectal cancers after neoadjuvant treatment: a prospective randomized trial with a 3-years minimum follow-up period. *Surg Endosc* 2005; 19(6): 751-756.

[19] Nivatongs S, Balcos EG, Schottler JL, Goldberg SM. Surgical management of large villous tumors of the rectum. *Dis Colon Rectum*. 1973 Nov-Dec;16(6):508-14

[20] Abir F, Alva S, Longo WE. The management of rectal cancer in the elderly. *Surg Oncol*. 2004 Dec;13(4):223-34.

[21] Kapiteijn E, Marijnen CA, Nagtegaal ID, Putter H, Steup WH, Wiggers T, Rutten HJ, Pahlman L, Glimelius B, van Krieken JH, Leer JW, van de Velde CJ; Dutch Colorectal Cancer Group. Preoperative radiotherapy combined with total mesorectal excision for resectable rectal cancer. *N Engl J Med*. 2001 Aug 30;345(9):638-46.

[22] Cataldo PA, O'Brien S, Osler T. Transanal endoscopic microsurgery: a prospective evaluation of functional results. *Dis Colon Rectum* 2005; 48(7): 1366-1371.

[23] Hemingway D, Flett M, McKee RF, Finlay IG. Sphincter function after transanal endoscopic microsurgical excision of rectal tumours. *Br J Surg* 1996; 83(1): 51-52.

[24] Kreis ME, Jehle EC, Haug V, Manncke K, Buess GF, Becker HD, Starlinger MJ. Functional results after transanal endoscopic microsurgery. *Dis Colon Rectum* 1996; 39(10): 1116-1121.

[25] Herman RM, Richter P, Walega P, Popiela T. Anorectal sphincter function and rectal barostat study in patients following transanal endoscopic microsurgery. *Int J Colorectal Dis* 2001; 16(6): 370-376.

[26] Kennedy ML, Lubowski DZ, King DW. Transanal endoscopic microsurgery excision: is anorectal function compromised? *Dis Colon Rectum* 2002; 45(5): 601-604.

[27] Banerjee AK, Jehle EC, Kreis ME, Schott UG, Claussen CD, Becker HD, Starlinger M, Buess GF. Prospective study of the proctographic and functional consequences of transanal endoscopic microsurgery. *Br J Surg* 1996; 83(2): 211-213.

[28] Rockwood TH, Church JM, Fleshman JW, Kane RL, Mavrantonis C, Thorson AG, Wexner SD, Bliss D, Lowry AC. Fecal Incontinence Quality of Life Scale: quality of life instrument for patients with fecal incontinence. *Dis Colon Rectum*. 2000 Jan;43(1):9-16; discussion 16-7.

[29] Doornebosch PG, Gosselink MP, Neijenhuis PA, Schouten WR, Tollenaar RA, de Graaf EJ. Impact of transanal endoscopic microsurgery on functional outcome and quality of life. *Int J Colorectal Dis*. 2008 Jul;23(7):709-13

[30] Doornebosch PG, Tollenaar RA, Gosselink MP, Stassen LP, Dijkhuis CM, Schouten WR, van de Velde CJ, de Graaf EJ. Quality of life after transanal endoscopic microsurgery and total mesorectal excision in early rectal cancer. *Colorectal Dis*. 2007 Jul;9(6):553-8.

[31] Beets-Tan RG, Beets GL. Rectal cancer: review with emphasis on MR imaging. *Radiology* 2004; 232(2): 335-346.

[32] Solomon MJ, McLeod RS. Screening strategies for colorectal cancer. *Surg Clin North Am* 1993; 73(1): 31-45.

[33] Suppiah A, Hunter IA, Cowley J, Garimella V, Cast J, Hartley JE, Monson JR. Magnetic Resonance Imaging Accuracy in Assessing Tumour Down-staging Following Chemo-radiation in Rectal Cancer. *Colorectal Dis.* 2008 May 29

[34] Gall FP, Hermanek P. Cancer of the rectum--local excision. *Surg Clin North Am* 1988; 68(6): 1353-1365.

[35] Hermanek P, Gall FP. [Significance of local control of colorectal cancer]. *Fortschr Med* 1985; 103(45): 1041-1046.

[36] Sengupta S, Tjandra JJ. Local excision of rectal cancer: what is the evidence? *Dis Colon Rectum* 2001; 44(9): 1345-1361

[37] Suppiah A, Maslekar S, Alabi A, Hartley JE, Monson JR. Transanal endoscopic microsurgery in early rectal cancer: time for a trial? *Colorectal Dis.* 2008 May;10(4):314-27; discussion 327-9

[38] Kikuchi R, Takano M, Takagi K, Fujimoto N, Nozaki R, Fujiyoshi T, Uchida Y. Management of early invasive colorectal cancer. Risk of recurrence and clinical guidelines. *Dis Colon Rectum* 1995; 38(12): 1286-1295

[39] Maslekar S, Pillinger SH, Sharma A, Taylor A, Monson JR. Transanl Endoscopic Microsurgery: (TEM) Costing in Rectal Tumours. *Colorectal Dis.* 2007 Mar;9(3):229-34

[40] Farmer KC, Wale R, Winnett J, Cunningham I, Grossberg P, Polglase A. Transanal endoscopic microsurgery: the first 50 cases. *ANZ J Surg* 2002; 72(12): 854-856.

[41] Serra-Aracil X, Vallverdú H, Bombardó-Junca J, Pericay-Pijaume C, Urgellés-Bosch J, Navarro-Soto S. Long-term follow-up of local rectal cancer surgery by transanal endoscopic microsurgery. *World J Surg.* 2008 Jun;32(6):1162-7.

[42] Bretagnol F, Merrie A, George B, Warren BF, Mortensen NJ. Local excision of rectal tumours by transanal endoscopic microsurgery. *Br J Surg.* 2007 May;94(5):627-33

[43] Guerrieri M, Baldarelli M, Morino M, Trompetto M, Da Rold A, Selmi I, Allaix ME, Lezoche G, Lezoche E. Transanal endoscopic microsurgery in rectal adenomas: experience of six Italian centres. *Dig Liver Dis* 2006; 38(3): 202-207.

[44] Floyd ND, Saclarides TJ. Transanal endoscopic microsurgical resection of pT1 rectal tumors. *Dis Colon Rectum* 2006; 49(2): 164-168

[45] Jotautas V, Strupas K, Poskus E, Seinin D. [Treatment of rectal tumors with transanal endoscopic microsurgery]. *Medicina (Kaunas)* 2005; 41(6): 470-476.

[46] Duek SD, Krausz MM, Hershko DD. Transanal endoscopic microsurgery for rectal cancer. *Isr Med Assoc J* 2005;7(7): 435-438.

[47] Suzuki H, Furukawa K, Kan H, Tsuruta H, Matsumoto S, Akiya Y, Shinji S, Tajiri T. The role of transanal endoscopic microsurgery for rectal tumors. *J Nippon Med Sch* 2005; 72(5): 278-284.

[48] Palma P, Freudenberg S, Samel S, Post S. Transanal endoscopic microsurgery: indications and results after 100 cases. *Colorectal Dis* 2004; 6(5): 350-355

[49] Stipa S, Lucandri G, Stipa F, Chiavellati L, Sapienza P. Local excision of rectal tumours with transanal endoscopic microsurgery. *Tumori* 1995; 81(3 Suppl): 50-56.

[50] Meng WC, Lau PY, Yip AW. Treatment of early rectal tumours by transanal endoscopic microsurgery in Hong Kong: prospective study. *Hong Kong Med J* 2004; 10(4): 239-243.

[51] Dafnis G, Pahlman L, Raab Y, Gustafsson UM, Graf W. Transanal endoscopic microsurgery: clinical and functional results. *Colorectal Dis* 2004; 6(5): 336-342

[52] Neary P, Makin GB, White TJ, White E, Hartley J, MacDonald A, Lee PW, Monson JR. Transanal endoscopic microsurgery: a viable operative alternative in selected patients with rectal lesions. *Ann Surg Oncol* 2003; 10(9): 1106-1111.

[53] Lloyd GM, Sutton CD, Marshall LJ, Baragwanath P, Jameson JS, Scott AD. Transanal endoscopic microsurgery--lessons from a single UK centre series. *Colorectal Dis* 2002; 4(6): 467-472.

[54] Lezoche E, Guerrieri M, Paganini AM, Feliciotti F. Long-term results of patients with pT2 rectal cancer treated with radiotherapy and transanal endoscopic microsurgical excision. *World J Surg* 2002; 26(9): 1170-1174.

[55] de Graaf EJ, Doornebosch PG, Stassen LP, Debets JM, Tetteroo GW, Hop WC. Transanal endoscopic microsurgery for rectal cancer. *Eur J Cancer* 2002; 38(7): 904-910.

[56] Demartines N, von Flue MO, Harder FH. Transanal endoscopic microsurgical excision of rectal tumors: indications and results. *World J Surg* 2001;25(7): 870-875.

[57] Benoist S, Taffinder N, Gould S, Ziprin P, Chang A, Darzi A. [Transanal endoscopic microsurgery: a forgotten minimally invasive technique]. *Gastroenterol Clin Biol* 2001; 25(4): 369-374.

[58] Azimuddin K, Riether RD, Stasik JJ, Rosen L, Khubchandani IT, Reed JF, 3rd. Transanal endoscopic microsurgery for excision of rectal lesions: technique and initial results. *Surg Laparosc Endosc Percutan Tech* 2000; 10(6): 372-378.

[59] Arribas del Amo D, Ramirez Rodriguez JM, Aguilella Diago V, Elia Guedea M, Palacios Fanlo MJ, Martinez Diez M. Transanal endoscopic surgery for rectal tumors. *Rev Esp Enferm Dig* 2000; 92(8): 526-535.

[60] Lev-Chelouche D, Margel D, Goldman G, Rabau MJ. Transanal endoscopic microsurgery: experience with 75 rectal neoplasms. *Dis Colon Rectum* 2000; 43(5): 662-667; discussion 667-668.

[61] Saclarides TJ. Transanal endoscopic microsurgery: a single surgeon's experience. *Arch Surg* 1998; 133(6): 595-598; discussion 598-599.

[62] Mentges B, Buess G, Effinger G, Manncke K, Becker HD. Indications and results of local treatment of rectal cancer. *Br J Surg* 1997; 84(3): 348-351.

[63] Said S, Muller JM. TEM--minimal invasive therapy of rectal cancer? *Swiss Surg* 1997; 3(6): 248-254

[64] Steele RJ, Hershman MJ, Mortensen NJ, Armitage NC, Scholefield JH. Transanal endoscopic microsurgery--initial experience from three centres in the United Kingdom. *Br J Surg* 1996; 83(2): 207-210.

[65] Smith LE, Ko ST, Saclarides T, Caushaj P, Orkin BA, Khanduja KS. Transanal endoscopic microsurgery. Initial registry results. *Dis Colon Rectum* 1996;39(10 Suppl): S79-84.

[66] Lirici MM, Chiavellati L, Lezoche E, Martelli S, Melotti G, Morino M, Guerrieri M, Selmi I, Stipa S, Angelini L. Transanal endoscopic microsurgery in Italy. *Endosc Surg Allied Technol* 1994; 2(5): 255-258.

[67] Buess G. Review: transanal endoscopic microsurgery (TEM). *J R Coll Surg Edinb* 1993; 38(4): 239-245.

[68] Buess G, Kipfmuller K, Ibald R, Heintz A, Hack D, Braunstein S, Gabbert H, Junginger T. Clinical results of transanal endoscopic microsurgery. *Surg Endosc* 1988; 2(4): 245-250.

[69] Wang HS, Lin JK, Yang SH, Jiang JK, Chen WS, Lin TC. Prospective study of the functional results of transanal endoscopic microsurgery. *Hepatogastroenterology* 2003; 50(53): 1376-1380.

Chapter V

STAGING AND TREATMENT OF EARLY RECTAL CANCER

G. Baatrup[1,2,*] and P. Pfeiffer[3,4]

[1]Haukeland University Hospital, N-5021 Bergen, Norway
[2]University of Bergen, N-5021 Bergen, Norway
[3]Odense University Hospital, DK-5000 Odense, Denmark
[4]University of Southern Denmark, Dk5 000 Odense, Denmark

ABSTRACT

Accurate preoperative staging of early rectal cancers is necessary in order to select those patients who will benefit from local resection or non-surgical treatment. Staging should combine inspection, digital examination, biopsy and transanal endoluminal ultrasonography. The patients' age and physical performance may also influence the decision.

Major surgery for early rectal cancer is followed by a long term cancer-specific survival of more than 90%. The overall mortality is largely due to the surgical trauma or causes other than the cancer disease. Some patients with high age or co-morbidity and rectal cancers of T stage 1 and 2, sometimes even 3 can be offered local resection without compromising long term survival.

The low risk T1 cancers can safely be treated with transanal endoscopic microsurgery. The long term results match those of major surgery. The long term results for high risk early cancers treated with radiotherapy and transanal endoscopic microsurgery may match those of major surgery, but prospective randomized trials are needed for a firm conclusion.

Local resection of high risk, early rectal cancers should be reserved for those with high age or co-morbidity or it should be combined with preoperative radiotherapy. In

---

[*] Correspondence concerning this article should be addressed to: Gunnar Baatrup chief consultant, ass. prof., dr. med. sci. Dept. of Surgery, Haukeland University Hospital, N-5021 Bergen, Norway. E-mail: gunnar.baatup @helse-bergen.no, telephone: 0047-55972727, fax: 0047-55972793.

cases of possible oncological compromise, the patient should decide how to prioritize short and long term survival, risk of complications and quality of life. The patient and the surgeon should be prepared for early rescue surgery after transanal surgery in case of staging errors.

The oncological safety of colonoscopic submucosal dissection is not clear and transanal endoscopic microsurgery is currently recommended for local resection of early rectal cancers.

Non-surgical treatment of early rectal cancers has gained renewed interest. The rate of complete oncological response is increasing as external radiotherapy is combined with modern chemotherapy and possible endocavitary radiotherapy. Combined oncological treatment induces a complete pathological response in 30% or more of the early cancers.

The frequency of early rectal cancers is low in areas without population screening programmes and the decision and planning of the treatment should be handled by a multidisciplinary team of dedicated specialists.

INTRODUCTION

The introduction of total mesorectal excision, of neoadjuvant chemo-radiation, multidisciplinary team handling, cylindrical extirpation of low cancers and more has improved the outcome for rectal cancer patients during the last 15 years. It is, however, primarily patients with more advanced cancers who have benefited from this development. The cancer specific survival after radical rectum resection for T1 and T2 rectal cancers is approximately 95 % [1] and deaths from other causes outnumber the deaths caused by cancer recurrence in these patients. It is therefore not possible to induce a significant improvement in long term outcome by refining surgical procedures or by introducing adjuvant or neoadjuvant chemo-radiation. Even improvements of the cancer specific survival by 50 % by some new technique will be very difficult to demonstrate by survival studies of patients treated for early rectal cancer. Major surgery is often regarded as the oncological safe treatment of rectal cancers, but it is followed by a high frequency of complications and side effects. Procedure related deaths occur in 2 – 4 % of the patients [2,3], and may increase to 8 % in patients over the age of 80 years [4] and may even be higher in patients with co-morbidity [2,4]. Approximately one third of patients operated by major procedures will experience a complication. Some of them are severe and some lead to permanent disabilities. Permanent conditions as impotency, disturbed urinary bladder function, reduced rectal compliance, fecal incontinence and permanent stomas may occur.

The combination of fecal incontinence and diarrhoea is troublesome, and common. Local resection can be performed with a low operative mortality and morbidity risk [5,6,7] and should therefore be offered to patients with low risk cancers if the long term survival is not compromised.

The term early rectal cancer is often used synonymous with T1 cancers, but low risk T2 cancers may be included also because the late oncological results after combined local treatment is no worse than those for high risk T1 cancers [4,8]. Preliminary results indicate that even high risk T2 cancers may be included as a candidate for local surgical treatment combined with adjuvant or neoadjuvant oncological treatment [8,9].

New methods for trans-anal surgery such as trans-anal endoscopic microsurgery (TEM) [10], endoscopic mucosa resection (EUS) [11,12] and endoscopic sub-mucosa dissection (ESD) [13,14] have been developed. New instruments with flexible tips and micro staplers are being developed and may be available in the clinic within a few years.

The alternatives to classic rectum resection are becoming more attractive and the decision of which method to use must be individualized. The surgeon therefore must be experienced in several different techniques of staging and treatment. The choice of treatment will depend on the tumour stage, tumour grade and patient characteristics. Intra-rectal ultrasound is mandatory in the preoperative evaluation. Postoperative rescue strategies in case of preoperative under-staging must also be a part of the strategy.

PREOPERATIVE STAGING AND SUBSTAGING OF EARLY RECTAL CANCERS

Introduction

Accurate preoperative staging of all rectal cancers is important because it defines the patient's prognosis. Grading is performed mainly from the resection specimen and may determine if further treatment is necessary.

No single method is sufficiently accurate for a precise preoperative T staging of rectum tumours [5,15,16]. The staging must rely upon a combination of inspection by proctoscopy, digital rectal examination if possible, biopsies and transanal ultrasound. MRI and CT may be useful in the N- and M-staging but are inaccurate in the T-staging of rectal cancers smaller than T3. The procedures supplement each other and are operator dependent. Inspection, palpation and ultrasound examination should be performed before biopsies are taken.

The following will discuss T-staging. N- and M-staging will be discussed at the end of this chapter.

Clinical Examination

The rigid 20 cm. proctoscope has been abandoned in most centres, but may still be useful in a first quick examination to determine the further diagnostic strategy. A comprehensive guide to the conduction of ano-rectal examination has been published by J. C. Golligher [17]. The demonstration of any neoplastic lesion in the rectum will dictate a later colonoscopy. Most small, benign lesions can be left to be resected during this later colonoscopy. Patients with tumours expected to be larger than T2 by clinical examination should have a MRI or multi-slice CT performed to determine optimal therapy by a multidisciplinary team. Rectal ultrasound is difficult in these cases and often not necessary. Less than 15 % of rectal tumours are potentially early rectal cancers on proctoscopy. They should be inspected through a video proctoscope or a flexible high-resolution sigmoidoscope. The surgeon looks for depressed areas, necrosis and areas of different colour within large sessile adenomas [14]. It is important to inspect the tumour with some magnification. New colonoscopes with magnification capacity of up till 100 times provide opportunities to investigate crypt patterns and may be advantageous, but this has not yet been demonstrated in clinical practice. Soluble dye as indigo carmine has also been described to help in demonstrating loss of the innominate grooves on the surface of adenomas which indicates malignancy [16]. These techniques have not yet become common practice.

Tumours that can be reached by a finger are investigated for in-homogeneity or hard foci. It is sometimes possible to determine if the tumour is freely movable over the lamina muscularis propria. Areas of rectal mucosa with pathological appearance, but with no apparent tumour are investigated for in-homogeneity and strain. The ability to discriminate benign and malignant tumours on digital rectal examination is, in some series, comparable to that of 7 – 10 MHz rectal ultrasound [5]. This means a positive predictive value of 65 – 73 % but the negative predictive value is lower [18]. The proportion of tumours that can be reached by the finger is examiner and patient dependent. The best position is the lithotomy-Trendelenburg position. In overweight patients this position will often add several cm to the proportion of the rectum accessible to digital examination.

The report from the clinical examination should include:

1. Endoscopic inspection:
    Distance between the outer anal verge and the tumour
    Largest diameter
    Position in the circumference (figure 1)
    Macroscopic appearance: polypoid, sessile, flat
    Benign/suspect/malignant

Marking the location of a rectal tumour for local resection

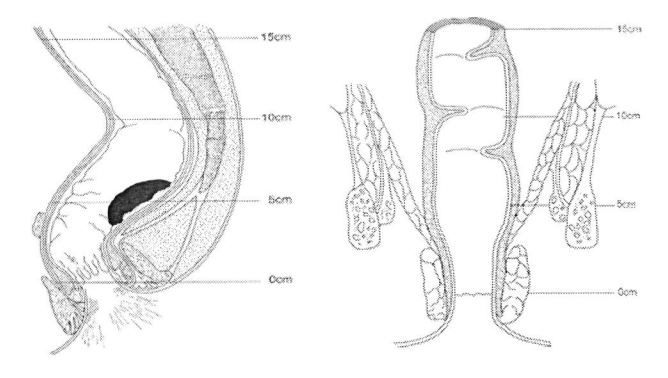

Figure 1. An accurate depiction of the location of a rectal tumour is important if local resection is planned.

2. Palpation:
    Consistency
    Homogeneity
    Distance to anal verge

Benign/suspect/malignant

3. Intraluminal ultrasound:
   Accessibility of all parts of the tumour
   T-stage and, if possible, T1 substage
   N-stage suggestion
   Relation to other organs (in the upper anterior aspect)

A conclusive suggestion is noted on the T-stage, N-stage, and resectability by local procedures and how the patient should be positioned during a local resection procedure.

A physical performance assessment is obtained if relevant, and the patient's preference is established. A history of anal continence, urinary bladder function and sexual capability is noted.

Transanal Ultrasound

Transanal ultrasound is accurate in T staging of rectal tumours [18,19]. It is the method of choice in the evaluation of large adenomas and small rectal cancers [18]. Large circumferential cancers might be difficult to investigate. They are more safely staged by MRI or multi-slice CT, which can give the distance from the tumour to the mesorectal fascia with high accuracy. Tumours that should be staged with transanal ultrasound and tumours that should be staged by MRI are easily identified by the initial clinical examination with proctoscopy and digital examination. Transanal ultrasound allows direct contact investigation of the tumours and high frequency ultrasound can therefore be applied to obtain a high resolution picture of the few centimetres in depth of interest in the T staging procedure (figure 2).

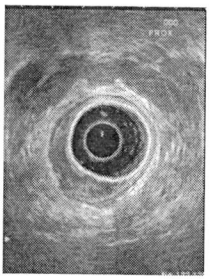

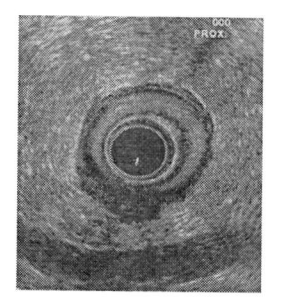

Figure 2. Transanal 16 MHz B-mode ultrasonography of rectal tumours for T-staging.

It has been claimed that even T1 sub-staging may be possible with 16 MHz intra-rectal ultrasound [20], but this has to be confirmed in larger series. The penetration of the muscularis mucosa defines a >T0 tumour and this layer is often lost in the ultrasound reflection that occurs in the zone between the mucosa and the submucosa (figure 3). Its position can be determined by indirect measures in common B-mode ultrasound. This makes accurate T1 sub-staging very difficult. The difference between visible ultrasound layers and anatomical layers are often confusing, and over-staging by B-mode ultrasound is common [21]. The discrimination between T1 and T2 cancers may be equally difficult because the border between the submucosa and the muscularis propria does not correspond to the layers seen by ultrasound. The T2/T3 cancers can often be discriminated quite easily. It is sometimes possible to demonstrate tumour budding by B mode ultrasound (figure 4). This indicating vascular or perineural invasion and is an important prognostic factor indicates that the tumour may be a high-risk cancer [20].

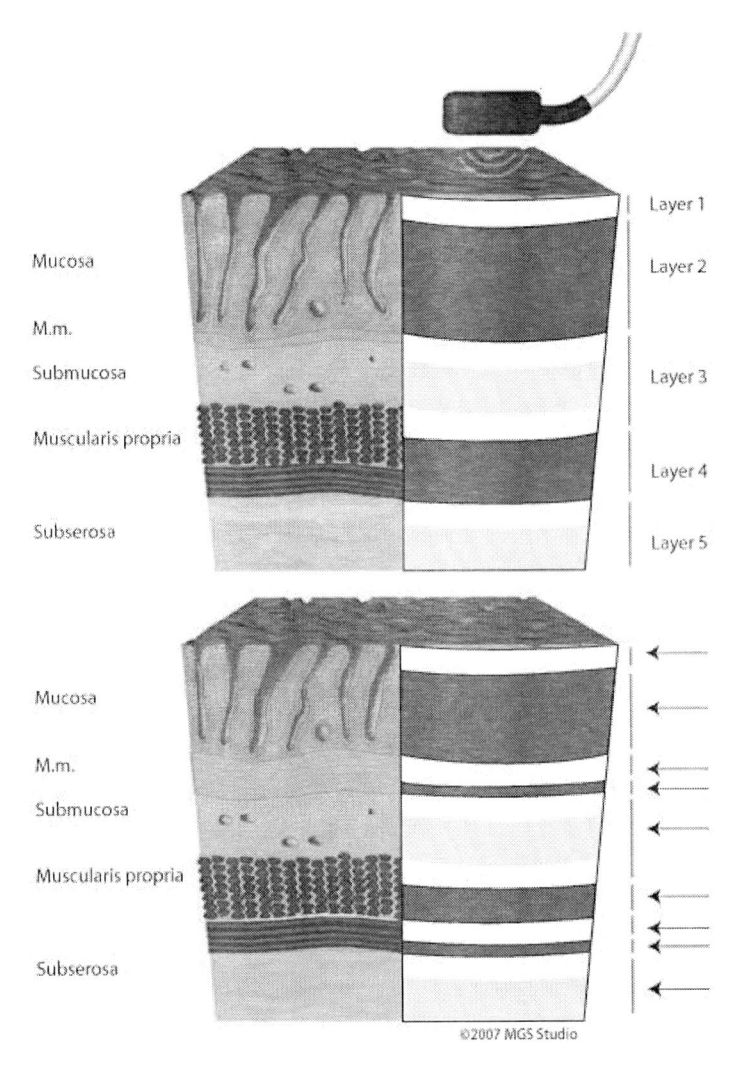

Figure 3. The B-mode ultrasonography picture shows the reflection zones between layers of different echogenicity. The relation of the ultrasound layers to anatomical layers is complex.
With kind permission from Prof. Svein Ødegaard.

Most systematic investigations of the relation between the B-mode ultrasound layers seen in the intestinal wall and the actual anatomical layers have been performed in the upper gastrointestinal tract, but we have good indications that the principles depicted in figure 3 is also valid for rectal wall anatomy. This has also been proven indirectly by the very high accuracy of preoperative staging by intraluminal ultrasound as compared to postoperative pathological examination obtained in dedicated centres [18].

Multicenter studies on T stage accuracy obtained with transanal high quality ultrasound equipment may reach 96 % [22], but results are investigator dependent and a high patient volume is necessary. Dedicated centres achieve both specificity and sensitivity in the discrimination between T0 and T1 and between T1 and T2 of more than 90%. Accuracy in the discrimination between T1 and T2 cancers is between 81 and 92 % [18]. Ultrasound has been compared to both digital rectal examination, pelvic CT and MRI in several studies, and come out better. The European Society of Gastrointestinal Endoscopy recommends transanal B-mode ultrasound for the staging of small rectal cancers.

Tumours in the lower two thirds of the rectum may be investigated with any rectal probe but a 16 MHz probe will increase the accuracy of T staging. A rotating 360° probe is advantageous. There is no evidence that 3D reconstruction increases the accuracy. Probes with crystals that move up and down in the probe at a defined speed; and of data storage can leave the data analysis until later and therefore shorten the time of investigation. Rigid rectal probes are the most commonly used as they are cost effective and reliable, but ultrasound colonoscopes and ultrasound miniprobes that fits into the biopsy channel of colonoscopes have been developed but not evaluated in clinical practice. Colonoscopic miniprobes with 20 MHz crystals provides excellent B-mode ultrasound pictures. It facilitates the investigation of all areas of the tumour because of the simultaneous colonoscopic visualization of the rectal wall.

In our experience one get better quality ultrasound pictures if one fills the rectum with water and uses the anal probe with a hard cone instead of using the rectal probe with a water-filled condom. The condom tends to trap air between the water and parts of the tumour or in the transition zone between the tumour and the normal rectal wall. It is often necessary to change the patients' position to have the tumour positioned downwards. A table, which can tip the patient in the anti-Trendelenburg position, will also help to prevent the water from moving upwards – to the sigmoid colon. Good contact with tumours in the upper third of the rectum may be difficult to obtain with the blindly introduced probe [19]. This problem can be overcome by passing a short, wide rectoscope as the video Rectolution® above the tumour and introduce the ultrasound probe through the rectoscope, and then retract the scope. A long ultrasound probe as the Hitachi 35 cm rectal probe is then necessary.

Newer ultrasound based visualization methods are being developed. They depict the rectal wall based upon other features than the simple ultrasound wave reflection. New software enhances the signal-to-noise ratio. Contrast enhanced ultrasound is being introduced in the evaluation of hepatic tumours [23], and may be introduced in the N-staging of rectal cancers also. Sonoelastography is another method that is now commercially available with probes for intra-rectal scans. It depicts the anatomical structures by their elasticity or strain pattern – that is the relative hardness of the tumour as compared to that of adjacent normal tissues [24] (figures 4 and 5). It has been proven useful in the diagnosis of malignant tumours in the breast, the prostate and in upper GI tract [25,26,27]. The tip of the rectal probe has a water filled balloon which can be in- and ex-sufflated with a syringe, creating rhythmic stress variation on the tissue. The strain (hardness) is depicted by a colour-scale which is superimposed upon an ordinary ultrasongram. Preliminary investigations in our clinic is promising as we can clearly demonstrate the anatomical layers including the muscularis mucosa (figure 6), and we have found a high accuracy in discriminating benign and malignant tumours in the rectum [28]. Further studies of the sensitivity of the method especially in demonstrating small malignant foci in larger adenomas are being conducted.

T3 cancer with tumour budding.

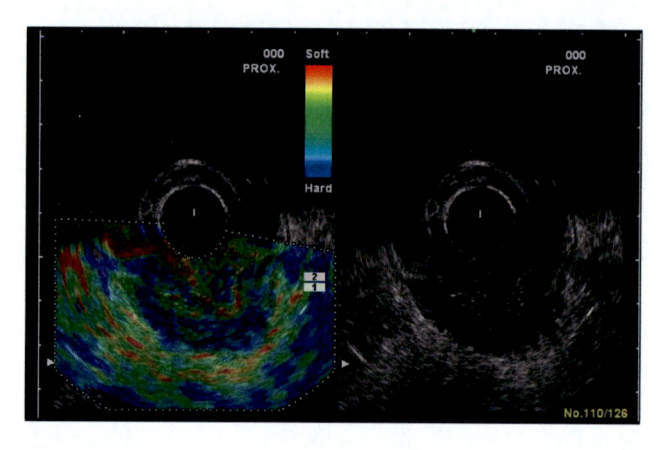

Figure 4. Cancer grading with B-mode ultrasound. The "budding" at the zone of invasion is a sign of high-grade malignancy.

T0 and T1 rectal tumour

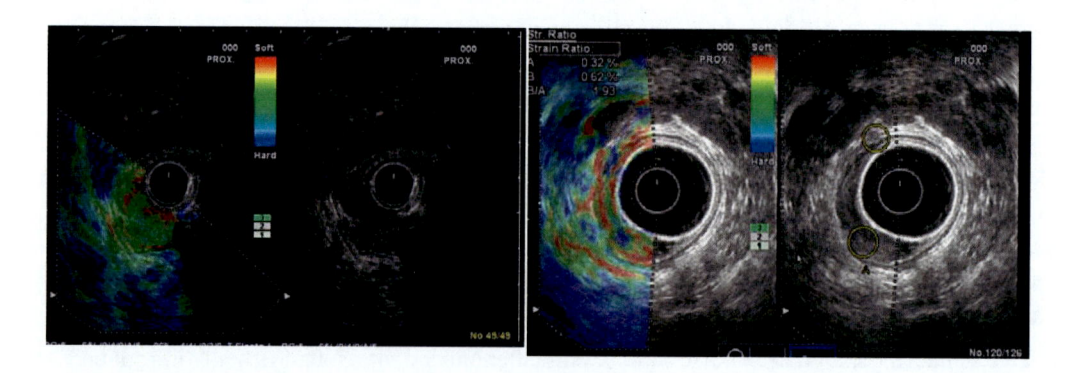

Figure 5. Sonoelastography of an adenoma to the left and a T1 cancer to the right. Note the colour scale in the elastogram. The small area of cancer within the large adenoma is marked by the A-circle in the B-mode picture.

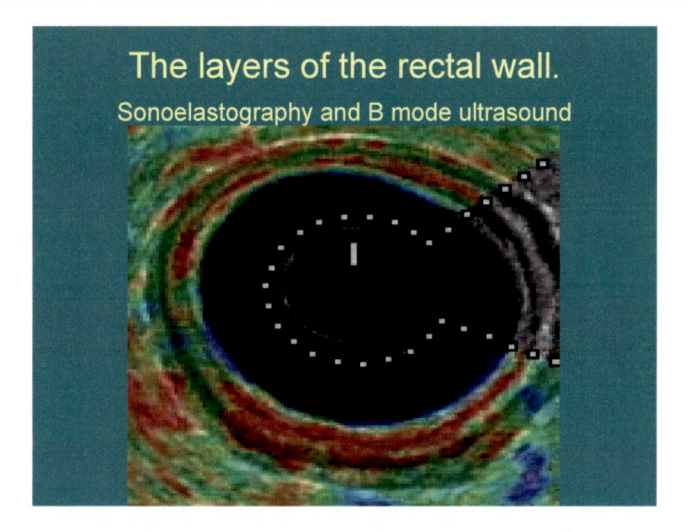

Figure 6. Sono-elastographic picture of a normal rectal wall. More different layers are demonstrable as compared to those of the B-mode picture.

MRI or CT Scanning

MRI is considered to be the gold standard for evaluating large T3 and T4 cancers. It is the method of choice to determine the distance between cancer and the mesorectal facia, and thus to determine the need for neoadjuvant chemo-radiation or radiation. New generations of high resolution spiral CT scanners may be comparable to 1.5 or 2.0 Tesla MRI scanners in sensitivity and staging but none of these modalities can discriminate T0, T1 and T2 tumours [29]. These methods are therefore not used in the staging of small rectal cancers. The accuracy of MRI in staging early tumours may be significantly improved by using intra rectal coils but it is expensive and time consuming and does not provide any advantage over rectal ultrasound. MRI staging of rectal cancers has been significantly improved by the new 3 Tesla MRI scanners, which have produced accuracy figures for T staging of more than 90 % [30]. The T staging by these third generation MRI scanners may thus be comparable to that of high quality endorectal ultrasound.

Endorectal ultrasound is still preferred by most centres because it can be performed during the first consultation without delay and because it is cost effective. The technical development of all these methods is fast and perhaps in the near future MRI will be preferred because it can execute the T-, N- and M-staging in one investigation.

The primary goal of T-staging in small rectal cancers is to identify malignant tumours which can be treated by local excision and to identify cancers for preoperative radio-chemotherapy.

N- and M-Staging

Preoperative N-staging is difficult but important as local resection in case of lymph node metastasis will lead to local recurrence in patients selected for local treatment of a low risk cancer. N-staging by intra luminal ultrasound and high quality MRI may be comparable [31] and the choice of method is discussed above. N-staging by ultrasound is time consuming, and has an accuracy of 62% - 82%. Lymph nodes in the mesorectum can easily be seen by MRI but the malignancy cannot be determined by size alone. A smallest diameter of 8 mm or more increases the risk of malignancy [18,32]. Spiculation, inhomogenety and indistinct borders are all indicators of malignancy [32]. The sensitivity for malignancy in lymph nodes may reach 85% and the specificity 95% in highly dedicated centres [18]. Contrast enhanced MRI using ultra-small super-para-magnetic iron oxide (USPIO) nano colloid particles has been evaluated in large randomized trials and came out with significant improvements of the lymph node staging [33]. USPIO were not approved for clinical use in the early spring of 2008. Mapping the lymph nodes of the mesorectum by MRI followed by intrarectal ultrasound with sonoelastography or biopsies may improve the accuracy. The current recommendations for TEM surgery in malignant tumours are based upon the statistical risk of lymph node metastasis as indicated by the T stage [20]. The risk of lymph node metastasis is up to 25 % in case of high risk T1 and T2 cancers [34,35,36,37]. This is considered too high for safe local resection, but the 75 % N0 patients with small T2 cancers suitable for local resection will have to risk a major surgical procedure. Development of accurate N-staging modalities therefore has high priority.

PET-CT probably has a low sensitivity in N-staging because the primary cancer will camouflage any nearby positive nodes. Several studies have investigated the possible use of sentinel node technique for N-staging of rectal cancers, but the results have been disappointing.

Preoperative M-staging is not mandatory as synchronous distant metastasis in early rectal cancers is rare. It may be conducted during and/or after the operation according to common guidelines for rectal cancer staging.

Biopsies

Biopsies obtained through an ordinary rigid proctoscope are unreliable to discriminate large adenomas from early cancers. False negative biopsies are common as the cancer focus may be small and because the introduction of the biopsy forceps into the rigid standard proctoscope lead to ex-sufflation of the air from the rectum. The view is therefore very poor during the procedure. A video-rectoscope or flexible endoscope with channels for forceps or membranes that allow biopsies to be taken while the rectum is expanded should be preferred. Multiple biopsies are necessary in large sessile adenomas [38,39]. The final evaluation of the preoperative TNM-stage is based upon results from the above mentioned investigations. It is important to have a logistic that ensures a fast and efficient preoperative evaluation to support the discussion with the patient on treatment options.

Treatment of Early Rectal Cancer

Surgical options include local tumour excision- and major rectum resection. Non surgical treatment includes radiotherapy alone (RT) or RT in combination with concomitant chemotherapy (radiochemotherapy – RCT). Long term survival without severe morbidity is the major goal. Indications listed in the following for each method follow the principles of highest possible cure rate with no compromises due to patient related risk factors, risk of complications, or patient's choice. The final choice of method or combination of methods may be more complex and some principles are described later.

Histology may reveal cancers different from adenocarcinoma. Evidence is accumulating that TEM for rectal carcinoid tumours with a diameter of 1 cm or less can be regarded as a definitive treatment whereas larger carcinoids should be treated with major resection [40,41]. Malignant melanomas may also be treated with local resection if radical resection can be achieved as the long term results from TEM in these patients seam to match those of more radical surgery [42]. Further discussion on histological rare cancers will not be discussed here.

It is important that the resected specimen is presented to the pathologist undamaged and that the surgeon and patient are prepared for further treatment in cases of unsuspected findings.

Surgical Treatment Local Resection

Simple Endoscopic Polypectomy

Indication: Simple polypectomy during flexible endoscopy is performed for pedunculated, apparently benign tumours and small sessile adenomas. Simple snare resection for known cancers in the rectum is not recommended. The usual scenario is a tumour removed in the assumption that it was benign [43]. The histology rapport reveals malignancy, and then what?

The risk of malignant foci in sessile or flat adenomas depends upon size [44]. The risk of high grade dysplasia or malignancy in adenomas larger then 1 cm is 39% [44,45] and cancer development is demonstrated in 79% of tumors larger then 4.2 cm [44,45].

Technique: Snares for rigid proctoscopes exists but should only be used in video proctoscopes with separate channels and air tight membranes for instrumentation in which the positive pressure can be sustained in the rectum to ensure god visibility during the procedure. As the identification of polyps in the rectum in most cases lead to a colonoscopy, it may be easier simply to postpone the resection until this.

A diathermy snare is used. The resection line should always be at the level of the rectal wall in polyps larger than 1 cm, not leaving any part of the stalk behind. The specimen should be secured for analysis and the resection line marked with ink for easy pathological evaluation. Deeper resection can be performed in the rectum by entrapping a small circular area around the polyp into the snare (figure 7). This can also be obtained by injecting a small saline or epinephrine-saline deposit into the submucosa beneath the polyp before resection.

Deeper snare resection is indicated in polyps larger than 2 cm because it may harbor a cancer [44].

Results: Benign tumors radically removed by the surgeon's judgment can be included into a follow up program with no further treatment regardless of the degree of dysplasia. The follow up protocol depends upon pathological features and is discussed later. If snare resection leaves a margin to the resection line of more than 2 mm, Haggits type 1 and 2 cancers may be regarded as radically removed and rescue procedures are not necessary [20].

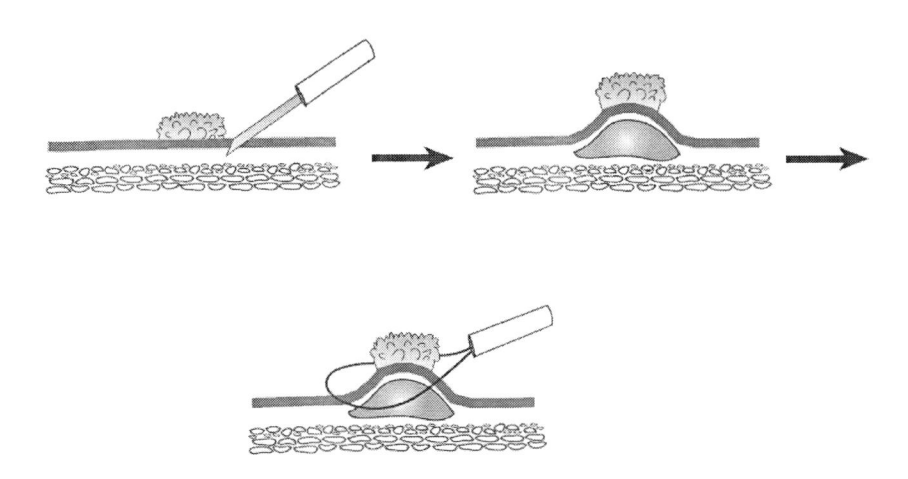

Figure 7. Lifting technique to ensure a radical resection by the snare technique.

The risk of perforation of the bowel wall is low and is, in the rectum, only a concern in the upper, anterior part. Polypectomy can be performed in patients treated with NSAID, but those treated with other anticoagulant drugs should discontinue the use from 3 days before the procedure, and receive heparin if they are in high risk of thrombosis. Polypectomy can be performed relatively safely with higher INR values if the indication is strong [46].

More Advanced Endoscopic Resection Techniques

Indication: Endoscopic mucosa resection (EMR) [47,48] or endoscopic submucosa dissection (ESD) (figure 8) [49] may be used for larger non-polypoid adenomas if malignancy is unlikely. Resection of large adenomas – larger than 3 cm - has been suggested but *en block* resection was obtained in only 38% of the cases [50]. Even early T1 cancer resection has been included in the indications for submucosal dissection [50,51] by this technique, but insufficient data has been published to support that this is safe [52].

Treatment of large adenomas in the colon and in the high anterior aspect of the rectum will probably be facilitated by these new techniques.

In the remaining rectum the indication is limited as the disadvantages' of whole wall resection by e.g. TEM are small [5,53] and the potential for an oncological unsafe result is high in large non-polypoid adenomas [20]. Advanced ESD may be indicated in patients with sub-clinical or tractable anal incontinence where TEM may precipitate a clinically significant condition, or in patients who will not accept or cannot be offered anesthesia or epidural analgesia necessary for the TEM procedure.

Technique: EMR and ESD are performed through a colonoscope with more channels for instrumentation and therefor do no harm to the anal sphincter. The different layers of the bowel wall are visible during dissection and the depth of resection is controlled. A variety of instruments have been developed for snare- or electro-needle dissection. The intended resection line is marked with diathermy needle before the resection is initiated. It is thus possible to obtain a well defined lateral resection margin. The lesion is lifted with a saline or epinephrine-saline injection. This also works as a test of cancer infiltration into the lamina muscularis propria, which may be demonstrated by unsuccessful lifting [54]. A controlled resection usually in the submucosa – muscularis propria transition zone can be obtained by the electro-needle technique. New instruments are being developed including a mini-stapling devise that can be introduced through the biopsy channel. This may allow for whole wall resection in the colon and upper anterior rectum.

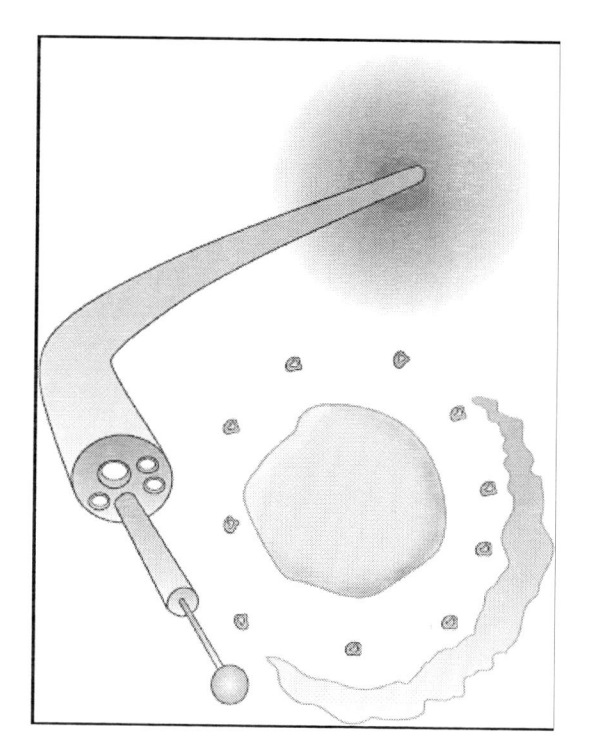

Figure 8. Endoscopic submucosal dissection of a large adenoma. The resection margin laterally and in depth may be controlled more accurately than by ordinary endoscopic procedures.

Results: The complication rate is low (1 – 5%) [55]. The most common complication is bleeding, which may be handled during the procedure with clips if recognised. Bleeding may occur as late as 1 – 2 weeks after the procedure [56]. Pain may sustain for 1 – 2 days, and perforation is usually recognised during the procedure. Small perforations may be handled by clips whereas large perforations demand immediate laparotomy in most cases. Large adenomas may need several consecutive procedures. Techniques involving piece meal resection should be avoided in larger adenomas. The recurrence rate of large adenomas after

EMD or ESD is 5 –30 % [57]. Polyp cancers of Haggits stage 1 and 2 can be considered as radically treated with ESR. Controversy exist on the Haggits stage 3 and sm1 and sm2 cancers in sessile adenomas. There is insufficient data to conclude on this and ESD should be regarded as insufficient in these cases [52].

The advantage of the procedures described in this chapter is that they are performed through flexible endoscopes with a small diameter. They can be performed with no risk of damage to the anal sphincter. Although the indication for EMR and ESR are few in the rectum, the fast technical development should be followed closely in the years to come.

Parks Transanal Procedure:

Indication: Transanal tumor excision with the aid of anal retractors is technically feasible for tumours located throughout the lower 2/3 of the rectum [58]. After the introduction of TEM Parks procedure is recommended only for the very low tumours where the TEM rectoscope cannot be positioned to ensure airtight closure around the rectoscope. These low tumours are also those where Parks procedure is easy.

Technique: The patient is positioned to ensure an inferior position of the tumour. The self-retracting Parks speculum is inserted after gentle anal dilatation. The technical challenge is to obtain a good vision and to avoid tearing of the specimen. The use of a harmonic scalpel will avoid annoying bleeding and smoke formation. Infiltration of the rectal wall with epinephrine-saline is therefore not necessary. Care should be taken when the specimen is retracted downwards to do the upper dissection without tearing it. Tumors are assessed under direct vision with fiber optic headlight or an external light source. Any damage to the anal sphincter is sutured immediately, and defects in the rectal wall larger than 50% of the circumference should be closed to reduce the risk of rectal stenosis.

Results: An all layer resection can be obtained with diathermy instruments or harmonic scalpel. The results are rather operator dependent. Complications are rare, the most common being strictures and bleeding and mortality low (0 - 5 %) [59,60]. The recurrence rates after resection of adenomas and cancers is 11 – 12 % [61,62] although lower figures were described in the initial rapports [59]. The rates of complications and recurrences are probably highly operator dependent and also dependent upon how high tumours one accepts for resection by this method. It has been claimed that one advantage of the Parks procedure is the possibility to retract parts of the mesorectum downward to palpate for possible pathologic lymph nodes [20]. His manoeuvre might lead to an undermining of the superior resection margin and the feared complication of ascending mesorectal infection and therefore it is not recommended (authors experience). Vision during dissection may be suboptimal and the lack of magnification may also be a problem. No touch technique is more difficult to do than during TEM. Large low adenomas may be excised by a combined method starting with Parks retractors for dissection of the lower part, and change to TEM instruments for continued dissection in the higher part of the rectum. Circumferential lesions can be excised without repositioning the patient during Parks procedure easier than during TEM. The use of Parks procedure is becoming seldom and is, in most cases, obsolete.

Transanal Endoscopic Microsurgery

Referred to as TEM or TEMS. TEM is used here as originally introduced by professor Buess, who invented and developed the technique for resection of adenomas in 1992 [5]. TEM provides excellent view through a stereo microscope for safe and accurate dissection within the layers one decides to follow. Advanced instruments for dissection and suturing have been developed and good access can be achieved to most parts of the rectum and lower sigmoid bowel (figure 9) [10,53].

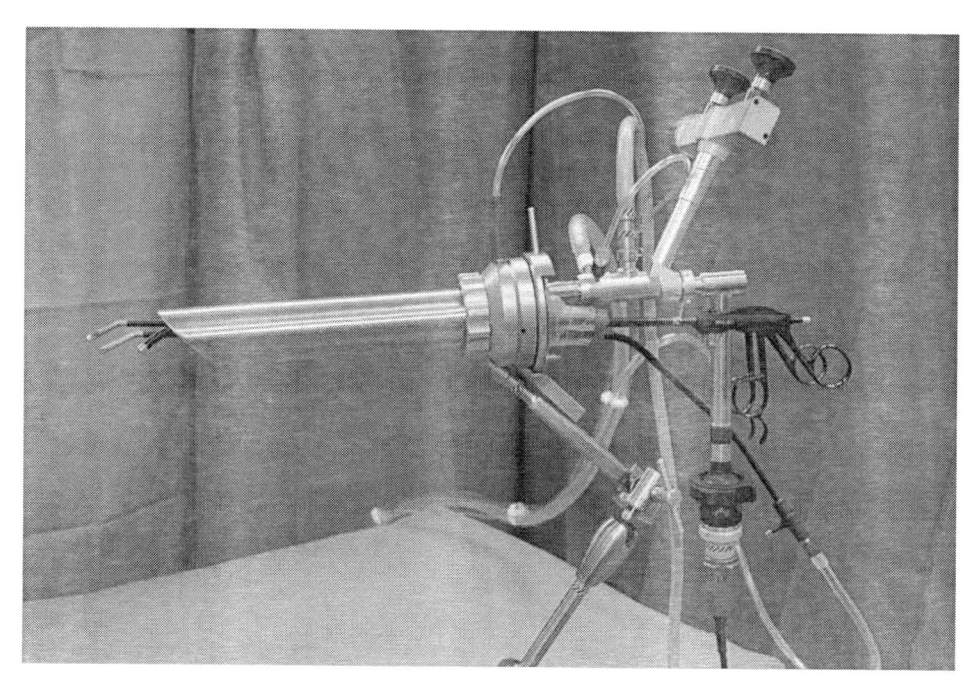

Figure 9. Equipment for transanal endoscopic microsurgery. A stereo microscope is used. The 4 cm wide rectoscope is air-tight ensuring a fully inflated rectum and a good view. The suction device removes smoke, blood and other liquids. A pump ensures a constant positive pressure in the rectum. The working channels allow for various instruments to be inserted, such as hook, forceps, needle holder, diathermy, harmonic scalpel etc.

Indication: The indications for TEM are sessile or flat adenomas not easily and safely removed by simple endoscopic procedures [63]. TEM can be performed as whole wall resection or submucosal resection. Successful resection of adenomas more than 10 cm in diameter has been described [63], and there is a general consensus that TEM is the preferred technique for larger sessile and flat adenomas in the rectum [20,63]. TEM has also been accepted for resection of small rectal cancers according to well-defined criteria [20,64]. TEM for cancer is often divided into TEM for cure; TEM for compromise and TEM for palliation [43]. TEM for cure means that the late oncological outcome must match that of a low anterior rectum resection or abdominoperineal rectum resection. TEM for compromise is offered to patients with poor performance status or high age. The predicted total long term survival is no worse than that of radical surgery due to the low operative mortality after TEM compared to radical surgery in "TEM for compromise". TEM for palliation is offered to patients with more advanced cancers that are not candidates for radical surgery. Although the use of TEM for palliation has not been investigated well, it should be remembered that small T3 cancers may be resected with up to 50% cure rate which is better than any non-operative palliative treatment. Palliative de-bulging has also been suggested to prevent obstruction or reduce pain. No data has been published on this, and it is not known if TEM provides any advantage over palliative RT or RCT when radical resection cannot be achieved. We have successfully treated a few patients with acute or urgent TEM for immediate release from obstruction and severe bleeding in our institution [65]. It seems obvious to take advantage of the TEM equipment and expertise in these situations if it is available.

There is general agreement that TEM should be regarded as the method of choice for T1, sm1 and sm2 cancers with low risk pathological features regardless of the patient's age and physical performance [20,64]. Some authors recommend TEM for all T1 cancers smaller than 3 cm. if the patient can be included in an intensive follow up program and accept later rescue surgery if necessary [43].

Larger cancers may be suitable for TEM combined with RT or RCT and this will be discussed later.

Technique: The patient should have a bowel preparation before the operation. A single dose of a long acting antibiotic is advised although it has not been proven to be necessary. The patient is positioned to ensure that the resection area is presented between 3 o'clock and 9 o'clock. The surgeon should have sufficient space between the patient's legs to allow for lateral movements during the procedure. The nurses should be well acquainted with the equipment and should have an illustrated manual accessible. The equipment with the suction system, pump, fiber-optics, the stereo-microscope and more is complicated and even experienced surgeons and nurses get frustrated sometimes during the preparation. The surgeon should be well educated in the function of all parts of the equipment, their connections and the usual causes of failure and he must be patient.

Cautious anal dilatation is performed before introducing the rectoscope. Whenever possible, the shorter 12 cm tube should be used as movements of the instruments are quite limited through the longer 20 cm tubes. A good view is ensured with a well-inflated rectum at a pressure of 10-15 cm H_2O and the rectoscope is fixed into the "Martins arm". The intended resection line, usually with a margin of 1 cm from the tumor is demarked with a harmonic scalpel or diathermy. We use a harmonic scalpel for the resection to prevent smoke and early as well as late bleeding complications. Injection of epinephrine is not necessary when the harmonic scalpel is used.

The resection is generally performed to include the muscularis propria in the case of larger adenomas. During the resection of proven cancers; half of the mesorectal fat (if present) should be included, but the mesorectal fascia must be preserved in the case that high risk T1 or T2 stage is demonstrated on later pathological examination [43]. Preservation of the mesorectal fascia during the following rescue/salvage surgery is not possible if it was included in the TEM resection. Care should be taken not to undermine the superior resection line. This may easily happen if one applies traction on the specimen while dividing the far most part of the rectal wall, often with limited vision in bulgy tumors. In the author's experience, this may lead to a serious ascending infection in the mesorectum [5].

The anterior rectal wall is closely related to the vagina/prostate and care should be taken to obtain the correct depth of resection. Re-TEM's in the anterior rectum is difficult and the risk of fistulas is high. In the upper anterior part, one should be prepared for a possible perforation to the peritoneal cavity [66].

The resulting defect in the rectal wall after TEM resection may be left open or may be sutured. Only one small randomized trial of 44 patients has been published dealing with this question [67]. They found no difference in outcome. In a non-randomized series of 144 whole wall resections, approximately one half was closed and the other half was left open. We found no significant difference in outcome (unpublished). Suturing the defect may lead to abscess formation and re-perforation of the suture line. This may cause fewer and delayed submission. It is, on the other hand important to obtain expertise in the suturing technique for those few cases of perforation to the peritoneum which unenviable will occur. Our practice is to suture defects larger than 50% of the circumference in an attempt to reduce the risk of postoperative rectal stenosis.

The specimen should be marked with a suture or a clip at its anal verge before it is completely freed to ensure correct orientation when it is pinned onto a cork plate (figure 10). The pinning should be performed with caution and should include all layers of the resected specimen. The more accurately it is performed, the less incomplete resections will be reported from the pathologist.

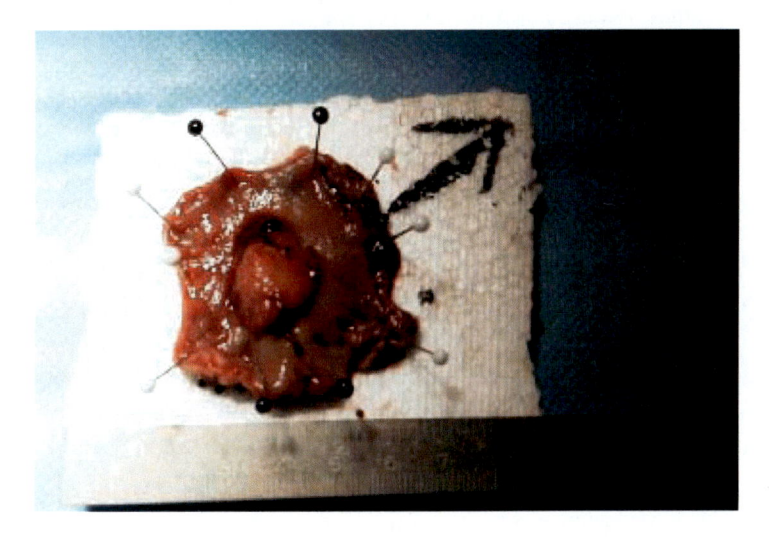

Figure 10. The specimen obtained by TEM technique is pinned and marked for an accurate pathological examination of the margins.

Equipment for gas-less TEM has been developed. It consists of a transparent plexiglas tube with a side-window. The idea is to place the side hole over the tumor and resect it while the tube keeps the rectum open for a good view [68].

Results: The short term results after TEM is good [5,69] compared to major rectal cancer surgery. Patients leave the hospital after 1-2 days depending on the protocol rather than physical well being. In a series of 144 TEM for cancer, 18 patients bleed more than 50 ml, two of which went back to the operating theatre for re-TEM with successful haemostasis. No patients needed transfusion. Eighteen patients had postoperative fever above 38 degree Celsius. Two patients had severe ascending infection into the mesorectum demanding laparotomy and a diverting stoma. One had acute myocardial infarction and one died within

30 days. This study consisted of very old patients with co-morbidity and the majority of the patients had TEM for compromise [6,43]. A 30 day mortality rate of 0 - 1% is reported for old patients without comorbidity in several studies. The frequency of perforation to the peritoneum depends on the attitude to TEM resection in the upper anterior rectum. In a study of 888 TEM procedures for rectal cancer performed by the UK TEM user group, The Mainz TEM group, The Danish TEM group and The Norwegian TEM users, 22 perforations were encountered (2%). As all perforations were sutured during the TEM procedure, and no patient had laparotomy or complications from this, it was regarded as a minor event [66]. Transient urinary retention occurs but is usually resolved within 24 hours. Transient anal incontinence occurs in up to 4% but long term incontinence is rare [70].

Long term oncological results after TEM for cancer depends upon selection of patients, design of the study (single- or multicenter), primary endpoint (local failure or recurrence rate or overall survival), experience of the surgeon and accuracy of the pathological staging. Most recent studies focus on the results after the combination of TEM and rescue and/or salvage surgery rather than after the TEM procedure alone [71,72,73].

Local recurrence after TEM for cancer may be due to incomplete resection of the primary tumour or to the presence of metastatic lymph nodes in the mesorectum. Pathological incomplete resection may occur in up to 35% of the cases when TEM is performed for adenomas of all sizes [74] but the recurrence rates are lower (2 - 13%) [18,20] indicating that the specimen is often presented to the pathologist in a poor condition. The recurrence rate is correlated to the size of the tumour [43] and this is the reason why a maximal diameter of 3 cm is defined as a criterion for low risk cancer. Less than 5% of low risk T1 cancers are lymph node positive and should be treated with a radical TEM [18,20]. Few data exist on the local recurrence rate of low risk rectal cancers removed by major or by local procedures. The local recurrence rate after major resection of T1 cancers is about 5% and after TEM between 0% and 26% in a large number of small studies [18]. It is evident that the local recurrence rate in high risk T1 cancers is higher after TEM than after major surgery. Up to 20% of high risk T1 cancers are lymph node positive. There are indications however that the long term total survival after TEM and later rescue surgery when needed, is comparable to that of major resection for unselected T1 cancers [71,73,74,75]. These data came from series where adjuvant or neoadjuvant oncological therapy was not part of the overall strategy.

At present it cannot be safely stated if survival after TEM for unselected T1 cancers is comparable to that after major surgery in fit young or middle aged patients. Cancer patients treated with TEM are in most centres selected, favouring old and co-morbid patients and no randomized studies have been performed.

The York Mason Technique

The posterior, trans-sphincteric approach was reinvented by York Mason in 1970 [77]. The patient is positioned in the lateral position and access to the tumour is obtained by a longitudinal trans-sphincteric and trans-rectal incision. It provides an excellent view of the low and medium height, anterior tumours and radical local resection of small rectal cancers may be easier by this technique than by any intra-rectal procedures. Unfortunately, complications are frequent and often severe. Anal incontinence and rectal fistulas are the most common complications. It may not qualify for the term; minimal invasive surgery. The York Mason technique is therefore not used for tumour surgery any longer.

Other Techniques of Local Surgical Treatment:

Both diathermy and argon laser has been described as methods for removing larger adenomas and recurrent adenomas or cancers in the rectum. Recurrences after TEM in the very fragile patients may be dealt with by these techniques if histology will have no consequence in the further handling of the patient.

Transrectal resection of tumours with a urologic resectoscope has described. The results are unknown as only a few small series have been published [77]. The pathological evaluation of radicallity and staging of the lesion is not possible. The arguments for using this technique have been inaccessibility to TEM equipment. It cannot be recommended as small lesions may be dealt with by simpler procedures and larger tumours always harbour the risk of malignancy. One possible exception might be the treatment of ileus due to a stenosing rectal cancer in the very fragile patient, but colon stents or TEM are usually used for that purpose, and resectoscopic resection may be a technical challenge.

Early Rescue Surgery

Indications: The preoperative staging and in particular T1 sub-staging may not be accurate and tumour grading can only be completed from postoperative evaluation of the resection specimen.

Average risk patients with cancers more advanced than low risk T1 and removed by local resection should be offered early rescue surgery. It is likely that the apparent higher cure rate from late salvage surgery after a TEM procedure compared to salvage after major surgery may change this recommendation, but this must await further confirmation. Some patients, who had TEM assuming that the tumour was benign, will also prefer rescue surgery for low risk T1 cancers, and this should be discussed with the patient. If intensive follow up is not acceptable or possible, rescue surgery might be the better choice.

Technique: Whenever local resections of larger adenomas are performed, final histology report must be accessible within a few days in order to prepare for a radical re-operation within weeks. The rescue surgery is performed as any other major rectum resection. One should take care in the dissection at the level of the tumour. In the anterior aspect of the rectum there is a high risk of scar formation and adherence to adjacent organs. Tearing of the mesorectal facia may be difficult to avoid. This may also be the case in cancers below 5 cm from the anal verge. Some authors claim that a preoperative TEM for low cancers may lead to more abdominoperineal resections and fewer low anterior resections [18].

Results: The long term results after TEM and rescue surgery is not completely determined, but increasing evidence is accumulating that it is comparable to primary major surgery [71,73-75]. The issue is important because preoperative sub-staging is difficult and some of the pathological features that allocate tumours to the high risk group (vascular and perineural invasion, differentiation at the invasive front) can not be determined from biopsies, but from the TEM specimen only. The strategy of using TEM as an excision biopsy in all small tumours without advanced preoperative staging is also based upon the assumption that

TEM and subsequent rectum resection is comparable to primary major resection. Local recurrence rates after TEM and rescue surgery when necessary is 0% - 5% [78,79].

Treatment of Local Recurrence (Salvage Surgery)

Little is known about the long term results after surgery for local recurrence after TEM. It may be regarded as any other local recurrence. The results may be comparable to that of surgery for local recurrence after major resection. There is no doubt that the results do not match those after early rescue surgery. The 5-year survival after surgery for recurrence after major surgery is between 20% and 40% in larger series. Small series rapport 55% long-term survival for recurrence surgery after TEM [18].

There are indications that R0 resection of local recurrence after TEM is possible in about 90% of the patients which is impressive compared to recurrence surgery after major surgery [18]. However it should be remembered that the results after TEM recurrences come from highly dedicated centres, and the patient populations and the surgical performance may not be comparable to data from large national databases on recurrences after major surgery.

The important questions to be answered in the future are: Why does local recurrence occur? Is it because malignant lymph nodes are left behind in the mesorectum? This may be counteracted by better preoperative N-staging procedures. Is it because of incomplete pathological resection? Most published series on TEM for cancer include tumours larger than 3 cm and therefore do not comply with the newly suggested protocols suggesting that all cancers larger than 3 cm are high risk cancers. Does no-touch technique prevent seeding of cancer cells during TEM? Do we need to improve our surgical technique in that aspect also? We don't know, but recurrences certainly have more causes. Our job is to quantify them and address them in order of importance.

Non-Surgical Treatment

Solid data – especially phase III data – on the efficacy of radiotherapy (RT) or radiochemotherapy (RCT) are deficient in patients with early rectal cancer (T1-2N0M0). In contrast, the usefulness of RT or RCT has been proven in many randomized studies in patients with T3-4N0M0 rectal cancer [80]. Before the era of total mesorectal excision (TME), local failure or recurrence rate (LFR) of more than 25 % was not unusual but the use of TME has reduced LFR considerable. During the past decade pre- or postoperative RT or RCT have reduced LFR to less than 10% and the survival is still increasing [80], however preoperative RCT is presently preferred for postoperative RCT because of reduced toxicity, a chance for increased sphincter preservation, and increased efficacy [81].

The aims of preoperative RCT in patients with resectable rectal cancer are to reduce the LFR, to improve survival, to increase the chance of a sphincter-sparing resection in low-lying cancers and to cause down-staging but also to cure selected patients in which resection is not otherwise possible [82].

RCT with 5-fluorouracil (5-FU) as the drug of choice improves the efficacy of RT and increases the chance of complete pathological remission (pCR) [82,83]. Continuous infusion of 5-FU is more effective than bolus injection [84]. Oral therapy with capecitabine [85] or tegafur [90,91] is convenient without the necessity of a central venous catheter and the plasma concentrations of 5-FU given in a 5/7 days schedule mimics that of CVI [85]. Adding chemotherapy to preoperative long-term RT decreases LFR and induce pathological complete response (pCR) in 10 to 30% of tumours [82]. Both short-course RT and long-course RCT reduce LFR in patients with resectable rectal cancer.

The most optimal preoperative radiation schedule has not been defined but most often long-term RCT with radiation dose of 45-50 Gy are recommended even though short-term RT is at least as effective in patients with resectable tumours [81]. Based on the evidence that higher radiation doses improve tumour regression and local control in other cancers [91], a dose-response relationship has also been evaluated and found in rectal cancer [87,88,89]. However, even with an optimal technique using conformal intensity-modulated radiotherapy, dose escalation in the pelvis is limited by rectal tolerance.

Endocavitary radiation is an attractive way to deliver a high dose in a very small volume. In a phase II study, external radiotherapy combined with a single 5 Gy endorectal boost resulted in a promising 27 % pCR in T3 rectal cancers [91]. In the Lyon R96-02 study [92], 88 patients with T2 or T3 rectal cancer were randomly assigned to preoperative external RT or the same RT with boost (extra 85 Gy in three fractions) using endocavitary contact x-ray. This dose escalation increased clinical (from 2% to 29%) and pathological (from 10% to 35%) complete response and sphincter preservation (from 44% to 76%) however without difference in terms of morbidity and two-year overall survival.

Oxaliplatin and irinotecan are excellent radiation sensitizers often used in combination with 5-FU infusions or the oral formulations, but these combinations have mostly been investigated in phase I or II studies. However, Hartley et al [89] have collected data from several studies with more than 3.000 patients and in a multivariate analysis they found that the use a second drug (often oxaliplatin or irinotecan) was associated with higher rates of pCR, which may be a surrogate marker for efficacy.

Modern preoperative RCT induce substantial regression of primary tumour and lymph node metastases and pathological complete remission (pCR) was found in 15 to 30% of patients even in patients with large non-resectable rectal cancer [87,81,91].

This opens the possibility of a non-surgical approach in selected patients [93,94]. Recently Habr-Gama et al published a study evaluating a non-surgical approach in patients with pCR, and this strategy seems appropriate [97]. This also opens the possibility of downstaging in patients with T2-T3 resectable rectal cancer followed by TEM resulting in decreased morbidity in this group of patients. Whether a short-course RT is as effective as long-course RT is not known but this important question is being investigated in a Swedish randomized phase III trial in which patients with resectable rectal cancer are randomized to RT with 25 Gy/5 fractions immediately followed by TME, 25 Gy/5 fractions followed by TME after 4 weeks or 45 Gy/25 fractions followed by TME after 4 weeks [98].

Local excision of distal rectal cancer is an established alternative surgical option for patients unfit for major surgery and patients unwilling to have a stoma. In low-risk patients (T1 adenocarcinoma, small size, G1-2, no vascular, lymphatic or perineural invasion) LFR is very low (3–5%), however in other patients local excision alone has an unacceptable LFR between 17 and 50% [100]. Fortunately, several studies have shown that neoadjuvant RCT can downstage primary tumour and sterilize lymph nodes.

In an excellent review, Borschitz et al presented data from 237 patients (collected from 7 papers) with primarily T2-3 rectal carcinoma who – for various reasons - received preoperative RCT before local excision [99]. RCT (36 to 52 Gy, most often combined with 5-FU) was carried out heterogeneously and therefore precluded an analysis of schedules. The proportion of clinical complete remission was almost 90% in these selected patients. A pCR (ypT0) was noted in 22% (53 of 237 patients) and a partial response at the submucosa level (ypT1) in 19% (45 of 237 patients). No patients with pCR (ypT0) experienced local recurrence and LFR was as low as 2% (0-6%) in patients with ypT1. In contrast, in patients with no response (ypT3) LFR was 21%.

A single randomized study [95,101] has compared TEM or laparoscopic resection in 70 patients with T2N0 low rectal cancer (G1-2, tumour less than 3 cm) after neoadjuvant RCT. Down-staging was observed for 34 patients (21 pT0 and 13 pT1). Three patients had LFR and three patients experienced metastases. The authors concluded that TEM and laparoscopic resection produce comparable results (LFR and survival) in selected patients pre-treated with RCT. In addition, postoperative morbidity and quality of life, and postoperative pain were lower after TEM. The authors sought an alternative to APR especially in elderly patients and therefore it is hard understand that they excluded patients above 70 years probably because of worry about chemotherapy but today, RCT in elderly patients is of no concern [91].

Follow Up

Pre- or peri-operative investigations include colonoscopy and radiological examination of liver and lungs before surgery. The main focus in follow up is on local recurrence. The early cancers treated for cure with TEM have little risk of distant metastasis, and those treated with TEM for compromise will usually not endure curative treatment for distant metastasis. There is however no evidence to support that follow up for liver and lung metastasis can be omitted. There is no evidence-based knowledge to support recommendations for a follow up regimen.

Local recurrence after TEM is usually seen within two years after the operation, but later recurrences occur [18]. Digital rectal examination, proctosopy and transanal ultrasound should to the author's opinion be performed with 3 months intervals during the 12 or 18 months, and thereafter with 6 months intervals. After 2 years, one should also consider the risk of metachrone colorectal tumours. The patients should be followed for possible recurrence with decreasing frequency for 5 years like all other colorectal cancer patients. The risk of metachrone tumours in the colo-rectum may dictate life long colonoscopic follow up. Follow up to detect liver and lung metastasis may follow the protocols for other rectal cancers.

The extramural local recurrences may be more frequent than after major surgery, and expert transanal ultrasound is important. PET-CT should be used if recurrence is suspected in patients who are candidates for intended curative treatment.

TEM surgery is often centralized to large tertiary referral hospitals. Old and co-morbid patients may not comply with a follow up programme if they have to travel far. Some kind of compromise may have to be arranged with his local hospital. In a larger series of Danish patients operated for cancer with TEM, only a small fraction was followed postoperatively according to the protocol [5]. This was in contrast to a high compliance amongst patients operated with major surgery.

INDIVIDUALIZED CHOICE OF TREATMENT:

An adequate preoperative evaluation of the patients' general health, physical performance and physiological age is mandatory before suggesting any treatment modality for rectal cancers. The pathological features of the cancer decide to what degree these parameters will influence the decision.

Most patients will choose the treatment recommended by the surgeon and most surgeons will suggest treatment modalities mastered by themselves. The safe choice will in most cases be a low anterior resection or abdominoperineal rectum resection even for early rectal cancers. This will ensure an oncological safe solution in most cases and is mastered by all colorectal surgeons. The only preoperative information needed on the primary tumour is its distance to the mesorectal fascia to determine on neoadjuvant oncological treatment. This policy is oncological safe but will lead to over-treatment and unnecessary complications and long term side effects in some patients. The operative mortality after major rectal surgery is 2-3% and major complications will occur in 30% or more (figure 11) [4]. About half the patients will have a temporary or permanent stoma. Impotence, urinary bladder paresis, disturbances of defecation and anal continence are common [4]. Further, the oncological safe choice will not always lead to the best chance of survival, as operative mortality in some subgroups of patients may be high [4,102].

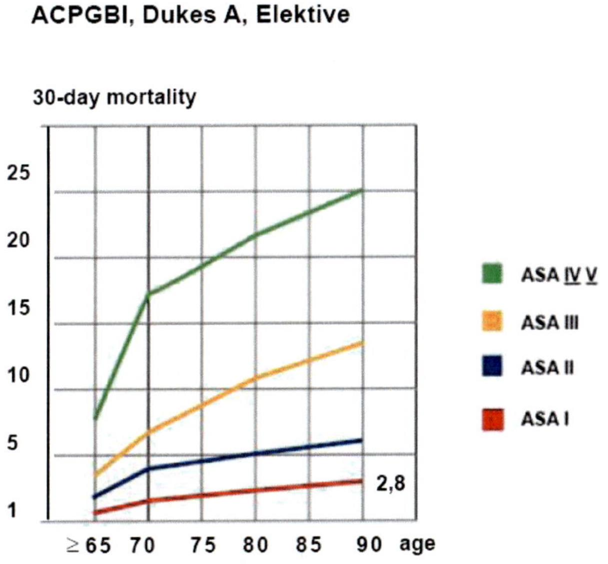

Figure 11. The 30-day mortality after major surgery for rectum cancer: The influence of age and physiological performance is illustrated. Based upon figures from the annual report from the Association of Coloproctology of Great Britain and Ireland.

Two essential questions should be discussed with the patient: Can local resection be performed without compromising long term survival, and if long term mortality is better after major resection: How much and at what cost?

Calculations of long term survival should compare total survival rates for major and local resection including supplementary oncological therapy, early rescue surgery and treatment for recurrences. Presently, these figures cannot be safely calculated before the operation, but some principles are becoming evident. Data from several trials indicate that elderly co-morbid patients with T1 cancers and low risk T2 cancers can be treated with primary TEM without compromising the long term survival [43]. This may also be true for all other patients if TEM for high risk T1 and all T2 cancers are combined with neoadjuvant RT or RCT. A close follow-up is mandatory. Early rescue surgery (or adjuvant RCT in patients without neo-adjuvant therapy) will be necessary for approximately 10% - 20% of the patients depending upon the quality of the preoperative staging. In other words, about 85% can avoid major surgery with no costs of long term total survival. Long term results from TEM followed by early rescue surgery may be comparable to those following primary major surgery.

Old age always comes out as a significant risk factor for complications and deaths after major surgery. This may be due to the close relation between age and co-morbidity, as high age per se does not increase the risk of operative complications. In the larger Scandinavian national databases the 30-day mortality after major surgery for rectal cancer is 2 – 3%. This increases to 8 – 10% for patients older than 80 years even though they are more carefully selected for intended curative surgery [4]. The 30-day mortality risk increases by a factor 1.8 for every 10 years increase in age [102]. Further; only about 50% of patients older than 79 years have major resection for cure as compared to 75% for patients younger than 80 years [4]. Appropriate use of TEM in the old patients may therefore lead to more intended curative treatments and may improve the survival.

The use of total survival rate rather than cancer specific survival is particularly important in the old patients as e.g. a healthy 86 year person has a statistical survival time of 6 years. This means that 30% - 50% of those patients who will experience a recurrence after rectal cancer treatment will die from other causes before they die from the cancer. This emphasizes the relative importance of achieving a low rate of 30-day mortality in old patients. An 86 year old patient will have an operative 30-day mortality risk of about 10% after major surgery and 0 - 1% after local resection. If he has only 6 years to compensate this 9% extra mortality from major surgery, he will, almost regardless of tumour stage and tumour grade, statistically be better off with a radical local resection followed by adjuvant treatment if necessary. The mean age of rectal cancer patients is more than 70 years in the developed countries and 25% are 80 years or older. These considerations therefore concern a high proportion of our patients.

Reduced physical performance will increase the risk of operative death. This extra risk should be quantified in patients with co-morbidity. An individual 30-day operative mortality risk can be calculated on http://www.riskprediction.org.uk. Some of the models for calculation of the risk adjusted operative mortality include parameters witch has to be estimated before the operation, as e.g. operative blood loss. Other calculators at this home-page as the ACPGBI include only parameters available prior to surgery.

It is therefore often necessary to choose treatment modalities which is not oncological optimal in order to optimise the total long term survival.

Trials where surgeons and patients are interviewed separately clearly demonstrate that the surgeon is more concerned about long-term survival than the patient is, and the patient is more concerned about quality of life than the surgeon [103]. Patients also become more concerned about quality of life a few months after the operation than they express before the operation. On the other hand, the quality of performance of a surgical department is judged by measurable parameters, and 5 years survival is *the* parameter by which we compare us with each other and – by which hospital owners and politicians compare themselves with other hospitals or countries. This may be one reason why health politicians and professional health care workers are more concerned about the 5 year survival rate than many patients are.

For most patients with rectal cancer these considerations imply no conflict. Patients with T3 and T4 cancers constitute the majority of rectal cancer patients and they must have major surgery if it can be performed without significantly increased risk of death from the operation. Patients with low risk T1 cancers also have no conflicts of choice as local resection by TEM provides an optimal oncological result. Individual risk assessment is necessary is those patients with high risk T1 cancers and T2 cancers. Some few severely co-morbid patients with small T3 cancers will also benefit from a local resection as more than half will be cured if radical resection is possible [43].

REFERENCES

[1] Påhlman L, Bohe M, Cedermark B et al. The Swedish rectal cancer registry. *Br. J. Surg.* 2007; 94: 1285-1292.

[2] Tekkis PP, Poloniecki JD, Thomson MR et al. Operative mortality in colorectal cancer: Prospective national study. *BMJ* 2003; 22: 196-201.

[3] Harling H, Büllow S, Kronborg O et al. Survival of rectal cancer patients in Denmark during 1994-99. *Colorectal Dis* 2004; 6: 153-7.

[4] Endreseth BH, Romundstad P, Myrvold HE et al, on behalf of the Norwegian Rectal Cancer Group. Rectal Cancer Treatment in the Older Population. *Colorectal Dis.* 2006; 8(6): 471-9.

[5] Baatrup G, Elbrønd H, Hesselfeldt P et al. Rectal adenocarcinoma and transanal endoscopic microsurgery: diagnostic challenges, indications and short term results. *Int J Colorectal Dis*, 2007; 22: 1347-52.

[6] Mentges B, Buess G, Effinger G. Indications and results of local treatment of rectal cancer. *Br J Surg* 1997; 84: 348 – 351.

[7] Lee W, Lee D, Choi S et al. Transanal endoscopic microsurgery and radical surgery for T1 and T2 cancer. *Surg. Endosc* 2003; 17: 1283 – 7.

[8] Lezoche E, Guerrieri M, Paganini AM et al. Long-term results of patients with pT2 rectal Cancer treated with radiotherapy and Transanal endoscopic microsurgical excision. *World J Surg* 2002; 49: 1185 – 90.

[9] Taylor RH, Hay JH and Larsson SN. Transanal local excision of selected low rectal Cancers. *Am J Surg* 1998; 175: 360 – 363.

[10] Buess G, Huttere F, Theiss J et al. A system for transanal endoscopic rectum operation. *Chirurg* 1984; 55: 677-680.

[11] Yamamoto H, Kawata H, Sunada K et al. Success rate of curative endoscopic mucosal resection with circumferential mucosal incision assisted by submucosal injection of sodium hyaluronate. *Gastrointest Endosc*, 2002; 56: 507-12.

[12] Ono H, Kondo H, Gotoda T et al. Endoscopic submucosal resection for treatment of early rectal. *Cancer. Gut*, 2001; 48: 225-9.

[13] Gotoda T, Yamamoto H, Soetikno RM. Endoscopic submucosal dissection of early rectal cancer. *J Gastroenterol*, 2006; 41: 929-42.

[14] Nusko, G., et al. Invasive carcinoma in colorectal adenomas: multivariate analysis of patient and adenoma characteristics. *Endoscopy*, 1997; 29: 626-31.

[15] Kudo, S, Kashida H, Nakajima T, et al. Endoscopic diagnosis and treatment of early colorectal cancer. *World J Surg*, 1997; 21: 694-701.

[16] Kudo, S, Rubio CA, Texeira CR, et al. Pit pattern in colorectal neoplasia: endoscopic magnifying view. *Endoscopy*, 2001; 33: 367-73.

[17] Golligher JC. *Surgery of the anus rectum and colon*, third ed. 1975; 75 – 85, Balliere Tindall, IBSN 0 70200519 3.

[18] Baatrup G, Endreseth B, Isaksen,V et al. Preoperative staging and treatment options in T1 rectal adenocarcinoma. *Acta Oncol.* 2009; 48: 328 - 42.

[19] Doornebosch PG, Bronkhorst PJ, Hop WC et al. The role in endorectal ultrasound in therapeutic decision-making for local vs transabdominal resection of rectal tumours. *Dis Colon Rectum*, 2008; 51: 38-42.

[20] Tytherleigh MG, Warren BF and Mortensen NJ McC. Management of early rectal cancer. *Br J Surg*, 2008; 95: 409-423.

[21] Akasu T, Sagihara K, Moriya Y et al. Limitations and pitfalls of transrectal ultrasonography for staging of rectal cancer. *Dis. Colon Rectum*, 1997; 40: 10-15.

[22] Akasu T, Kondo H, Moriya Y et al. Endorectal ultrasonography and treatment of early stage rectal cancer. *World J Surg*, 2000; 24: 1061-8.

[23] Forsberg F, Shi WT, Knauer MK et al. Real-time excitation ultrasound contrast imaging. *Ultrason Imaging*, 2005; 27: 65-74.

[24] Ophir J, Alam SK, Garra B et al. Elastography: imaging the elastic properties of soft tissue with ultrasound. *J Med Ultrasonics*, 2002; 29: 155-171.

[25] Samani A and Plewes D. An inverse problem solution for measuring the elastic modulus of intact ex vivo breast tumours. *Phys Med Biol*, 2007; 52: 1247-60.

[26] Pallwein L, Aigner F, Faschingbauer R et al. Prostate cancer diagnosis: value of real-time elastography. *Abdominal Imaging*, 2008; 33: 729 - 35.

[27] Giovannini M, Hookey LC, Borries E et al. Endoscopic ultrasound elastography: the first step towards virtual biopsy? Preliminary result in 49 patients. *Endoscopy*, 2006; 38: 344-348.

[28] Baatrup G, Havre RF and Ødegaard S. Intra-rectal sono-elastography for the evaluation of rectal tumours.*Colorectal Dis*, 2008; 10, suppl 2. abstract O012.

[29] Brown G, Radcliffe AG, Newcombe RG et al: Preoperative assessment of prognostic factors in rectal cancer using high-resolution magnetic resonance imaging. *Br J Surg* 2003; 90:355-364.

[30] Kim CKK, Kim SH, Chun HK et al: Preoperative staging of rectal cancer: accuracy of 3-Tesla magnetic resonance imaging. *Eur Radiol.*2006;16:972-980

[31] Bipat S, Glas AS, Slors FJM et al: Rectal cancer: Local staging and assessment of lymph node involvement with endoluminal us, CT, and MR imaging- a meta-analysis *Radiology* 2004; 232:773-783.

[32] Brown G, Richards CJ, Bourne MW et al: Morphologic predictors of lymph node status in rectal cancer with use of high-spatial-resolution MR imaging with histopathologic comparison. *Radiology* 2003; 227:371-377.

[33] Koh DM, Brown G, Temple L et al: Rectal cancer: mesorectal lymph nodes at MR imaging with USPIO versus histopathologic findings--initial observations. *Radiology* 2004; 231:91-99.

[34] Huddy SP, Husband EM, Cook MG et al. Lymph node metastasis in early rectal cancer. *Br J Surg*, 1993; 80: 1457-58.

[35] Kikuchi R, Takano M, Fujimoto N et al. Management of early invasive colorectal cancer. Risk of recurrence and clinical guidelines. *Dis Colon Rectum*, 1995; 38: 1286-95.

[36] Yamamoto S, Watanabe M, Hasegawa H. The risk of lymph node metastasis in T1 colorectal carcinoma. *Hepatogastroenterology*, 2004; 51: 998-1000.

[37] Sitzler, PJ, Seow-Choen F, Ho YH. Lymph node involvement and tumor depth in rectal cancers: an analysis of 805 patients. *Dis Colon Rectum*, 1997; 40: 1472-76.

[38] Gondal G, Grotmol T, Hofstad B et al. Biopsy of colorectal polyps is not adequate for grading of neoplasia. *Endoscopy*, 2005; 37: 1193-97.

[39] Nesbakken A, Løvig T, Lunde OC et al. Staging of rectal carcinoma with transrectal ultrasonography. *Scand J Surg*, 2003; 92: 125-129.

[40] Maedak K, Maruta M, Utsumi T et al. Minimal invasive surgery for carcinoid tumours in the rectum, *Biomed Pharmacother*; 55 suppl 1: 222-226.

[41] Laundry CS, Brook G, Scoggins CR et al. A proposed staging system for carcinoid tumours based on an analysis of 4701 patients. *Surgery*, 2008; 144: 460-466.

[42] Nilsson PJ and Ragnarsson-Olding BK. Anorectal malignant melanoma: clear resection margins of importance irrespective of surgical approach.*Colorectal Dis*, 2008; 10 suppl. 10, abstract O011.

[43] Baatrup G, Breum B, Qvist N et al. Transanal endoscopic microsurgery in 143 consecutive patients with rectal adenocarcinoma. Results from a danish multicenter study. *Colorectal Dis*, 2008; 11: 270 - 75.

[44] Nusko G, Mansmann U, Altendorf-Hofmann A et al. Risk of invasive carcinoma in colorectal adenomas assessed by size and site. *Int J Colorectal Dis*, 1997; 12: 267-271.

[45] Gschwanter M, Kriwanek S, Langner E et al. High-grade dysplasia and invasive carcinoma in colorectal adenomas; a multivariate analysis of the impact of adenoma and patient characteristics. *Eur J Gastroenterol Hepatol*, 2002; 14: 183-188.

[46] Lauren B, Gage BF, Owens DK et al. Effect and outcome of the ASGE guidelines on the periendoscopic management of patients who take anticoagulants. *AJG*, 2000; 95: 1717-24.

[47] Yamamoto H, koiwai H, Yube T et al. A succesful single-step endoscopic resection of a 40 millimeter flat-elevated tumor in the rectum: endoscopic mucosal resection using sodium hyaluronate. *Gastrointest Endosc*, 1999; 50: 701-704.

[48] Yamamoto H, Yube T, Isoda N et al. A novel method of endoscopic mucosal resection using sodium hyaluronate. *Gastrointest Endosc*, 1999; 50: 251-256.

[49] Tanaka S, Oka S, Kaneko I et al. Endoscopic submucosal dissection for colorectal neoplasia: possibility of standardization. *Gastrointest Endosc*, 2007; 66: 100-107.

[50] Stergiou N, Riphaus A, Lange P et al. Endoscopic snare resection of large colonic polyps: how far can we og? *Int J Colorectal Dis*, 2003; 18: 131-135.

[51] Tanaka S, Haruma K, Oka S et al. Clinicopatologic features and endoscopic treatment of superficially spreding colorectal neoplasms larger than 20 mm. *Gastrointest Endosc*, 2001; 54: 62-66.

[52] Kantsevoy SV, Douglas G, Adler DG et al on behalf of the ASGE Technology Committe. Endoscopic mucosal resection and endoscopic submucosal dissection. *Gastrointest Endosc*, 2008; 68: 11-18.

[53] Darwood RJ, Wheeler JM and Borley JM. Transanal endoscopic microsurgery is a safe and reliable technique even for complex rectal lesions. *Br J Surg*, 2008, 95: 915 - 18.

[54] Kato H, Haga S, Endo S et al. Lifting of lesions during endoscopic mucosal resection (EMR) of early rectal cancer: implication for the assessment of resectability. *Endoscopy*, 2001; 33: 568-573.

[55] Rembacken BJ, Gotoda T, Fujii T el al. Endoscopic mucosal resection. *Endoscopy*, 2001; 33: 709-718.

[56] Morales TG, Sampliner RE, Garewal HS et al. The difference in colon polyp size before and after removal. *Gastrointest Endosc*, 1996; 43: 25-28.

[57] Brooker JC, Saunders BP, Shah SG. Treatment with argon plasma coagulation reduces recurrence after piecemeal resection of large sessile colonic polyps: a randomized trial and recommendations. *Gastrointest Endosc*, 2002; 55: 371-375.

[58] Parks AG. A technique for excising extensive villous papillomatous change in the lower rectum. *Proc R Soc Med*, 1968; 61: 441-442.

[59] Parks AG and Stuart AE. The management of villous tumours of the large bowel. *Br J Surg*, 19973; 60: 688-695.

[60] Welch JP and Welch CE. Villous adenomas of the colorectum. *Am J Surg*, 1976; 131: 185-191.

[61] Southwood WFM. Villous tumours of the large intestine: their pathogenesis, symptomatology, diagnosis and management. *Ann R Coll Surg Engl*, 1962; 30: 791-797.

[62] Quan SHO and Castro EB. Papillary adenomas (villous tumours) a review of 215 cases. *Dis Colon Rectum*, 1971; 14: 267-280.

[63] Røkke O, Iversen KB, Øvrebø K et al. Local resection of rectal tumors by transanal endoscopic microsurgery: experience with the first 70 cases. *Dig Surg*, 2005; 22: 182-189.

[64] DeGraaf EJ, Doornebosch PG, Stassen LP et al. Transanal endoscopic microsurgery for rectal cancer. *Eur J Surg*, 2002; 38: 904-910.

[65] Baatrup G, Svendsen R and Ellensen V. Benign rectal strictures managed with transanal resection and advancement plasty in six patients. A novel application for Transanal Endoscopic Microsurgery. *Colectroal Dis*. In press

[66] Baatrup G, Borschitz T, Cunningham C et al. Perforation into the peritoneal cavity during transanal endoscopic microsurgery for rectal cancer is not associated with major complications or oncological compromise. *Surg. Endosc*. 2009; E-pub ahead of print, PMID 19172355.

[67] Ramirez JM, Aguilella V, Arribas D et al. Transanal full-thickness excision of rectal tumours: should the defect be sutured? A randomized controlled trial. *Colorectal Dis*, 2002; 4: 51-55.

[68] Kanehira E, Yamashita Y, Omura K et al. Early clinical results of endorectal surgery using a newly designed rectal tube with a side window. *Surg Endosc*, 2002; 16: 14-17.

[69] Azimuddin K, reither RD, Stasik JJ et al. Transanal endoscopic microsurgery for excision of rectal lesions: technique and initial results. *Surg Laparosc Percutan Tech*, 2000; 10: 372-378.

[70] Buess FG and Heike R. Transanal endoscopic microsurgery. *Surgcal oncology clinics of north america*, 2001; 10: 709-731.

[71] Borschitz T, Haintz A and Junginger T. Transanal endoscopic microsurgical excision of pT2 rectal cancer: results and possible indications. *Dis Colon Rectum*, 2007; 50: 292-301.

[72] Whitehouse PA, Armitage JN, Tilney HS et al. Transanal endoscopic microsurgery: local recurrence rate following resection of rectal cancer. *Colorectal Dis*, 2008; 10: 187-193.

[73] Borschitz T, Kneist W, Gockel I et al. Local excision for more advanced tunors. *Acta Oncol*, 2008; 47: 1140-7.

[74] Endreseth BH, Myrvold HE, Romundstad P et al. Transanal excision vs. Major surgery for T1 rectal cancer, *Dis Colon Rectum* 2005; 48: 1380-88.

[75] Mentges B, Buess G, Effinger G et al. Indications and results of local treatment of rectal cancer. *Br J Surg*, 1997, 84; 348-351.

[76] Mason AY. Surgical acess to the rectum: a trans-sphincteric exposure. *Proc R Soc Med*, 1970; 13 (suppl 1).

[77] Beattie GC, Paul I and Calvert CH. Endoscopic transanal resection of rectal tumours using a urological resectoscope – still has a role in selected patients. *Colorectal Dis*, 2005; 7: 47-50.

[78] Lee W, Lee D, Choi S et al. Transanal endoscopic microsurgery and radical surgery for T1 and T2 cancers. *Surg Endosc*, 2003; 17: 1283-87.

[79] Stipa F, Burza A and Luciandri G. Outcomes for early rectal cancer managed with transanal endoscopic microsurgery: a 5-year follow-up study. *Surg Endosc*, 2006; 4: 541-545.

[80] Glimelius B, Holm T, Blomqvist L. Chemotherapy in addition to preoperative radiotherapy in locally advanced rectal cancer - a systematic overview. *Rev Recent Clin Trials* 2008; 3: 204-11.

[81] Glimelius B, Gronberg H, Jarhult J, Wallgren A, Cavallin-Stahl E. A systematic overview of radiation therapy effects in rectal cancer. *Acta Oncol* 2003; 42: 476-92.

[82] Glimelius B. Chemoradiotherapy for rectal cancer - is there an optimal combination? *Ann Oncol* 2001; 12: 1039-45.

[83] Frykholm GJ, Påhlman L, Glimelius B. Combined chemo- radiotherapy vs. radiotherapy alone in the treatment of primary, nonresectable adenocarcinoma of the rectum. *Int J Radiation Oncology Biol Phys* 2001; 50: 427-34.

[84] O'Connell MJ, Martenson JA, Wieand HS, et al. Improving adjuvant therapy for rectal cancer by combining protracted-infusion fluorouracil with radiation therapy after curative surgery. *N Engl J Med* 1994; 331: 502-7.

[85] Liauw SL, Minsky BD. The use of capecitabine in the combined-modality therapy for rectal cancer. *Clinical colorectal cancer* 2008; 7: 99 -104.

[86] Sadahiro S, Suzuki T, Kameya T, et al. A pharmacological study of the weekday-on/weekday-off oral UFT schedule in colorectal cancer patients. *Cancer Chemother Pharmacol* 2001; 47: 447-50.

[87] Mohiuddin M, Regine WF, John WJ, et al. Preoperative chemoradiation in fixed distal rectal cancer: Dose time factors for pathological complete response. *Int J radiat Oncol Biol Phys* 2000; 46: 883-8.

[88] Glimelius B, Isacsson U, Jung B, Påhlman L. Radiotherapy in addition to radical surgery in rectal cancer: Evidence for a dose-response effect favouring preoperative treatment. *Int J Radiat Oncol Biol Phys* 1997; 37: 281-7.

[89] Hartley A, Ho KF, Mcconkey C, Geh JI. Pathological complete response following pre-operative chemoradiotherapy in rectal cancer: analysis of phase II/III trials. *Br J Radiology* 2005; 78: 934-8.

[90] Pfeiffer P. High-dose radiotherapy and concurrent UFT plus l-leucovorin in locally advanced rectal cancer: A phase I trial. *Acta Oncol* 2005; 44: 224-29.

[91] Vestermark LW, Jacobsen A, Qvortrup C, Hansen F, Bisgaard C, Baatrup G, Rasmussen P, Pfeiffer P. Long-term results of a phase II trial of high-dose radiotherapy (60 Gy) and UFT/l-leucovorin in patients with non-resectable locally advanced rectal cancer (LARC). *Acta Oncol.* 2008; 47(3): 428-33.

[92] Pollack A, Zagars GK, Starkschall G, et al. Prostate cancer radiation dose response: results of the M.D.Anderson phase III randomized trial. *Int J Radiat Oncol Biol Phys* 2002; 53: 1097-105.

[93] Glynne-Jones R, Wallace M, Livingstone JIL, Meyrick-Thomas J. Complete clinical response after preoperative chemoradiation in rectal cancer: is a "wait and see" policy justified? *Dis Colon Rectum* 2008; 51: 10-9.

[94] O'Neill BD, Brown G, Heald R, Cunningham D, Tait DM. Non-operative treatment after neoadjuvant chemoradiotherapy for rectal cancer. *Lancet Oncol* 2007; 8: 625–33.

[95] Gerard JP, Chapet O, Nmoz C, et al. Improved sphincter preservation in low rectal cancer with high-dose preoperative radiotherapy: the LYON R96-02 randomized trial. *J Clin Oncol* 2004; 22: 2404-9.

[96] Jacobsen A, Mortensen JP, Bisgaard C, et al. Preoperative chemoradiation of locally advanced T3 rectal cancer combined with an endorectal boost. *Int J Radiat Oncol Biol Phys* 2006; 64: 461-5.

[97] Habr-Gama A, Perez RO, Proscurshim I, et al. Patterns of failure and survival for nonoperative treatment of stage c0 distal rectal cancer following neoadjuvant chemoradiation therapy. *J Gastrointest S*urg 2006; 10: 1319-28.

[98] Glimelius B. Rectal cancer irradiation. long course, short course or something else? Editorial. *Acta Oncol* 2006; 45: 1013-17.

[99] Borschitz T, Gockel I, Kiesslich R, Junginger T. Oncological Outcome After Local Excision of Rectal Carcinomas. *Ann Surg Oncol*. 2008, 15: 3101 - 08.

[100] Lezoche E, Guerrieri M, Paganini AM, et al. Transanal endoscopic vs total mesorectal laparoscopic resections of T2–N0 low rectal cancers after neoadjuvant treatment A prospective randomized trial with a 3-year minimum follow-up period. *Surg Endosc* 2005; 19: 751–6.

[101] Lezoche G, Baldarelli M, Guerrieri M, et al. A prospective randomized study with a 5-year minimum follow-up evaluation of transanal endoscopic microsurgery versus laparoscopic total mesorectal excision after neoadjuvant therapy. *Surg Endosc* 2008; 22: 352–8.

[102] TekkisPP, Poloiecki JD, Thompson MR et al. Operative mortality in colorectal cancer: Prospective national study. *BMJ*, 2003; 22: 1196-1201.

[103] Pieterse AH, Baas-Thijssen MC, Marijnen CA et al. Clinician and cancer patient views on patient participation in the treatment decision-making: a quantitative and qualitative exploration. *Br J Cancer*, 2008; 16: 875-882.

In: Rectal Cancer: Etiology, Pathogenesis and Treatment ISBN 978-1-60692-563-8
Editors: Paula Wells and Regina Halstead © 2009 Nova Science Publishers, Inc.

Chapter VI

TRANSANAL ENDOSCOPIC MICROSURGERY OF RECTAL TUMOR A REVIEW

Damian Casadesus[†]
Hospital Calixto Garcia, Havana, Cuba.

ABSTRACT

In 1984, G. Buess introduced transanal endoscopic microsurgery (TEM). Since this time the frequency of such procedure has been increasing for rectal adenoma resection and selected cases of rectal cancer. For the purposes of this review, Medline literature search was performed in order to locate articles on the indications, clinical and functional results of TEM. Emphasis was placed on reports from the past decade. Perusal of the literature reveals that TEM is a safe technique in the treatment of rectal adenomas with better outcomes compared with other techniques. TEM appears to be an effective method of excising selected T1 carcinomas of the rectum. The place of this technique in the resection of advanced carcinomas has yet to be properly evaluated; however its use has produced better results compared with radical techniques. In conclusion, TEM is a safe procedure and can achieve good results in terms of local tumor resection, with lower recurrences rates, fewer complication and higher survival rates than those of radical techniques.

INTRODUCTION

Different alternative techniques have been developed for the removal of the high number of early-stage rectal cancers and benign adenomas that are not amenable to removal during colonoscopy. In the lower rectum, transanal excision of benign lesions is a common

---

[†] Correspondence concerning this article should be addressed to: Dr. Damian Casadesus, Hospital Calixto Garcia, J and University, Plaza, Havana, Cuba. Email: dcasadesus@hotmail.com.

procedure. It has also been offered to selected patients with a malignant lesion of the lower rectum for decades, with low morbidity and mortality, but with high local recurrence rates for T2 lesions in some series [1,2]. In the middle and upper thirds of the rectum, benign and malignant lesions are difficult to reach transanally and standard radical surgical options, such as low–anterior resection, posterior trans–sphincteric or trans–sacral approach and abdominoperineal resection, with or without sphincter preservation, are traditionally offered to the patient. Nevertheless, these procedures are associated with significant mortality and high morbidity, including anastomotic leakage, sexual dysfunction, fecal and urinary incontinence, and the rejection of colostomy by the patient.

New horizons in the treatment of middle and upper rectal neoplasms were opened up with the introduction of transanal endoscopic microsurgery (TEM) technique by Professor Buess in 1984 [3]. It was proposed that TEM would enable local excision of adenomas up to 24 cm from the anal verge and could be used to excise suitable early–stage rectal cancers, offering a minimally invasive alternative to transanal excision and radical surgery, with superior endoscopic magnification, accurate and complete resection with secure suture closure.

TEM AND BENIGN RECTAL LESIONS

The risk of carcinoma developing in a colorectal polyp that is 1 cm or larger is 2.5% at 5 years and 8% at 10 years, [4] and this potential for malignancy is an indication for the excision of such polyps. The first–line treatment of adenomatous colorectal polyps is endoscopic removal during the diagnostic procedure, which is associated with low mortality and morbidity rate. Different transanal approaches are used to remove adenomatous polyps in the lower rectum when the size and/or location of the tumor limits standard endoscopic resection, but adenomas in the middle or upper rectum are difficult to remove using the standard transanal excision instruments. If TEM was not available, these inaccessible neoplasms might require trans–sphincteric or trans–sacral resection, or low–anterior resection.

TEM has produced satisfactory results with low recurrence rates and low morbidity and mortality. In a large series of 286 cases of adenoma resection using TEM, [5] the authors reported a 3.4% early postoperative complication rate and 1.2% and 7% recurrence rates after 1 year and 5 years, respectively. In a review of 1780 adenoma resection procedures from 19 studies (Table 1), the residual adenoma rate in the surgical margin was 10% and the recurrence rate was less than 6% after a minimum available follow up of 20 months.

In terms of local recurrence after adenoma resection, histological positive resection margin has been considered highly significant. Galandiuk et al. [25] found that adenoma recurred in 34% of tumors with positive resection margins, compared with only 3% of tumors with negative resection margins. Dafnis et al. [26] found adenoma recurrence in 11% of patients after TEM resection in a series of patients in whom the resection had been classified as "not microscopically radical" in 19% of patients and "of uncertain microscopical radicality" in 23%. Six studies reported a frequency rate of between 10 and 40% of adenoma extending to the surgical margin of locally excised polyps (Table 2); however, it is remarkable that, with such high positive residual margin rates, the recurrence rates in these cases was less than 5.6%, lower than the rates reported in some series with lower positive residual margin rates.

In five studies comparing adenoma resection with TEM and another procedure (Table 3), the lower recurrence rates, the residual tumor and the early complication rates favor TEM resection. Late complication rates were higher after TEM, probably due to the increased incidence of transient incontinence in the postoperative period [29,30].

Table 1. Adenoma resected by transanal endoscopic microsurgery

First author (reference)	No. of Lesions	Residual adenoma in surgical margin (%)	Local recurrence (%)	Follow up (months)
Lloyd et al. [6]	68	9	5.9	28.7
Ganai et al. [7]	82	10	15	44
Steele et al. [8]	77	9	5.1	7.4
Farmer et al. [9]	36	25	5.6	33
Nakagoe et al. [10]	9	0	0	dno
Cocilovo et al. [11]	56	1.7	3.5	dno
Neary et al. [12]	21	0	4.7	dno
Katti et al. [13]	58	7	10	34
Vorobiev et al. [14]	113	-	8.3	29.5
Bretagnol et al. [15]	148	14.9	7.6	33
Endreseth et al. [16]	64	20	13	24
Zacharakis et al. [17]	48	4.2	6.3	37
Schafer et al. [18]	33	18	12	36.4
Rokke et al. [19]	56	10	0	12
Guerrieri et al. [20]	530	-	4.3	44
McCloud et al. [21]	75	37.3	16	31
Whitehouse et al. [22]	146	5.5	4.8	39
Platell et al. [23]	62	-	2.4	24
Moore et al. [24]	40	17	3	20

dno data no obtained.

Table 2. Adenoma recurrence in incomplete excised lesions

First author (reference)	No. patients	Incomplete excised Lesion (%)	Recurrence (%)	Follow up (months)
Farmer et al. [9]	36	25	5.6	33
Enderseth et al. [16]	64	37.7	4.3	24
Rokke et al. [19]	56	10	0	12
McCloud et al. [21]	75	46	3	31
Whitehouse et al. [22]	146	25	3.7	39
Morschel et al. [27]	238	30.7	3.6	67.5

Table 3. Adenoma resection with transanal endoscopic microsurgery and other methods

First author (reference) Procedures	No. Patients	Complications (%)	Recurrence
Nakagoe et al. [10]			
TEM	9	22	0
PA	4	0	0
Moore et al. [24]			
TEM	40	dno	1
TA	30	dno	12
Winde et al. [28]			
TEM	98	14	6
PSE	90	23	20
Naggy et al. [29]			
TEM	80	11.2	2
RR	16	25	4
TP	8	25	-
Madhala et al. [30]			
TEM	16	10	0
SE	14	14	3

TEM Transanal endoscopic microsurgery, PSE perianal submucosal excision, RR radical resection, TP transanal polypectomy, PA conventional posterior approach, TA transanal excision, SE submucosal excision.

TEM AND CARCINOID RECTAL TUMOR

Carcinoid tumors are very rare neuroendocrine neoplasm found most often in the gastrointestinal tract with a very variable 5 year survival. The therapy depends on the histopathologic features, the localization and the stage of the tumor at the time of the diagnosis. In the gastrointestinal tract it is most frequently detected in the small intestine, the appendix and the rectum. Rectal carcinoid tumors are incidentally found at endoscopy at an early stage without lymph node invasion or metastasis, and they are often suitable for local resection with curative intent.

TEM has also been used in the treatment of carcinoid tumor with good results [31-35]. Peerbooms and coworkers [31] resected a small highly differentiated carcinoid tumor in 5 patients with no morbidity, mortality and recurrence. In the largest study I found using TEM in the treatment of rectal carcinoid tumors, Kinoshita et al. [32] performed 14 resections of primary carcinoid tumors and 13 resections as completion surgery after incomplete resection by endoscopic polypectomy. In all their cases both deep and lateral surgical margins were completely free of tumors, minor morbidities were present in 2 cases, and no recurrences were reported after more than 70 months of follow up.

TEM AND MALIGNANT RECTAL LESIONS

Different studies advocate the use of TEM for treating cancers that are smaller than 3 cm, well to moderately differentiated on previous biopsy, situated up to 25 cm from the anal verge, located in the extraperitoneal portion of the rectum, without lymphatic and vascular invasion, or infiltrating as far as the submucosa on endoanal ultrasound [18,36,37,38]. Nevertheless, the preoperative tumor extension in the rectal wall and lymph node invasion are often impossible to determine by endoluminal ultrasound because of destruction or stricture of the rectal wall caused by the tumor, or by scarring from a previous operation, multiple biopsy, or fulguration, and only the specimen resected is useful to know the tumoral stage.

Authors have strongly recommended TEM resection for the treatment of patients with low-risk T1 tumors because survival rates are higher with TEM than they are with other treatment techniques in such patients. Heintz et al. [39] compared the treatment of high-risk and low-risk T1 carcinomas by resection with local excision (TEM and Park's resection) with treatment by radical excision. In terms of 5-year survival, they found no difference between local excision and radical surgery in either T1 carcinoma group, but patients with low-risk T1 carcinoma had better survival rates than patients with high-risk T1 carcinoma.

Studies of T2 carcinomas resected by TEM had enrolled very heterogeneous groups of patients who had followed different radiotherapy and/or chemotherapy plans before or after TEM making difficult to evaluate the treatment of T2 rectal tumors by TEM alone [10,40,41]. Saclarides based on his results in 73 patients, however, considered TEM alone as an inappropriate resection method to use in patients with T2 tumors [42].

Table 4. Recurrence of rectal tumor after TEM according to tumoral T stage

First author (reference)	Tis	T1	T2	T3
Ganai et al. [7]	0	19	50	0
Bretagnol et al. [15]	-	9.6	11.8	75
Endreseth et al. [16]	-	0	20	50
Zacharakis et al. [17]	-	7.1	42.8	66.6
Schafer et al. [18]	-	5	-	-
Mentges et al. [38]	-	4.1	0	14.2
Lee et al. [41]	-	4.1	19.5	-
Saclarides et al. [42]	15.3	25	80	-
Lev-Chelouche et al. [43]	-	0	20	22.2
Suzuki et al. [44]	0	0	0	-
Demartines et al. [45]	-	8.3	0	-
Smith et al. [46]	-	10	40	66
Helgstrand F et al. [47]	-	15	16	-
Whitehouse et al. [48]		26	22	0

Local and distant recurrences have a great bearing on survival rates. Lymph node metastases, the depth of mural infiltration, and the full-thickness tumor resection are important factors in the development of recurrence. Unfortunately, studies reporting recurrence rates according to the stage of the tumor (Table 4) have not had similar follow-up periods, many have been single descriptive investigations, they have not had similar numbers of patients in each stage group to allow for a detailed analysis, the patients had followed different postoperative treatment according to the criteria set out by each surgeon or institution, and they show different and contradictory recurrence rates.

Most authors avoided much discussion about TEM and T3-stage rectal cancer treatment, some authors not even mentioning it. Survival rates of between 59% and 69% indicate that TEM is not a valid option in this situation, but these results are similar to the results described in studies of T3 rectal cancer treated by anterior resection and mesorectal excision [49]. TEM has been used in the palliative treatment of T3-stage rectal cancer. It has a clear role in patients with rectal cancer in who age, extent of disease, or concurrent illnesses preclude conventional surgical resection. This technique allows complete excision of the tumor, reduces the chance of recurrence, and improves the quality of remaining life at home, with their family, with comfort and good symptom control [50,51]. Other standard treatments for advanced rectal cancer are often only suitable for small lesions, can result in inaccurate tumor destruction, often require multiple applications, and are associated with high mortality and morbidity compared with TEM.

Studies Comparing TEM with Radical Surgery

Only three studies have compared the resection of T1 and T2 cancers by TEM and resection using other radical procedures [10,28,41]. They advocated the use of TEM for resecting T1 lesions because of the lower complication rate and better long-term survival rate after TEM. Heintz et al. [39] compared local excision with radical surgery in 103 patients. The complication rate and mortality were higher for radical resection than for TEM, but the local recurrence rate was lower and there was no difference in 5-year survival between both treatment groups. In addition, when Langer et al. [52] compared abdominal or abdominoperineal resection, conventional transanal resection, and TEM, they also showed that radical resection gave excellent results with respect to recurrence and residual tumor. Compared with radical resection, however, TEM was associated with a lower complication rate and lower perioperative mortality and afforded to patients a better quality of life. In the same study, TEM also showed better results than conventional transanal excision in terms of recurrence rate, residual margin infiltration, and complication rate.

Moore et al. [24] in a recent study compared rectal tumor excision with TEM and transanal excision (TE) and concluded that TEM is more effective than the other technique because they found significant higher rate of clear margin and significant less fragmented specimen after TEM than after TE, with low complications and low recurrence rate in TEM.

TEM and Preoperative Radiotherapy

Several studies have described treatment with a combination of radiotherapy and/ or chemotherapy and TEM; however, no details were given of these patients' subsequent management, morbidity, and mortality and they followed up different pre or post-operatory programs, making impossible accurate analysis. The combination of preoperative radiotherapy with TEM for the treatment of rectal tumors appears to be feasible, safe, and effective in terms of preserving anal sphincter function, but the survival rates after this type of treatment have been found to be similar or lower than after TEM without radiotherapy. Three series (with probably some double recording of patients) from University of Ancona, Italy, using radiotherapy and TEM, reported similar results [20,53,54] and they are also similar to results of treatment with TEM alone.

In one preliminary study with different treatment groups that did not undergo similar follow-up regimens, authors had found that similar cancer specific survival rates were reported for surgery alone (92%), radiotherapy or chemotherapy followed by surgery (94%), surgery followed by radiotherapy (96%), and radical radiotherapy alone (96.6 %), masking the apparent advantages of the radiotherapy and TEM combination [55]. If preoperative radiotherapy can lead to downgrading of tumor stage, shrinkage of tumors, induction of complete tumoral remission or an improvement in loco regional disease, TEM has an important role to play after radiotherapy according to oncological principles of local resection in well-selected and followed-up patients without compromising their possibility of cure. In this regard, endoscopy and endorectal ultrasound scans are mandatory in the follow-up regimen during radiotherapy, the group must be homogeneous for proper analysis, a minimum of 5 years' follow-up is necessary in all patient series for accurate analysis, and patients should be correctly selected without compromising their chance of cure. Sufficient numbers of patients could probably be accrued in the setting of a multicenter international trial for further randomized studies comparing TEM with and without radiotherapy and chemotherapy.

TEM AND RETRORECTAL TUMORS

Zoller and coworkers first described the resection of retrorectal tumor by TEM in 3 cases [56]. These are rare entities within the retrorectal space, frequently find on routine physical examination or the patients most frequently present rectal pain, recurrent abscesses, fistulas, and constipation. Tumors were resected completed, without recurrence and complications.

TEM COMPLICATIONS

In a review of 19 studies involving a total of 1484 patients (Table 5), complications were recorded in 206 patients (13.8 %), with more than 50% of these being urinary retention and temporary incontinence. Anal incontinence is the most common complication reported, however, it is transient, mainly to flatus and most of the patients improve in the first month postoperative. This transient incontinence observed after TEM can be explained by changes in rectoanal perception and coordination, and electrosensitivity of the anal mucosa. Manometric results before and after TEM have identified the main risk factors of anal dysfunction after TEM as: preoperative anal disorders in older patients or caused by the tumor, postoperative internal sphincter defects, the extent and the depth of the tumor excision, the anal mucosa loss, and the duration of the procedure [63,64,65]. The increase in bowel frequency observed after the TEM procedure is probably related to low rectal compliance after full-thickness or circumferential excisions with significant reduction of the rectal diameter. To assure a correct quality of life in these patients after rectal tumoral resection, it is important to emphasize not only the results in terms of oncology outcomes, operation time, and technical improvements, but also the functional results after what is considered a sphincter preserving operation.

Table 5. TEM complications
(Postoperative fever, pelvic pain and myocardial infarction were not included)

First author (reference)	No. of Patients	Total No. of complications	Incontinence	Bleeding	Urinary retention
Steele et al. [8]	100	9	2	-	-
Farmer et al. [9]	49	2	-	1	1
Neary et al. [11]	40	8	-	7	1
Katti et al. [13]	65	10	2	2	6
Vorobiev et al. [14]	128	3	2	1	-
Bretagnol et al. [15]	200	28	-	10	2
Endreseth et al. [16]	79	11	5	-	-
Schafer et al. [18]	33	10	4	-	-
Rokke et al. [19]	70	8	-	2	-
Whitehouse et al. [22]	146	24	3	6	6
Saclarides [42]	73	13	4	2	1
Lev-Chelouche et al. [43]	75	18	5	4	4
Demartines et al. [45]	50	13	6	-	-
Swastrom et al. [57]	27	5	2	3	-
Arribas del Amo et al. [58]	42	8	6	1	-
De Graff et al. [59]	76	15	1	4	2
Platell et al. [60]	113	31	1	4	26
Araki et al. [61]	217	12	12	-	-
Meng et al. [62]	31	8	2	1	1
Total	1614	236	57	48	50

Urinary retention accounted for 50 patients (24.2%) half of them in only one study; it occurred occasionally in the early postoperative period and few patients subsequently required surgery or catheterization to resolve it. Sexual problems have not yet been reported following TEM. Bleeding was the third most common complication, but few patients required blood transfusion or another surgical intervention to control it. Other complications, such as perforation, rectovaginal fistula or wound leakages are less common.

Mortality associated with TEM is rare and only two studies reported one death associated directly with the procedure. In one of the study a patient died of multi-organ failure 10 days after a partial thickness resection of a rectal adenoma with an undetected perforation treated with open repair and stoma [22]. The other patient had a retroperitoneal phlegmon which occurred after TEM resection of a rectal adenoma, who died in septic shock after 28 days [66].

ADVANTAGES OF TEM

Although results are not expressed uniformly, 1871 TEM procedures that were reported in seventeen studies showed other important advantages (Table 6). There were only 27 patients (3.7 %) in who attempted TEM procedures were unsuccessful or had to be converted to radical surgery or conventional transanal resection as a result of inadequate exposure, difficulties with the neumorectum, inability to see the complete lesion, perforation, or for reasons related to the oncological risk. The mean hospital stay was less than 6 days with the maximum being 51 days in one study. The recurrence rate was very low with only 69 (3.7%) recurrences. The short duration of the procedure and the low blood loss, which obviates the need for blood transfusion, are also important advantages of this procedure.

Table 6. Features of transanal endoscopic microsurgery

First author (reference)	No. of Procedures	Duration of TEM procedure (range) minutes	Blood loss (range), ml	No. converted to other procedure	Hospital stay (range) days	No. of cases with recurrence
Steele et al. [8]	100	79* (30-240)	-	8	4† (1-21)	6
Farmer et al. [9]	50	67* (20-175)	24* (0-300)	3	3.6* (1-11)	2
Neary et al. [11]	40	91* (35-175)	-	-	3.2* (1-6)	1
Vorobiev et al. [14]	128	60* (10-190)	25.2 (0-155)	-	-	-
Bretagnol et al. [15]	202	45† (10-180)	-	-	3* (1-20)	19
Endreseth et al. [16]	79	110† (45-240)		2	4† (1-25)	10
Zacharakis et al. [17]	76	80.6* (38-180)		2	3.2* (1-51)	9
Rokke et al. [19]	70	105† (30-455)		1	2† (1-16)	1
Guerrieri et al. [20]	588	105† (90-120)		3	.5† (4-6)	
Lev-Chelouche et al. [43]	75	-	-	7	5.5* (2-13)	8
Suzuki et al. [44]	26	96* (40-235)	40* (0-150)	0	13.5* (5-37)	1
Swastrom et al.[57]	27	127* (49-280)	20* (5-150)	-	1.7* (0-5)	1
Arribas del Amo et al. [58]	42	85* (25-180)	100* (10-350)	-	4* (2-15)	3
Araki et al. [61]	217	63*	-	7	5.8*	2
Meng et al. [62]	31	95† (45-200)	-	-	4† (2-10)	1
Toreson et al. [67]	20	85† (55-140)	-	-	3† (1-5)	0
Palma et al. [68]	100	98* +/- 24	-	2	5.5† (3-21)	5

† Median, * Mean.

Others advantages of TEM include: complete resection and secure suture closure; a shorter time to the patient being able to walk, sit, take solid food, and defecate; less postoperative pain and use of analgesia; and the avoidance of a major abdominal operation and colostomy.

DISCUSSION

The cost of the instrument had limited the extension of TEM to a few institutions, but the many advantages of this technique can cover the high capital cost. The TEM instruments are technically demanding, the operation and the manipulation of the instruments are performed in parallel, and there is no facility for counter traction from an assistant or another port. Different modifications to the instruments such as the use of standard laparoscopic instruments, low pressure insufflations and conversion to video TEM had an important role in the extension of the technique. Other modifications of the instruments will have an important role in the future if they make the technique easier to learn, and if they conserve the low morbidity and mortality associated with the TEM technique.

It is difficult to go back doing rectal neoplasms resection in the old-fashioned way, once you have learned how to use TEM and after experiencing its good results. Nevertheless, favorable outcomes have also been obtained with other techniques, such as minimally invasive transanal surgery, endoscopic transanal resection, and transanal resection. These are also good options for treatment that should not be forgotten in both our daily practice and in training the new generation of surgeons.

REFERENCES

[1] Mellgren A, Sirivongs P, Rothenberger DA et al. Is local excision adequate therapy for early rectal cancer? *Dis Colon Rectum* 2000; 43: 1064-1074.

[2] Minsky BD, Rich T, Recht A et al. Selection criteria for local excision with or without adjuvant radiation therapy for rectal cancer. *Cancer* 1989; 63: 1421-1429.

[3] Buess G, Hutterer F, Theiss J et al. A system for a transanal endoscopic rectum operation [in German]. *Chirurg* 1984; 55: 677-680.

[4] Gordon PH, Nivatvongs S. *Principles and practice of surgery for the colon, rectum, and anus*. 2nd edn. New York: Marcel Dekker, 1999.

[5] Said S, Stippel D. Transanal endoscopic microsurgery in large, sessile adenomas of the rectum: a 10−year experience. *Surg Endosc* 1995; 9: 1106-1112.

[6] Lloyd G. M, Sutton CD, Marshall LJ, Baragwanath P, Jameson JS, Scott AD. Transanal endoscopic microsurgery – lessons from a single UK centre series *Colorectal Dis* 2002; 4: 467–472.

[7] Ganai S, Kanumuri P, Rao Roshni, Alexander A. Local recurrence after transanal endoscopic microsurgery for rectal polyps and early cancers. *Ann Surg Oncol* 13: 547-556.

[8] Steele RJC, Hershman MJ, Mortensen NJ et al. Transanal endoscopic microsurgery: initial experience from three centers in the United Kingdom. *Br J Surg* 1996; 83: 207-210.

[9] Farmer KC, Wale R, Winnet J et al. Transanal endoscopic microsurgery: the first 50 cases. *ANZ J Surg* 2002; 72: 854-856.

[10] Nakagoe T, Sawai T, Tsiju T et al. Local rectal tumor resection results: gasless, video-endoscopic transanal excision versus the conventional posterior approach. *World J Surg* 2003; 27: 197-202.

[11] Cocilovo C, Smith LE, Stahl T, Douglas J. Transanal endoscopic excision of rectal adenomas. *Surg Endosc* 2003; 17: 1461-1463.

[12] Neary P, Makin GB, White TJ et al. Transanal endoscopic microsurgery: a viable operative alternative in selected patients with rectal lesions. *Ann Surg Oncol* 2003; 10: 1106-1111.

[13] Katti G. An evaluation of transanal endoscopic microsurgery for rectal adenoma and carcinoma. *JSLS* 2004; 8: 123±126.

[14] Vorobiev GI, Tsarkov PV, Sorokin EV. Gasless transanal endoscopic surgery for rectal adenomas and early carcinomas *Tech Coloproctol* 2006; 10: 277-281.

[15] Bretagnol F, Merrie A, George B, Warren BF, Morten NJ. Local excision of rectal tumours by transanal endoscopic microsurgery *Br J Surg* 2007; 94: 627-633.

[16] Endreseth BH, Wibe A, Svinsas, Marvik R, Myrvold HE. Postoperative morbidity and recurrence after local excision of rectal adenomas and rectal cancer by transanal endoscopic microsurgery. *Colorectal Dis* 2005; 7: 133-137.

[17] Zacharakis E, Freilich S, Rekhraj S, Athanasiou T, Paraskeva, Zirpin P, Darzi A. Transanal endoscopic microsurgery for rectal tumors: the St. Mary's experience. *Am J Surgery* 2007; 194: 694-698.

[18] Schafer H, Baldus SE, Gasper F, Holscher AH. Submucosal infiltration and local recurrence in pT1 low-risk rectal cancer treated by transanal endoscopic microsurgery. *Chirurg* 2004; 76: 379-384.

[19] Rokke O, Iversen KB, Maartmann-Moe H, Skarstein A, Halvorsen JF. Local resection of rectal tumors by transanal endoscopic microsurgery: Experience with the first 70 Cases. *Dig Surg* 2005; 22:182-190.

[20] Guerrieri M, Feliciotti F, Baldarelli M et al. Sphincter-saving surgery in patients with rectal cancer treated by radiotherapy and transanal endoscopic microsurgery: 10 years' experience. *Dig Liver Dis* 2003; 35: 876-880.

[21] Mc Cloud J. M, Waymont N, Pahwa N et al. Factors predicting early recurrence after transanal endoscopic microsurgery excision for rectal adenoma. *Colorectal Dis* 2005; 8: 581-585.

[22] Whitehouse P. A., Tilney HS, Armitage JN, Simson JNL. Transanal endoscopic microsurgery: risk factors for local recurrence of benign rectal adenomas. *Colorectal Dis* 2006; 8: 795-799.

[23] Platell C, Denholm E, Makin G. Efficacy of transanal endoscopic microsurgery in the management of rectal polyps. *J Gastroenterol Hepatol* 2004; 19: 767-772.

[24] Moore JS, Cataldo PA, Osler T, Hyman NH. Transanal endoscopic microsurgery is more effective than traditional transanal excision for resection of rectal masses. *Dis Colon Rectum* 2008; 51: 1026-1031.

[25] Galandiuk S, Fazio VW, Jagelman DG et al. Villous and tubulovillous adenomas of the colon and rectum: a retrospective review, 1964- 1985. *Am J Surg* 1987; 153: 41-47.

[26] Dafnis G, Pahlman L, Raab Y et al. Transanal endoscopic microsurgery: clinical and functional results. *Colorectal Dis* 2004; 6: 336-342.

[27] Morschel M, Heintz A, Bussmann M, Junginger T. Follow-up after transanal endoscopic microsurgery or transanal excision of large benign rectal polyps. *Langenbeck's Arch Surg* 1998; 383: 320-324.

[28] Winde G, Nottberg H, Keller R et al. Surgical cure for early rectal carcinoma (T1): transanal endoscopic microsurgery vs. anterior resection. *Dis Colon Rectum* 1996; 39: 969-976.

[29] Nagy A, Kovacs T, Berki C, Jano Z. Surgical management of villous and tubulovillous adenomas of the rectum. *Orv Hetil* 1999; 140: 2215- 2219.

[30] Madhala O, Lelcuk S, Rabau M. Transanal endoscopic microsurgery for local excision of rectal neoplasms. *Harefuah* 1995; 129: 236-237.

[31] Peerbooms JC, Simons JL, Tetteroo GWM, De Graaf EJR. Curative Resection of Rectal Carcinoid Tumors with transanal endoscopic microsurgery. *J Laparoendosc Adv Surg Tech* 2006; 16: 435-438.

[32] Kinoshita T, Kanehira E, Omura K, Tomori T, Yamada H. Transanal endoscopic microsurgery in the treatment of rectal carcinoid tumor. *Surg Endosc* 2007;21: 970-4.

[33] Maeda K, Maruta M, Utsumi T, Sato H, Masumori K, Matsumoto M Minimally invasive surgery for carcinoid tumors in the rectum. *Biomed Pharmacother* 2002; 56: 222-226.

[34] Araki Y, Isomoto H, Shirouzu K. Clinical efficacy of video-assisted gasless transanal endoscopic microsurgery (TEM) for rectal carcinoid tumor. *Surg Endosc.* 2001; 15: 402-404.

[35] Kwaan MR, Goldberg JE, Bleday R. Rectal carcinoid tumors: review of results after endoscopic and surgical therapy. *Arch Surg* 2008;143: 471-5.

[36] Mentges B, Buess G, Effinger K et al. Indications and results of local treatment of rectal cancer. *Br J Surg* 1997; 84: 348-351.

[37] Buess GF, Raestrup H. Transanal endoscopic microsurgery. *Surg Oncol Clin N Am* 2001; 10: 709-731.

[38] Mentges B, Buess G, Schafer D et al. Local therapy of rectal tumors. *Dis Colon Rectum* 1996; 39: 886-892.

[39] Heintz A, Mörschel M, Junginger T. Comparison of results after transanal endoscopic microsurgery and radical resection for T1 carcinoma of the rectum. *Surg Endosc* 1998; 12: 1145-1148.

[40] Stipa F, Lucandri G, Ferri M et al. Local excision of rectal cancer with transanal endoscopic microsurgery (TEM). *Anticancer Res* 2004; 24: 1167-1172.

[41] Lee W, Lee D, Choi S, Chun H. Transanal endoscopic microsurgery and radical surgery for T1 and T2 rectal cancer. *Surg Endosc* 2003; 17: 1283-1287.

[42] Saclarides TJ. Transanal endoscopic microsurgery: a single surgeon's experience. *Arch Surg* 1998; 133: 595-599.

[43] Lev-Chelouche D, Margel D, Goldman G, Rabau MJ. Transanal endoscopic microsurgery: experience with 75 rectal neoplasms. *Dis Colon Rectum* 2000; 43: 662-667.

[44] Suzuki H, Furukawa K, Kan H et al. The role of transanal endoscopic microsurgery for rectal tumors. *J Nippon Med Sch* 2005; 72: 278-284.

[45] Demartines N, von Flüe MO, Harder FH. Transanal endoscopic microsurgical excision of rectal tumors: indications and results. *World J Surg* 2001; 25: 870-875.

[46] Smith LE, Ko ST, Saclarides TJ et al. Transanal endoscopic microsurgery: initial registry results. *Dis Colon Rectum* 1996; 39: 79-84.

[47] Helgstrand F, Iversen E, Bech K. Transanal endoscopic microsurgery. The latest 5 years' experience in Roskilde County. *Ugeskr Laeger*. 2007;169: 1784-8.

[48] Whitehouse PA, Armitage JN, Tilney HS, Simson JN. Transanal endoscopic microsurgery: local recurrence rate following resection of rectal cancer. *Colorectal Dis.* 2008;10:187-93.

[49] Pacelli F, Giorgio A, Papa V et al. Preoperative radiotherapy combined with intraoperative radiotherapy improves results of total mesorectal excision in patients with T3 rectal cancer. *Dis Colon Rectum* 2004; 47: 170-179.

[50] Turler A, Schafer H, Pichlmaier H. Role of transanal endoscopic microsurgery in the palliative treatment of rectal cancer. *Scand J Gastroenterol* 1997; 32: 58-61.

[51] Dickinson AJ, Savage AP, Mortensen NJ, Kettlewell MG. Long-term survival after endoscopic transanal resection of rectal tumors. *B J Surg* 1993; 80: 1401-1404.

[52] Langer C, Liersch T, Süss M et al. Surgical cure for early rectal carcinoma and large adenoma: transanal endoscopic microsurgery (using ultrasound or electrosurgery) compared to conventional local and radical resection. *Int J Colorectal Dis* 2003; 18: 222-229.

[53] Lezoche E, Guerrieri M, Feliciotti F et al. Local excision of rectal cancer by transanal endoscopic microsurgery (TEM) combined with radiotherapy: new concept of therapeutic approach. *Przegl Lek* 2000; 57 Suppl 5: 72-74.

[54] Lezoche E, Guerrieri M, Paganini AM, Feliciotti F. Long-term results of patients with pT2 rectal cancer treated with radiotherapy and transanal endoscopic microsurgical excision. *World J Surg* 2002; 26: 1170-1174.

[55] Hersman MJ, Sun Myint A, Makin CA. Multi-modality approach in curative local treatment of early rectal carcinomas. *Colorectal Dis* 2003; 5: 445-450.

[56] Zoller S, Joos A, Dinter D, Back W, Horisberger K, Post S, Palma P. Retrorectal tumors: Excision by transanal endoscopic microsurgery. *Rev Esp Enferm Dig* 2007; 99: 547-550.

[57] Swanstrom LL, Smiley P, Zelko J, Cagle L. Video endoscopic transanal rectal tumor excision. *Am J Surg* 1997; 173: 383-385.

[58] Arribas del Amo D, Ramirez Rodriguez JM, Aguilella Diago V et al. Transanal endoscopic surgery for rectal tumors. *Rev Esp Enferm Dig* 2000; 92: 526-535.

[59] De Graaf EJR, Doornebosch PG, Stassen LPS et al. Transanal endoscopic microsurgery for rectal cancer. *Eur J Cancer* 2002; 38: 904-910.

[60] Platell C, Denholm E, Makin G. Efficacy of transanal endoscopic microsurgery in the management of rectal polyps. *J Gastroenterol Hepatol* 2004; 19: 767-772.

[61] Araki Y, Isomoto H, Shirouzu K. Video-assisted gasless transanal endoscopic microsurgery: a review of 217 cases of rectal tumors over the past 10 years. *Dig Surg* 2003; 20: 48-52.

[62] Meng WCS, Lau PYY, Yip AWC. Treatment of early tumours by transanal endoscopic microsurgery in Hong Kong: prospective study. *Hong Kong Med J* 2004; 10: 239-243.

[63] Herman RM, Richter P, Walega P, Popiela T. Anorectal sphincter function and rectal barostat study in patients following transanal endoscopic microsurgery. *Int J Colorectal Dis* 2001; 16: 370-376.

[64] Kreis ME, Jehle EC, Haug V et al. Functional results after transanal endoscopic microsurgery. *Dis Colon Rectum* 1996; 39: 1116-1120.

[65] Kennedy ML, Lubowski DZ, King DW. Transanal endoscopic microsurgery excision. Is anorectal function compromised? *Dis Colon Rectum* 2002; 45: 601-605.

[66] Klaue HJ, Bauer E. Retroperitoneal phlegmon after transanal endoscopic microsurgery excision of rectal adenoma. *Chirurg* 1997; 68: 84.

[67] Toreson JE, Marvik R, Sahlin Y, Myrvold HE. Transanal endoscopic microsurgery. *Tidsskr Nor Laegeforen* 1996; 116: 52-53.

[68] Palma P, Freudenberg S, Samel S, Post S. Transanal endoscopic microsurgery: indications and results after 100 cases. *Colorectal Dis* 2004; 6: 350-355.

In: Rectal Cancer: Etiology, Pathogenesis and Treatment
Editors: Paula Wells and Regina Halstead

ISBN 978-1-60692-563-8
© 2009 Nova Science Publishers, Inc.

Chapter VII

CORRELATION BETWEEN METABOLIC ENZYMES OF NUCLEIC ACID IN COLORECTAL CANCER PATIENTS AND FRNA/TSIR, PROGNOSTIC FACTORS[*]

Kenji Katsumata[*], Tetsuo Sumi, Daisuke Matsuda, Shoji Suzuki, Masayuki Hisada, Yasuharu Mori, Tatehiko Wada, Akihiko Tuchida and Tatsuya Aoki

Department of Surgery, Tokyo Medical University, Japan.

ABSTRACT

This study examined metabolic pathway of 5-fluorouracil (5-FU) in cancer and non-cancer sites of colorectal cancer patients including: 16 patients who received 500 mg/day 5-FU drip infusion for 3 days (group R), and 19 patients who received 500 mg/day 5-FU continuous venous injection (groupC). The metabolic pathway was examined in both groups as non-cancerous group (No) and cancerous group (Ca), focusing on the relationship between nucleic acid metabolizing enzymes and 5-FU incorporation into RNA (FRNA) as well as tymidylate synthetase inhibition rate (TSIR). Of the enzyme concentrations in non-cancer and cancer sites, no difference was observed with dyhydropyridine (DPD) at the either site, whereas significantly higher concentrations were detected with orotate phosphoribosyl transferase (OPRT), thymidine phosphorylase (TP), uridine phosphorylase (UP), and tymidine synthetase (TS) free at cancerous than non-cancerous sites ($p<0.0005$). Among the enzymes, correlations were found between

---

[*] A version of this chapter was also published in *Cancer Metastases Research*, edited by Akira Watanabe, published by Nova Science Publishers, Inc. It was submitted for appropriate modifications in an effort to encourage wider dissemination of research.

[*] Correspondence concerning this article should be addressed to: Kenji Katsumata, M. D. Department of Surgery, Tokyo Medical University, 6-7-1, Nishi-Shinjyuku, Shinjyuku-ku, Tokyo, 160-0023, Japan. E-mail:k-katsu@tokyo-med.ac.jp; Tel: 81-03-3342-6111.

TP and UP in No (p=0.01), and, in Ca, correlations were seen TP and UP (p=0.01) and between DPD and TS free (p=0.05). There was no correlation between the enzymes in group R-No, whereas in group R-Ca, correlations were found between FRNA and OPRT (p=0.01), and between TSIR and OPRT as well as TS free (p=0.05); in group C-No, correlations were seen between FRNA and UP as well as TS free (p=0.05), and TSIR and TS free (p=0.05); and, in group C-Ca, correlations were observed between FRNA and DPD (p=0.05), and between TSIR and TS free (p=0.05). These findings indicated that 5-FU metabolism in the large intestine differed at non-cancer or cancer sites and by different 5-FU administration methods.

And we examined the correlation among immunostaining metabolic enzyme of nucleic acid and clinicopathologic factors, prognosis. Result showed TP staining positive cases had a higher incident of progression (p=0.0403) and those with TS staining (p=0.0324). These cases had lower 5-year survival rates. But DPD had no incidence of these factors. These findings suggested that TP and TS are prognostic factors of colorectal cancer patients.

Keywords: Colorectal cancer, Preoperative 5-fluorouracil, Metabolic enzymes of nucleic acid, FRNA/TSIR, prognostic factor.

INTRODUCTION

Chemotherapy against colorectal cancer often includes 5-FU to increase efficacy and to decrease adverse drug reactions. Nevertheless, some patients with colorectal cancer show have ineffective clinical responses. In order to select the patients in whom regimens with 5-FU are effective and to establish tailor-made treatments, it is necessary to predict the metabolic pathway of 5-FU. It is necessary to examine the all not just some of the enzymes relating to 5-FU metabolism, and to investigate the enzymes thought that the different enzymes may be involved in such different lesions as non-cancer and cancer sites and according to different administration regimens of 5-FU. Thus, in the present study, we employed the following procedures: 1) 5-FU was administered by either drip infusion or continuous venous injection; 2) enzymes related to 5-FU metabolism were measured, i.e., OPRT, TP, UP, TS and DPD, together with TSIR and FRNA, in both the non-cancer and cancer sites; 3) 5-FU metabolism pathway was analyzed; and 4) prediction of treatment efficacy and adverse reaction of 5-FU were investigated.

And it was reported that these enzymes were correlation with clinicopathogic factors and prognosis. Especially TP staining was strongly correlation with colorectal prognostic factors, not enzyme activities. Further immunostaining investigation may clarify correlations between enzymes and clinicopathologic factors or prognosis of colorectal cancer. We examined correlation between TP, TS, DPD staining and prognosis of colorectal cancer.

MATERIALS AND METHODS

The present study employed 35 patients with colorectal cancer. The patients included: 22 men and 13 women (mean age, 64.4). Cancer stages were: stage I, one patient; stage II, 18; stages IIIA and IIIB, 9; and stage IV, 7. The 35 patients were divided into 2 groups: those given preoperative 5-FU, 500 mg/day for 3 days, over 2 hours by drip infusion (group R); and those given preoperative 5-FU, 500 mg/day, by continuous venous injection (group C). Then, we measured the concentrations of nucleic acid metabolizing enzymes and FRNA in the cancer and non-cancer sites in groups R and C.

Group R included: 11 men and 5 women (mean age, 66.7). Cancer stages were: stage II, 7 patients; stages IIIA and IIIB, 4; and stage IV, 5. Group C included: 11 men and 8 women (mean age, 62.5). Cancer stages were: stage I, one patient; stage II, 11; stages IIIA and IIIB, 5; and stage IV, 2.

Measuring Methods

The enzymes activities were measured as follows. Resected specimens were immediately washed with physiological saline, and 0.5 g of each specimen, from the cancer and non-cancer sites were stored at -80°C.

OPRT was assayed using Parker Disk method [1]. The specimens were added by the extracted enzyme solution (including 1.5 mM $Mgcl_2$, 2.0 mM dithiothreitol, and 50 mM Tris-Hcl buffer, pH 7.5), homogenized and centrifuged (105,000 x g, one hour, 4°C), and the supernatant was collected. The supernatant was added to a substrate of [^{3}H]-5-FU and incubated at 37°C, and the solutions were separately collected at 5, 10 and 15 minutes after starting the incubation. Each of the solutions of were warmed in a hot water bath at 100°C to stop the reaction and then centrifuged to obtain the reacted solutions. The preparations were put on DEAE-cellulose/ion-exchange filter paper to be washed repeatedly to remove non-reacted [^{3}H]-5-FU. [^{3}H]-FUMP, absorbed to the filter paper, was added by liquid scintisole to measure radioactivity of the resulting products. The enzyme activities were measured based on the reaction rates obtained by both the reaction time and concentration of the resulting products. OPRTase activity (n mol/min/mg protein) per protein was calculated based on the separately measured protein concentration.

As for TP and UP measurements, the test tissues were homogenized and added to 10 μM [^{14}C]-5-FU and 4 mM dRibl-P (TP), or 4 mM Ribl-P (UP) and 50 mM Tris-HCl buffer (pH 7.4), and reacted for 30 minutes, and added by 2M perchloric acid solution, to stop the reaction. The reacted solution was cooled in ice water to be centrifuged, and the degenerated protein was excluded. The supernatant was neutralized by 2 N KOH to be pasted on a thin-layer chromatography (TLC) plate, and the preparation was developed at room temperature using a development solvent of chloroform ethyl acetate ethanol. Then, FUra was extracted under a ultraviolet lamp. The preparation in a vial was added by 10 mL scintillator to be measured the radioactivity using scintillation counter. Radioactivities of TP and UP were shown by n mol of 5-FU that had been reduced during one minute under the reaction above [2].

TS was measured using Radio-binding assay [3]. In concrete, the test tissue was added by extracted solution of the enzyme (50 mM KH_2PO_2, pH 7.4) to be homogenized and centrifuged, and the resulting supernatant was divided into 2 parts. Then, concentrations of both the TS total (a complex of TS and TS-FdUMP-CH_2FH_4) and TS free (TS), and TSIR was calculated using a formula of [1-(TS free/TS total)] x 100.

DPD activity was measured using RI-HPLC [4]. In particular, the test tissue was added by extracted solution of the enzyme to be homogenized and centrifuged (105,000 x g, one hour, 4°C), and the supernatant was collected. The supernatant of 250 µL was added by both 12.5 µL of 6.25 mM NADPH solution and 50 µL of [^{3}H]-5-FU solution (125 µM 25 µCi-mL), incubated at 37°C, and the solutions were separately collected 10, 20 and 30 minutes after the incubation. Each of the preparations was added by an equal volume of 5% $HClO_4$ solution to be stopped the reaction. The resulting solutions were added by 140 µL of the mobile phase (20mM NaH_2PO_4, pH 3.5 to be centrifuged, and the supernatant was analyzed using RI-HPLC. The reaction rate was calculated basing on the generated quantities of both 5-FU and its metabolites such as DHFU, FUPa and FBAL. And DPD enzyme activity per protein (p mol/min/mg protein) was calculated basing on the protein concentrations separately assayed.

FRNA was measured using capillary gas chromatography-mass spectrometry [5]. In concrete, the test tissue was added to 200-500 mL water, homogenized and added to ice-cooled 10% trichloroacetic acid (TCA), centrifuged and removed the supernatant to collect the precipitation. The precipitation was washed each one time by 70% and 95% ethanol, then washed twice by ethanol diethyl ether. And resulting precipitation was added by 0.3 N potassium hydroxide to be hydrolyzed for 20 hours at 37°C. The preparation was added by 60% perchloric acid to finally obtain 0.5 N perchloric acid. This solution was centrifuged to collect the supernatant to be neutralized by 3 N potassium hydroxide, and removed newly produced precipitation to obtain mononucleotide solution. To this solution were added equal volume of 12 N hydrochloric acid and further added, as an intrinsic standard substance, a constant volume of 1, 3-bis- [^{15}N]-5-FU to be hydrolyzed for 20 hours at 100°C to collect solution of nucleic acid bases. The solution was washed by chloroform to collect the upper layer to be concentrated and dried using nitrogen purging, to which was added 1 M buffer solution of phosphoric acid (pH 4.0) to be extracted using ethyl acetate. The extracted solution was concentrated and dried to be purified using silica gel column method, the same method as to measure 5-FU being liberated in the test tissue, and 5-FU fragment was obtained. The preparation was concentrated to be added solution of N_2O-bis (trimethylsilyl)-trifluoroacetamide/etyl acetate (3/1), and was trimethylsilyed for 30 minutes at 75°C. Then, 5-FU concentration in mononucleotide solution was assayed by gas chromatography-mass spectrometry (GC-MS).

Using aliquot of this mononucleotide solution, RNA reduced concentration was assayed by orcinol method employing yeast-derived RNA as the standard substance. Thus, concentrations of 5-FU in both the test specimens and the RNA.

Regarding preoperative 5-FU administration, the patients were given informed consent that the preoperative administration of 5-FU was performed for a purpose to predict efficacy and adverse drug reaction. As for statistical analysis, T-test was used to compare both the test subjects and the enzyme activities, and Spearman's coefficient was employed to analyze correlations between each metabolic enzyme and TSIR as well as FRNA. And $p<0.05$ was regarded as significance.

The subjects of immunostaining were 82 patients with colorectal cancer. The mean age was 63.7. Cancer stages were: stage I, 10 patients; stage II, 32; stages IIIA and IIIB, 26; and stage IV,14.

The immunostaining was done using anti-dThd-pase mouse monoclonal antibody (Roche-654-1). Tissue samples were sectioned into 3μm slice and placed on vectabond (Vector,Burlingame,CA,USA) coated glass slides. The deparaffinized sections were placed in 0.1 M citrate buffer (pH6.0) and heated in a microwave over for a 5 min twice (500W). After being washed with phosphate buffered saline (PBS), the sections were treated with 3%(w/v) skim milk in PBS at room temperature and incubated with the primary 654-1(1μm/ml) were further incubated with biotinylated anti-mouse IgG for 30 min at room temperature. Thereafter, the sections were treated with 1 mg/ml periodic acid in PBS for 10 min to block endogenous peroxide activity. After being washed again with PBS, the sections were incubated with Avidine-Biotin Complex, Vectastain ABC Kit, (Vector, Burlingame, CA, USA) for 30 min at room temperature, and developed with 1 mg/ml diaminobezidine tetrahydro-chloride in PBS containing 0.003% (v/v) hydrogen peroxide. The sections were also counterstained with methylgreen and mounted.

The immunostaining of TS was done using anti-recombinant TS specific antibody RTSSA. The immunostainig of DPD was done using anti-DPD polyclonal antibody.

TP classification according to results of staining ratio for cancer cells included: negative 10% below, positive over 10%. TS classification according to results of staining ratio for cancer cells included: negative 30% below, positive over 30%. DPD classification according to results of staining ratio for cancer cells included: negative 70% below, positive over 70%.

RESULTS

1. Comparison between Metabolic Enzymes' Activities in Non-Cancer and Cancer Sites

Table 1. Correlation between cancer and non-cancer sites of metabolic enzymes of nucleic acid in colon cancer patient

		cancer site	non-cancer site	significant difference
DPD	n=25	28.2±3.2	26.0±3.0	0.586
OPRT	n=27	0.24±0.03	0.11±0.02	*0.0005>
TP	n=27	15.7±1.4	3.7±0.5	*0.0005>
UP	n=22	7.6±1.0	1.5±0.3	*0.0005>
TSf	n=27	12.5±1.8	4.4±0.9	*0.0005>

The significant difference was seen for OPRT, TP, UP and TS free.

Results included: OPRT in non-cancer site, 0.11±0.002 n mol/min/mg; OPRT in cancer site, 0.24±0.03 n mol/min/mg; TP in non-cancer site, 3.75±0.52 n mol/min/mg; TP in cancer site, 15.09±1.41 n mol/min/mg; UP in non-cancer site, 1.57±0.28 n mol/min/mg; UP in cancer site, 5.18±2.30 n mol/min/mg; TS free in non-cancer site, 4.42±0.86 p mol/g; TS free in cancer site, 12.48±1.79 p mol/g; DPD in non-cancer site, 26.04±3.00 p mol/min/mg; DPD in cancer site, 28.2±3.21 pmol/min/mg.

DPD showed no difference between non-cancer and cancer sites though, OPRT, TP, UP and TS free showed significant differences between the both sites (p<0.0005) (Table1). As for correlations between the test enzymes, TP and UP showed correlation in non-cancer site (p=0.01), and, in cancer site, correlations were found between TP and UP (p=0.01) and between DPD and TS free (p=0.05) (Table2).

Table 2. Correlation of metabolic enzymes of nucleic acid for cancer and non cancer sites in colon cancer patients

non-cancer site	DPD	OPRT	TP	UP	TSf
DPD	----	----	----	----	----
OPRT	0.286	----	----	----	----
TP	0.081	- 0.049	----	----	----
UP	- 0.004	- 0.230	0.937**	----	----
TSf	- 0.022	- 0.024	0.132	0.309	----
cancer site	DPD	OPRT	TP	UP	TSf
DPD	----	----	----	----	----
OPRT	- 0.076	----	----	----	----
TP	0.106	- 0.059	----	----	----
UP	0.156	- 0.105	0.905**	----	----
TSf	- 0.588**	- 0.204	0.089	-0.049	----

Spearman 's test * P>0.05 **P>0.01.

2. Assessment of Correlation between the Test Enzymes and FRNA as well as TSIR

Table 3. Correlation between metabolic enzymes of nucleic acid and FRNA/TSIR for cancer and non-cancer sites in rapid venons infusion group (n=16)

	cancer site		non-cancer site	
	FRNA	TSIR	FRNA	TSIR
OPRT	0.945**	-0.588*	0.056	0.413
TP	-0.176	0.406	-0.209	0.100
UP	-0.429	0.405	0.36	0.190
TSf	-0.214	-0.587*	0.054	-0.034
DPD	-0.190	-0.213	-0.611	-0.033

Spearman 's test *P>0.05 **P>0.01.

(1) In group R-No, no enzyme showed correlations to FRNA or TSIR.
(2) In group R-Ca, correlations were observed between FRNA and OPRT (p=0.01) and between TSIR and OPRT (p=0.05); and negative correlation was seen between TSIR and TS free (p=0.05) (Table3).
(3) In group C-No, correlations were found between FRNA and UP as well as TS free (p=0.05), and negative correlation was seen between TSIR and TS free (p=0.05).
(4) In group C-Ca, negative correlations were observed between FRNA and DPD (p=0.05) and between TSIR and TS free (p=0.05) (Table4).

Table 4. Correlation between metabolic enzymes of nucleic acid and FRNA/TSIR for cancer and non-cancer sites in continuous venons infusion group (n=19)

	cancer site		non-cancer site	
	FRNA	TSIR	FRNA	TSIR
OPRT	-0.287	0.254	-0.138	0.126
TP	0.041	0.147	0.497	-0.281
UP	-0.017	-0.011	0.665*	-0.281
TSf	0.427	-0.706**	0.606*	-0.601*
DPD	-0.619*	-0.215	-0.168	-0.011

Spearman's test *P>0.05 **P>0.01.

3. Correlation between Immunostaining Enzymes and Clinicopathologic Factor, Prognosis

(1) TP staining positive cases had a higher incidence of vascular invasion (p=0.007) and progression (p=0.040). TP staining positive cases had low 5-year survival rate. The positive group was 67.9%, negative group was 80.0% (p=0.008) (Table5).

Table 5. Correlation between TP staining and pathological factors

TP Staining			> 10%	10% ≤	
Invasion to the wall	- mp		9	3	
	ss -		32	38	
Lymph node metastasis	negative		25	18	
	positive		16	23	
Vascular permeation	negative		30	17	p=0.0074
	positive		11	24	
Stage	Dukes	A	8	2	
		B	17	15	p=0.0403
		C	13	13	
		D	3	11	

(2) TS staining positive cases had a higher incident of progression (p=0.032). TS staining positive cases had low 5-year survival rate. The positive group was 67.5%, negative group was 88.9% (p=0.081) (Table6).

(3) There was no significant difference between DPD positive staining group and negative group (Table7).

Table 6. Correlation between TS staining and pathological factors

TP Staining			> 30%	30% ≤	
Invasion to the wall	- mp		9	3	
	ss -		21	49	
Lymph node metastasis	negative		15	28	
	positive		14	25	
Vascular permeation	negative		22	25	
	positive		7	28	
Stage	Dukes	A	7	3	
		B	9	23	p=0.0324
		C	10	16	
		D	4	10	

Table 7. Correlation between DPD staining and pathological factors

DPD Staining			> 70%	70% ≤
Invasion to the wall	- mp		8	3
	ss -		36	34
Lymph node metastasis	negative		25	17
	positive		20	19
Vascular permeation	negative		25	21
	positive		19	16
Stage	Dukes	A	6	3
		B	18	14
		C	13	13
		D	7	7

DISCUSSION

5-FU is phosphorylated to develop anti-tumor activity. Enzymes for this phosphorylation in the cancer site are reportedly TP, UP and OPRT [6]. These enzymes play a role to generate; FRNA causing RNA impairment, and to generate FdUMP performing TS inhibition resulting in the DNA impairment [6]. It is also reported that DPD decomposes 5-FU into fluoro-βalanine, an inactivated product of 5-FU [7]. Basing on administration method of 5-FU, mechanism of anti-tumor cell of 5-FU reportedly includes 2 modalities such as higher concentrations of 5-FU resulting in shorter activities and lower concentrations of the drug resulting in longer activities [8], both of which may cause impairments of the RNA and DNA.

There are few reports indicating 5-FU metabolism in non-cancer site resulting in lesser finding of the adverse drug reaction. Whereas, basing on findings obtained by numerous studies of 5-FU metabolism in cancer site, anticancer drugs such as: to inhibit DPD activity to prohibit 5-FU degradation; to increase the drug concentration in tumor tissues; to inhibit OPRT activity in the digestive tract mucous membrane resulting in lesser adverse drug reaction [9]. These circumstances led us to a thought that metabolic pathway of 5-FU in non-cancer site should be urgently clarified.

In the present study with colorectal cancer patients, we measured enzymes such as OPRT, TP, UP and DPD, as well as FRNA. The patients preoperatively received 5-FU by either intravenous drip infusion or continuous venous injection. And basing on findings of the DNA impairment resulting from TSIR [6] and of the RNA impairment resulting from FRNA [10], we examined correlations between the enzymes and the DNA and RNA impairments in cancer and non-cancer sites. We employed such preoperative 5-FU administration as reported by Jacob et al. [11] that: 500 mg/body was effective; and 3 days dosing periods for purposes to ensure a short half-life of 5-FU metabolism resulting in neither adverse drug reaction nor reduction of umbalanced concentrations in the tumor tissue.

As for the enzyme concentrations in non-cancer and cancer sites, results in the present study showed that the enzymes except DPD were higher in the cancer site than in the non-cancer site as previously reported [12]. The present study also revealed correlations between such enzymes in non-cancer site as TP and UP, while, in cancer site, between TP and UP as well as DPD and TS free. A high level correlations between TP and UP in the both sites suggests that the 2 enzymes cooperatively work in the both sites. Correlation between DPD and TS free was supposedly resulted from inactivation of 5-FU by the enzymes. This supposedly results from a fact that DPD with a high concentration results in decreasing TSIR and increasing TS free activity.

Although 5-FU supposedly produces FRNA through the pathways of OPRT, TP and UP resulting in the RNA impairment, a pathway of OPRT is suggestively important [13]. It is also reported that anti-tumor efficacy of 5-FU depends on the pathway to inactivate the drug by DPD causing 85% degradation of 5-FU [14]. This corresponds to a finding that high concentrations of DPD and TS cause a reduction of TSIR resulting in an insufficient efficacy of 5-FU [15].

Results of our present study showed that drip infusion of 5-FU revealed significant positive correlation between FRNA and OPRT in the carcinoma. Although it has been reported that OPRT concentration is essentially low, the phosphorylated aliquot exists in a high concentration suggesting an important role of OPRT. Results of the present study support and prove the finding above. The present study also shows positive correlation between OPRT and TSIR to indicate an importance of the pathway through OPRT, i.e, from FUDP to FdUDP and FdUMP. This finding coincides a report by Fukushima et., al. [16], whereas no tendency was found in correlations between the substances. In non-cancer site, this may result from a fact that the enzymes are in lesser qualities in the non-cancer site.

With continuous administration of 5-FU, results of the present study showed a significant negative correlation in the cancer site. This supposedly resulted from previous finding that:

continuous venous injection of 5-FU primarily results in efficacy against the DNA though, a certain anti-RNA efficacy of the drug is also found; 5-FU has a primary pathway from FUDP to FdUMP; thus, continuous venous injection of 5=FU is supposedly much more influenced by DPD, an inactivating enzyme against 5-FU, than in case of venous drip infusion of the drug. And, in the pathway, FU nucleotide is slowly generated and is capably produced by any of the pathway. Thus, no definite pathway is definitely proven.

In the non-cancer site, DPD showed less influence, and TS free as well as UP correlate to FRNA. This may indicates that, unlike in case of cancer site, UP plays a role in the pathway to generate FRNA, and UP correlates to TS free, and that the pathway from FUTP to FdUMP is not the primary route. While 5-FU given by continuous venous injection capably interrupts the FUTP pathway to decrease the adverse drug reaction. Lesser clinical significance of TS free is controversial, i.e, is this results from an assumption that TS free has lesser ribonucleotide reductase or that TS free essentially has different metabolic pathway from other enzymes. It is also suggested that, in non-cancer site, metabolic pathway of UP is important. For example, UP has a secondarily significant role following to that of OPRT for 5-FU metabolism [17]. Results of our present study supports this report above.

Findings above suggest that: in cancer site, 5-FU by drip infusion is primarily metabolized through OPRT pathway resulting in strong relationships to FRNA generation and TSIR; and 5-FU by continuous venous injection is intensively metabolized through DPD pathway. These are conceivably supported by clinical fields.

Whereas, no constant tendency was seen by 5-FU drip infusion against non-cancer site. Neither constant tendency was observed by continuous venous injection of 5-FU, although FRNA showed relationship to UP and TS free. This supposedly results from a finding reported by Philip [18] et al. that 5-FU is primarily absorbed through the small intestine, but is hardly absorbed through the large intestine.

Recently FOLFOX is used as a world standard treatment for advanced and recurrent colon cancer [19,20]. The rate of effectiveness is high, and the treatment has done in Japan two years ago. However, this is not a habitual treatment in Japan for the following reasons: complication in the introduction of CV, catheter troubles, neurotoxicity, characterized side effects of L-OHP [21], side effects such as allergic reaction, which later cause problems [23], and continuous administration of a high dose of 5-FU. Nevertheless, supportive therapy for these was devised, and in this institution as well, several supportive therapies have been tried and are going well. However, continuous administration of a high dose of 5-FU caused a new problem. It is hyperammonaemia, which was considered to be caused by the continuous administration of a high dose of 5-FU was observed. We have experienced two cases (2.4%). Yeh *et al* [24], speculated the cause as a high amount of fluoroacetate, production of intermediate products of 5-FU, damaged citric acid cycle related to ATP production, which caused lactic acidosis, damaging the urea cycle and thereby elevating ammonia. According to Matsubara *et al.* [25], 5-FU converts into fluorocitric acid or fluoroacetate *in vivo*. Citrate converts into aconitic acid in the TCA cycle, which is necessary as an enzyme aconitase. Fluorocitric acid or fluoroacetate inhibits this aconitase and accumulates citrate in said damaged urea cycle from α-ketoglutaric acid, which appeared as ammonia accumulation [26]. On the other hand, Valik [27] mentioned the factors as DPD deficiency and stress induced in an abnormal urea cycle due to a mitochondrial disorder.

However, according to Lin YC et al [28], after this same treatment has combined with CDDP, the incidence rate of hyperammonaemia was 9%, and renal function fell due to CDDP, which should be considered as one factor. From the above point of view, it was suggested correlations with DPD, which has 5-FU catabolism. DPD is a catabolic enzyme, and it is well known that 5-FU side effects are exacerbated when DPD levels are low [29]. The intestinal tract and carcinoma DPD are almost normal, and metabolism is predictable *in vivo* from carcinoma DPD [30]. It is considered somewhat relevant to DPD but does not show any significant difference. The only point of difference is the condition of performance. Reports from Europe and U.S.A. were not found as far as we have researched, so, influence dependent on race is also thinkable. As hyperammonaemia does not always relapse, the cause may not be unitary [31]. There are patients with light hyperammonaemia who present no clinical symptoms, so there is a possibility of the occurrence of impaired consciousness in the course of therapy. It is necessary to measure ammonia levels in the blood during administration and DPD, bearing in mind possible side effects.

And metabolic enzymes of nucleic acid have important prognostic factors [32,33]. They are correlated with clinicopathologic factors, prognosis and efficacy of postoperative adjuvant chemotherapy [34]. Especially TP and TS are prognostic factors of colorectal cancer and DPD combined with either TS or TP indicated the efficacy of postoperative adjuvant chemotherapy. Metabolic enzymes of nucleic acid in colon cancer are important factors with 5-FU metabolism, predict of efficacy and side effect and prognosis.

REFERENCES

[1] Laskin JD, Evance RM, Hakala MT, et al: Basis for natural variation in sensitivity to 5-FU in mouse and human cells in culture. *Cancer Res. 39*; 1-10, 1979.

[2] Horiuchi T, Suga S, Kimura K, et al: A fundamental study on clinical application of pyrimidine fluoride compounds — Metabolism of pyrimidine fluoride in cancer patients (No. 1). Rinsho Yakuri *Japanese Journal of Clinical Pharmacology 16*; 475-487, 1985.

[3] Spears CP, Gustavssoon BG, Mitchel MSS, et al: Thymidine synthetase inhibition in malignant tumors and normal liver of patients given intravenous 5-FU. *Cancer Res. 44*; 4144-4150, 1984.

[4] Harris BE, Song RR and Diasio RB: Relationship between DPD activity and plasma levels with evidence for circadian variation of enzyme activity and plasma levels in cancer patients receiving 5-FUby protracted continuous infusion. *Cancer Res. 50*; 197-201, 1990.

[5] Masuike T, Kikuchi K, Saitoh A, et al: Assay of 5-fluorouracil incorporated into RNA of the tissues using gas chromatography-mass spectrometry. Kagakuryoho no Ryoiki *Antibiotics and Chemotherapy 11*; 162-167, 1995.

[6] Takeda S, Uchida J, Yuda y, et al: Correlation between inhibition of thymidine synthase and anti-tumor efficacy of pyrimidine fluoride anticancer drugs. Gan To Kagakuryoho. *Japanese Journal of Cancer and Chemotherapy.15*; 2125-2129,1988.

[7] Choong YS and Lee SP: The degradation of 5'-deoxy-5-fluoridine by pyrimidine nucleoside phosphorylase and cancer tissue. *Clin. Chem. Acta 149*; 175-183, 1985.

[8] Hanatani Y, Kodaira S, Asagoe T, et al: Anti-tumor efficacy of 5-fluorouracil according to administration schedules — A study using nude mice grafted human gastric cancer strains. *Chemotherapy 42*; 1015-1020, 1994.

[9] Shirasaka T, Tsukuda m, Inuyama M, Taguchi t: A new trial with oral administration of TS-1 (S-1) — From the conception to clinical application. Gan To Kagakuryoho. *Japanese Jornal of Cancer and Chemotherapy. 28*; 855-864, 2001.

[10] Ikenaka K, Tanaka h, Kawai M, et al: a study on action mechanism of 5-fluoriuracil (5-FU) — Focusing on abnormal metabolism of RNA. Gan To Kagakuryohou. *Japanese Jornal of Cancer and Chemotherapy. 10*; 227-231, 1983.

[11] Lokich J J, Ahlgren J D, Gullo J J, et al: A prospective randomized comparison of continuous infusion fluorouracilwith a conventional bolus schedule in metastatic colorectal carcinoma. A Mild-Atlantic *Oncology Program Study Journal of Clinical Oncology* t; 425-432, 1989.

[12] Etienne MC, Cheradame S, Fischel J L, et al: Response to fluorouracil therapy in cancer patients — he role of tumoral dihydroprimidine dehydrogenase activity. *Journal of Clinical Oncology 13*; 1663-1670, 1995.

[13] Uchida M and Nakamura T: 5-fluorouracil metabolism in tumor cells. *Purine and Pyrimidine Metabolism 15*; 112-118, 1991.

[14] Etinen MC, Ohe'radame S, Fischel JL, et al: Response to fluorouracil therapy in cancer patients — the role of tumoral dihydropyrimidine dehydrogenase activity. Journal of Clinical Oncology *13*; 1663-1670, 1995.

[15] Patric G J, Heinz-Josef L, Cynthia GL, et al: Thymidylate synthasegene and protein expression correlate and are associated with response to 5-fluorouracil in human colorectal cancer. *Cancer Research*; 1407-1412, 1995.

[16] Fukushima M, Nomura Y, Murakami Y, et al: Analysis of phosphorylation pathway with 5-fluorouracil. Gan To kagakuryouho. *Japanese Journal of Cancer and Chemotherapy 6*; 721-731, 1996.

[17] Jeffrey D, Laskin R, Mark E, Harry K S, et al: Basis for natural variation in sensitivity to 5-fluorouracil in mouse and human cells in culture, *Cancer Research 39*; 383-390, 1979.

[18] Smith P, Mirabelli C, Fondacaro J, Ryman F, and Dent J: Intestinal 5-fluorouracil absorption — Use of Using chambers to assess transport and metabolism. *Pharmaceutical Research 5*; 598-603, 1988.

[19] de Gramont, A. Figer, M. Seymour, M. Homerin, A. Hmissi, J. Cassidy, C. Boni, et al. Leucovorin and Fluorouracil With or Without Oxaliplatin as First-Line Treatment in Advanced Colorectal Cancer. *J. Clin. Oncol.* 2000; 18 2938-2947.

[20] Richard M. Goldberg, Daniel J. Sergeant, Roscoe F. Morton, Charles S. Fuchs, Ramesh K. Ramanathan, Stephen K. Williamson, et al. A Randomized Controlled Trial of Fluorouracil Plus Leucovorin, Irinotecan and Oxaliplatin Combinations in Patients With Previously Untreated Metastatic Colorectal Cancer. *J. Clin. Oncol.* 2004; 22 23-30.

[21] Axel Grothey: Oxaliplatin-Safety Profile: Neurotoxicity. *Seminars in Oncology* 2003; 30 5-13.

[22] Frederique Maindrault-Goebel, Thierry Andre, Christophe Tourhigand, Christophe Louvet, Nathalie Perez-Stauz, Nora Zeghib, et al. Allergic-Type Reactions to Oxaliplatin: Retrospective Analysis of 42 patients. *Eur. J. Cancer* 2005; 41 2262-2267.

[23] Laurence Gamelin, Michele Boisdron-Celle, Remy Delva, Veronique Guerin-Meyer, Norbert Ifrah, Alain Morel, et al. Prevention of Oxaliplatin-Related Neurotoxicity by Calcium and Magnesium Infusion: A Retrospective Study of 161 Patients Receiving Oxaliplatin Combined with 5-Fluorouracil and Leucovorin for Advanced Colorectal Cancer. *Clin. Cancer Res.* 2004; 10 4055-4061.

[24] K H Yeh and AL Cheng: High-Dose 5-Fluorouracil Infusional Therapy is Associated with Hyperammonaemia, Lactic Acidosis and Encephalopathy. *Brit. J. Cancer* 1997; 75 464-465.

[25] Matsubara I, Kamiya J, Imai S: Cardiotoxic Effects of 5-Fluorouracil on the Guinea Pig. Jpn J pharmacol 30: 871-879, 198011) D Valik: Encephalopathy, Lactic Acidosis, Hyperammonaemia and 5-Fluorouracil Toxicity. *Brit. J. Cancer* 1998;77 1710-1712.

[26] Robert K. Murray, Daryl K. Granner, Peter A. Mayes and Victor W. Rodwell: Chapter 18. *The Citric Acid Cycles: The Catabolism of Acetyl-Coa. Harper's Biochemistry.* 25th Edition 196-204.

[27] D Valik: Encephalopathy, Lactic Acidosis, Hyperammonaemia and 5-Fluorouracil Toxicity. *Brit. J. Cancer* 1998; 77 1710-1712.

[28] Yung-Chang Lin, Jen-Shi Chen, Cheng-Hsu Wang, Hung-Ming Wang, Hseng-Kun Chang, Chi-Ting Liau, et al. Weekly High-Dose 5-Fluorouracil (5-FU), Leucovorin (LV) and Bimonthly Cisplatin in Patients with Advanced Gastric Cancer. *Jpn. J. Clin. Oncol.* 2001; 31 605-609.

[29] Dennis Salonga, Kathleen D. Dannenberg, Martin Johson, Ralf Metzger, Susan Groshen, Denice D.Taso-Wei, et al. Colorectal Tumors Responding to 5-Fluorouracil Have Low Gene Expression Levels of Dihydropyrimidine Dehydrogenase, Thymidylate Synthase, and Thymidine Phosphorylase. *Clin. Cancer Res.* 2000; 6 1322-1327.

[30] Katsumata K, Sumi T, Murohashi T, et al. Analysis of Colon Cancer Salvage System Nucleic Acid Synthetic Route Enzyme. *Jpn. J. Cancer Chemother.* 2000; 27 1415-1420.

[31] Chuang-Chi Liaw: Transit Hyperammonaemia Related to Chemotherapy with Continuous Infusion of High-Dose 5-Fluorouracil. *Anti-Cancer Drug* 1993; 4: 311-315.

[32] Yamachika T, Nakanishi H, Inada K, et al.: A new prognostic factor for colorectal carcinoma, thymidylate synthase, and its therapeutic significance. *Cancer* 82: 71-77, 1998.

[33] Katsumata K, Sumi T, Yamashita S, et al: The significance of thymidine phosphorylase expression in colorectal cancer. *Oncol. Rep.* 8: 127-130, 2001.

[34] Katsumata K. Sumi T, Wada T: et al: *Prognosis and Efficacy of Postoperative Adjuvant Chemotherapy in Colorectal cancer Correlates with Nucleic Acid Metabolizing Enzymes* 2004; 31: 1357-1360.

In: Rectal Cancer: Etiology, Pathogenesis and Treatment
Editors: Paula Wells and Regina Halstead

ISBN 978-1-60692-563-8
© 2009 Nova Science Publishers, Inc.

Chapter VIII

GERMLINE AND SOMATIC MUTATIONS IN COLORECTAL CANCERS FROM PATIENTS WITH HEREDITARY NONPOLYPOSIS COLORECTAL CANCER[*]

Michiko Miyaki[1,†], *Tatsuro Yamaguchi*[1,2] *and Takeo Mori*[2]
[1]Hereditary Tumor Research Project, [2]Department of Surgery, Tokyo Metropolitan Komagome Hospital, Tokyo, Japan

ABSTRACT

Hereditary nonpolyposis colorectal cancer (HNPCC) is one of the most common hereditary colon cancer syndromes. The causative genes of HNPCC are DNA mismatch repair genes, and inactivation of these genes triggers HNPCC tumors.

We detected germline mutations of the hMSH2, hMLH1 and hMSH6 genes in Japanese HNPCC families. These mutations included single-base substitutions and frameshifts, both resulting in truncated proteins, a mutation at the splice donor site of exon 5, and a 2kb genomic deletion encompassing exon 5. The coexistence of germline and somatic mutations of DNA mismatch repair genes was observed in colorectal and extracolorectal cancers. The majority of somatic mutations were frameshift, one was a mutation at the splice donor site of exon 5, and two were loss of the normal allele. All HNPCC cancers exhibited high microsatellite instability. Sixty-four % of HNPCC colorectal cancers included somatic mutations of either the APC or ß-catenin gene, whereas only 13% of the cancers had p53 mutations and none of the cancer cases showed the BRAF mutation. The loss of heterozygosity at tumor suppressor regions

---

[*] A version of this chapter was also published in *New Developments in Mutation Research*, edited by Charles L. Valon, published by Nova Science Publishers, Inc. It was submitted for appropriate modifications in an effort to encourage wider dissemination of research.

[†] Correspondence concerning this article should be addressed to: Michiko Miyaki; Hereditary Tumor Research Project, Tokyo Metropolitan Komagome Hospital, 3-18-22 Honkomagome, Bunkyo-ku, Tokyo 113-8677, Japan; Tel: +81-3-3823-2101 (ext. 4425), Fax: +81-3-3823-5433, E-mail: mmiyaki@opal.famille.ne.jp.

(chromosomes 5q, 8p, 17p, 18q and 22q) was not observed. We also detected frequent somatic frameshift mutations of growth-related genes with coding repeats in HNPCC colorectal cancers. Mutation frequencies at these repeats were 77% at TGFßRII(A)$_{10}$, 55% at hMSH3(A)$_8$, 52% at CASP5(A)$_{10}$, 48% at BAX(G)$_8$, 48% at RIZ(A)$_8$ and (A)$_9$, 45% at RAD50(A)$_9$, 45% at MBD4(A)$_{10}$, 36% at hMSH6(C)$_8$, 23% at BLM(A)$_9$, 19% at IGFIIR(G)$_8$ and 19% at PTEN(A)$_6$.

The present data have the following implications: Inactivation of DNA mismatch repair genes through germline and somatic mutations causes genetic instability resulting in somatic mutations in various growth-related genes. Disruption of the WNT signaling pathway by mutations of the APC or ß-catenin gene and disruption of the TGF-ß signaling pathway by alteration of the TGFßRII gene seem to largely contribute to the development of HNPCC colorectal cancer via adenomas. Moreover, inactivation of apoptosis-related genes, such as the BAX, CASP5 and RIZ genes, may also contribute to the development, and inactivation of the IGFIIR and PTEN genes play a role in the progression of HNPCC colorectal cancer.

INTRODUCTION

Colorectal cancer comprises hereditary and non-hereditary types. Hereditary colorectal cancer with an autosomal dominant mode of inheritance includes familial adenomatous polyposis (FAP), with numerous colonic polyps, and hereditary nonpolyposis colorectal cancer (HNPCC), without multiple colonic polyps. HNPCC cancer develops at an early age (mean of approximately 45 years) and accounts for 3%-6% of all colorectal cancers [1]. HNPCC also develops into extracolonic cancer, such as cancer of the endometrium, ovaries, stomach, small intestine, and hepatobiliary and urinary tracts. HNPCC results from germline mutations of DNA mismatch repair genes, including hMSH2 [2,3], hMLH1 [4,5], hMSH6 [6,7], hPMS1 [8] and hPMS2 [8]. Detection of germline mutations of mismatch repair genes is important in identifying HNPCC patients and in the follow up of patients with both colorectal and extracolorectal cancer, and is also significant in identifying non-carriers in HNPCC families.

Inactivation of these mismatch repair genes through germline and somatic mutations leads to mutations at microsatellite regions (microsatellite instability or replication error) [9,10] and frameshift mutations of repeated sequences in coding regions of various tumor-related genes [11], which triggers the development of HNPCC tumors. These properties in HNPCC patients are distinct from those in FAP and the majority of sporadic cancer patients. In the latter two cases, colorectal cancers develop via an adenoma-carcinoma sequence [12,13] by mutations of tumor suppressor genes, such as APC, p53 and Smad4, and oncogenes such as K-ras. To clarify the mechanisms of HNPCC colorectal carcinogenesis, it is necessary to determine the extent of the contribution of frameshift mutations in growth-related genes, as well as the mutations in tumor suppressor genes and oncogenes. In this study we analyzed germline and somatic mutations of DNA mismatch repair genes, as well as mutations in various tumor-related genes in HNPCC cancer.

MATERIALS AND METHODS

Clinical Characterization of HNPCC Families

Pedigrees of independent Japanese families that include multiple patients with colorectal cancer were clinically analyzed. HNPCC families that fit the Amsterdam criteria II [14] were selected for DNA analysis. The criteria are: (a) at least three relatives must have a cancer associated with HNPCC (colorectal, endometrial, stomach, ovary, ureter or renal-pelvis, brain, small-bowel, hepatobiliary tract, or skin), (b) one must be a first-degree relative of the other two, (c) at least two successive generations must be affected, and (d) at least one of the relatives with cancer associated with HNPCC should have received the diagnosis before the age of 50 years.

Samples and DNA Preparation

Tumor tissues, corresponding normal tissues and peripheral blood were obtained after full informed consent, and analysis of these samples was approved by the Komagome Hospital Review Committee. DNA was prepared from each sample using SDS-proteinase K and phenol-chloroform. RNA was extracted using the guanidine thiocyanate method.

Analysis of Germline Mutations of DNA Mismatch Repair Genes

Analysis of germline mutations of the hMSH2, hMLH1 and hMSH6 genes by PCR-SSCP was performed as follows: The PCR reaction mixture (6 µl) contained 300 ng of genomic DNA from normal tissue, 0.2 µM of each primer, 25 µM each of four dNTPs, 1 X PCR buffer, Taq polymerase and [α-^{32}P]dCTP. PCR conditions were: 5 min at 97 °C once; 1 min at 94 °C, 1 min at 58 °C and 1 min at 72 °C for 35 cycles; and 10 min at 72 °C once. Primers used to amplify the 16 coding exons of the hMSH2 gene were the same as those previously reported [15,16], and primers used to amplify the 19 exons of the hMLH1 gene were the same as those previously described [4,5] and primers for the 10 exons of the hMSH6 gene were designed based on the reported sequence [17]. PCR products were diluted with formamide-dye solution, heated for 5 min at 80 °C, and applied to 5% polyacrylamide gel containing 5% glycerol. The gel was then exposed to X-ray film. Aberrant single-strand DNA fragments were extracted with water from the corresponding band on SSCP gel. The extracted DNA fragments were amplified through asymmetrical PCR, purified using a purification kit, and then sequenced with dideoxy chain-termination reaction using T7 Sequenase V 2.0.

Analysis of germline genomic deletions of the hMSH2 gene by Southern blot hybridization was performed as follows: Probes for Southern blot hybridization were prepared by RT-PCR using total RNA from human normal tissue and a primer set (primer for probe A involving exons 1-5, for probe B involving exons 4-11 or for probe C involving exons 9-16 of the hMSH2 gene) under the conditions previously described [18]. RT-PCR products were subcloned in plasmids, and then confirmed by direct sequencing. Purified plasmids containing hMSH2 cDNA were labeled with Dig (Roche), and used for probes. For Southern blot hybridization, 5 µg genomic DNA from normal tissue of the patients was digested by 25 units of a restriction enzyme (*Eco*RI, *Hind*III or *Nsi*I) for 20 hr at 37 °C, electrophoresed in agarose gel for 20 hr at 20 V, and transferred to nylon membrane. The membrane was pre hybridized for 4 hr at 42 °C, and hybridized with Dig-labeled cDNA probe for 20 hr at 42 °C. After hybridization the membrane was washed at 65 °C, and exposed to X-ray film. Confirmation of a deleted exon of the hMSH2 gene was performed by RT-PCR-sequencing using total RNA from normal tissue of the patients.

Analysis of Somatic Mutations of DNA Mismatch Repair Genes

DNA samples of tumors were analyzed for somatic mutations of the hMSH2, hMLH1 ans hMSH6 genes by PCR-SSCP-sequencing under the same conditions as those for the analysis of germline mutations.

Analysis of Mutations at Repeated Sequences

DNA samples from tumors and corresponding normal tissues were amplified by PCR. The reaction mixture (6 µl) contained 300 ng of genomic DNA, 0.2 µM of ^{32}P-labeled forward primer, 0.2 µM of unlabeled reverse primer, 25 µM concentrations of each of four dNTPs, 1 X PCR buffer, and Taq polymerase. PCR was performed under the same conditions as those previously described [19]: 5 min at 97 °C once; 1 min at 94 °C, 1 min at 55 °C and 1 min at 72 °C for 35 cycles; and 10 min at 72 °C once. PCR products were diluted with formamide-dye solution and heated for 5 min at 80 °C, then applied to 6% polyacrylamide gel containing 7 M urea. The gel was then exposed to X-ray film. Primer sets used for the analysis of microsatellite instability were BAT25, BAT26, D2S123, D5S346 and D17S250 [20]. Primers used for repeated sequences in the coding region of tumor-related genes were the same as those previously reported: TGFßRII [11], IGFIIR [21], BAX [22], hMSH3 [23], hMSH6 [23], CASP5 [24], PTEN [25], MBD4 [26], RIZ [27], BLM [28] and RAD50 [29].

Analysis of Mutations of Tumor Suppressor Genes and Oncogenes

DNA samples of tumors were analyzed for mutations of the APC, ß-catenin, p53, K-ras and BRAF genes by PCR-SSCP-sequencing under the same conditions as those previously described [30-33]. Primers used were the same as those previously reported: APC [34], p53 [31], ß-catenin [35], K-ras [19] and BRAF [36].

Analysis of Loss of Heterozygosity

To analyze LOH in tumors, Southern blot hybridization was performed as described previously [37].

RESULTS

Germline Mutations of DNA Mismatch Repair Genes

The PCR-SSCP-sequencing method detected 6 hMSH2, 3 hMLH1 and 1 hMSH6 germline mutations in 10 independent Japanese HNPCC families (Table 1). The six hMSH2 mutations included 3 frameshifts and 2 single-base substitutions, both resulting in truncated proteins, and a mutation at the splice donor site of exon 5, resulting in deletion of exon 5. The three hMLH1 mutations included a frameshift mutation and a single-base substitution, resulting in truncated and extended proteins, and a deletion of one amino acid. The mutation of the hMSH6 gene was a frameshift mutation resulting in a truncated protein.

Table 1. Germline mutations of hMSH2, hMLH1 and hMSH6 genes in Japanese HNPCC families

HNPCC family	Gene	Exon	Codon	DNA change	Protein change
HNP1	hMSH2	3	136	TTT to TT	Truncation at codon 173-174
HNP4	hMSH2	4	227-229	AGAAAAAAA to AGAAAAAAAA	Truncation at codon 230-231
HNP2	hMSH2	7	419	CAG to TAG	Truncation at codon 419
HNP3	hMSH2	14	811	TTA to TGA	Truncation at codon 811
HNP5	hMSH2	15	877-878	AGAGAG to AGAG	Truncation at codon 880-881
HNP7	hMSH2	5	265-314	G/gta to G/gtt	Deletion of exon 5
HNP15	hMSH2	5	2 kb	Genomic deletion	Deletion of exon 5
HNP19	hMLH1	11	343	TAC to TAA	Truncation at codon 343
HNP8	hMLH1	16	616-618	AAGAAGAAG to AAGAAG	Deletion of a lysine
HNP20	hMLH1	19	712	TGG to TG	Extension of COOH terminus
HNP13	hMSH6	4	534	AAC to AA	Truncation at codon 570-571

In one HNPCC family a germline mutation of the hMSH2 gene could not be detected by the PCR-SSCP method, although this family fulfills the Amsterdam criteria and tumors from two affected individuals showed microsatellite instability, somatic mutations of the hMSH2 gene and a high frequency of alterations at repeated sequences of tumor-related genes. These characteristics of tumors and the presence of somatic hMSH2 mutations in tumors in this family were suggestive of the existence of a germline mutation in the same gene. The Southern blot hybridization method was then applied to detect this germline mutation. Genomic DNA from normal mucosa of an affected individual was digested by the restriction enzymes *Eco*RI, *Hind*III and *Nsi*I, respectively. These genomic digests were hybridized to three different hMSH2 cDNA probes, probe A involving exons 1-5, probe B involving exons 4-11 and probe C involving exons 9-16. The *Nsi*I digest of this patient's DNA exhibited an aberrant restriction fragment of 8.6 kb in addition to the normal fragment of 10.6 kb when hybridized with probe B. The same aberrant fragment was also observed in the hybridization with probe A. These patterns suggested the presence of a heterozygous 2 kb genomic deletion encompassing exon 4, 5 or 6, when referred to the reported restriction patterns of the hMSH2 gene [38]. Sequencing of the RT-PCR product of total RNA from the patient revealed the loss of exon 5 sequences. These results confirmed that the patient's germline mutation was a 2 kb genomic deletion encompassing exon 5 [18] (Table 1). An aberrant *Nsi*I fragment was also detected in the genomic DNA of normal tissue from the other patient but was not detected in healthy family members, which indicated that the 2 kb genomic deletion is pathogenic. The frequency of such a large genomic deletion is not so high, since 10 of 11 germline mutations detected in Japanese HNPCC families were frameshift, nonsense and alternative splicing mutations. The percentage of HNPCC families fulfilling the Amsterdam criteria and carrying the hMSH2 genomic deletion/rearrangement has been estimated to be nearly 10 % [39].

Table 2. Tumors produced in HNPCC families with hMSH2 and hMSH6 germline mutations

Tumor	hMSH2 No. of patient	(7 families) Mean age at diagnosis (yrs)	hMSH6 No. of patient	(1 family) Mean age at diagnosis (yrs)
Colorectal cancer	33/37 (89%)	42	1/6 (17%)	52
Endometrial cancer	7/21 (33%) [a]	44	3/4 (75%) [a]	58
Ovarian cancer	4/21 (19%) [a]	37	1/4 (25%) [a]	61
Gastric cancer	5/37 (14%)	52	0	
Urinary tract cancer	1/37 (3%)		0	
Prostate cancer	1/16 (6%) [b]	70	0	
Brain tumor	1/37 (3%)	49	0	
Skin cancer	1/37 (3%)	49	0	
Pancreatic cancer	0		1/6 (17%)	68
Multiple cancer	17/37 (46%)		2/6 (33%)	

a, female patient; b, male patient.

With respect to the effect of germline mutations on cancer pathogenesis, differences were observed between hMSH2 and hMSH6 (Table 2). Among patients in HNPCC families with hMSH2 germline mutations, 33 of the 37 patients (89%) were affected by colorectal cancers, with a mean age at diagnosis of 42. Of 21 female patients 7 (33%) had endometrial cancer at about the age of 44. In addition to these two most common types, there were ovarian (19%), gastric (14%), brain (3%), skin (3%), prostate (6%), and urinary tract (3%) cancers. In 17 cases (46%), a second, third, or even fourth primary cancer occurred in each patient [40]. In contrast to HNPCC families with hMSH2 mutations, the family with the hMSH6 mutation predominantly produced endometrial (75%) and ovarian (25%) cancers, with colorectal cancers being 17% [6]. The mean age of cancer formation in the family with the hMSH6 mutation was 58 years old, which is later than the mean age of 44 years for the appearance of cancer in families with hMSH2 mutations. Such clinical aspects suggest that the effect of germline mutations of the hMSH6 gene on cancer pathogenesis may be different from that of the hMSH2 mutation. A predominance of endometrial cancer and delayed cancer onset has also been reported for HNPCC families with hMSH6 mutations [41].

Table 3. Somatic mutations of hMSH2, hMLH1 and hMSH6 genes in HNPCC cancers

Tumor		Somatic mutation			Germline mutation
	Gene	Exon	Codon	DNA change	Gene
HNP1 CoCa	hMSH2	5	311-312	AACCTT to AACTT	hMSH2
HNP3 CoCa	hMSH2			Loss of normal allele	hMSH2
HNP4 CoCa	hMSH2	12	661	AAA to AAAA	hMSH2
HNP5 CoCa1	hMSH2	2	82-83	AAAATG to AAAAATG	hMSH2
HNP5 CoCa2	hMSH2	3	173-176	CTAGGACTGTGT to A	hMSH2
HNP7 CoCa1	hMSH2	13	690-691	CAAATT to CAATT	hMSH2
HNP7 CoCa2	hMSH2	5	311-312	AACCTT to AACTT	hMSH2
HNP15 DuoCa	hMSH2	4	227-229	AGAAAAAAA to AGAAAAAA	hMSH2
HNP15 GaCa	hMSH2	1	21	CGC to CAGC	hMSH2
HNP2 EnCa	hMSH2	5	265-314	G/gta to G/gtt	hMSH2
HNP8 CoCa	hMLH1			Loss of normal allele	hMLH1
HNP13 CoCa	hMSH6	2	128	CGT to CG	hMSH6
HNP13 EnCa	hMSH6	5	1085-1087	ACCCCCCCC to ACCCCCCC	hMSH6

CoCa, colorectal cancer; DuoCa, duodenal cancer; GaCa, gastric cancer; EnCa, endometrial cancer.

Somatic Mutations of DNA Mismatch Repair Genes

PCR-SSCP-sequencing analysis of genomic DNA from HNPCC tumors revealed somatic mutations of DNA mismatch repair genes. To determine whether these mutations were caused by a somatic mutation or a germline mutation, genomic DNA from corresponding normal tissues was also examined using PCR-SSCP. The coexistence of somatic and germline mutations in the same DNA mismatch repair gene was observed in HNPCC tumors. Inactivation of the hMSH2, hMLH1 and hMSH6 genes through germline plus somatic mutations occurred in 13 tumors, including colorectal, duodenal, gastric and endometrial cancers (Table 3). Somatic mutations included six 1-bp deletions, one 11-bp deletion, three 1-bp insertions, and one mutation at the splice donor site of exon 5. Of these eleven somatic mutations, ten mutations led to stop codons resulting in truncated proteins and one mutation led to a deletion of exon 5. Two other tumors showed loss of the normal allele, which was confirmed by the absence of normal bands in the SSCP pattern showing abnormal bands of germline mutation.

Microsatellite Instability

The fidelity of DNA replication is maintained by a system that recognizes DNA mismatched sequences, excises and corrects the mismatch. Mismatches are caused by incorrect base pairings and by the slippage of DNA polymerase on the template strand containing repeated sequences. hMSH2 and hMSH6 proteins produce a heterodimeric complex that binds to mismatches, and hMLH1 and hPMS2 bind the hMSH2-hMSH6 plus heteroduplex DNA complex. This complex participates in mismatch repair [42]. Microsatellite regions are repeating sequences that are distributed throughout the human genome, most commonly $(A)n/(T)n$ and $(CA)n/(GT)n$, located within non-coding DNA sequences. Inactivation of DNA mismatch repair genes causes genomic instability, as shown by a 100-700 fold increase in slipped-strand mismatches of $(CA)n$ repeats [43]. Such genomic instability (replication error or microsatellite instability) is one aspect of the remarkable nature of tumors from HNPCC patients.

We analyzed microsatellite instability in 31 colorectal cancers from 23 HNPCC patients in at least 5 microsatellite regions, such as BAT25, BAT26, D2S123, D5S346 and D17S250, including mononucleotide repeats and dinucleotide repeats. All cancers showed a high frequency (more than 4/5) of microsatellite instability (Figure 1). Such microsatellite instability was also observed in duodenal, gastric and endometrial cancers from HNPCC patients.

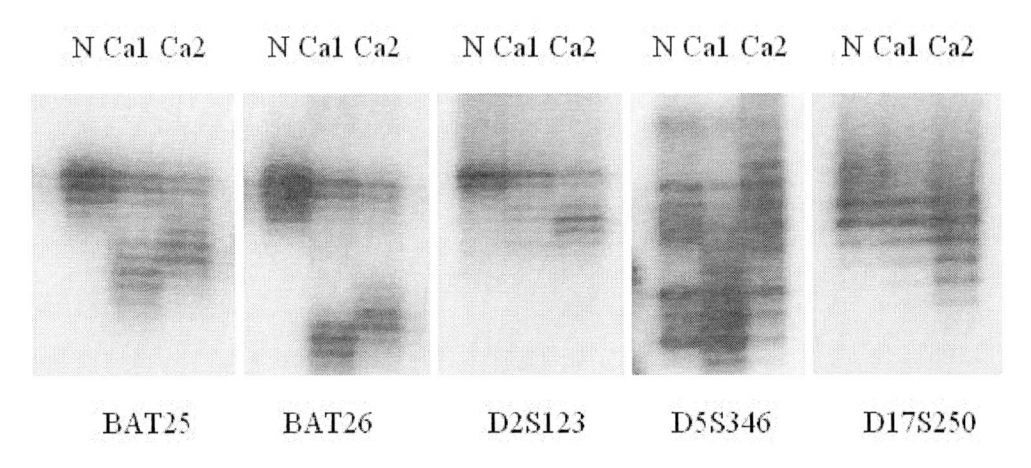

Figure 1. Microsatellite instability in HNPCC colon cancer. N, normal tissue; Ca, colon cancer. In these two cancers, 5 of 5 regions are altered.

Frameshift Mutations in Coding Repeats

Most microsatellite instability occurs in repeated sequences in non-coding DNA which is assumed to have no effect on protein function. However, there are many genes that have repeated sequences in their coding regions. Replication errors (frameshift mutations) at coding repeats frequently occur in tumors with microsatellite instability. Frameshift mutations of coding repeats of tumor suppressor genes form stop codons leading to the inactivation of proteins, which propagate growth advantages to tumors. To clarify the significance of frameshift mutations in HNPCC colorectal carcinogenesis, we analyzed the frequencies and accumulation profiles of frameshift mutations of 11 genes in 31 HNPCC colorectal cancers.

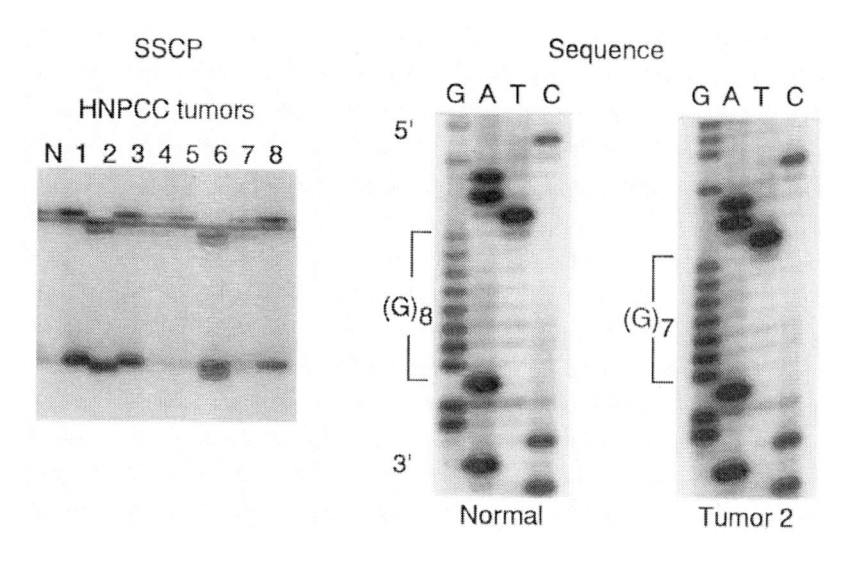

Figure 2. Framashift mutation at $(G)_8$ region of BAX gene in HNPCC colon cancer. N, normal tissue; 1-8, colon cancers. In Tumor 2, $(G)_8$ is changed to $(G)_7$.

Table 4. Frameshift mutations in HNPCC colorectal cancers

Gene	Function	Mutation frequency (%)
TGFβRII $(A)_{10}$	growth factor receptor	77.4
hMSH3 $(A)_8$	mismatch repair	54.8
CASP5 $(A)_{10}$	proapoptotic factor	51.6
BAX $(G)_8$	proapoptotic factor	48.4
RIZ $(A)_8$, $(A)_9$	cell cycle arrest	48.4
RAD50 $(A)_9$	DNA repair	45.2
MBD4 $(A)_{10}$	DNA repair	45.2
hMSH6 $(C)_8$	mismatch repair	35.5
BLM $(A)_9$	DNA repair	22.6
IGFIIR $(G)_8$	growth factor receptor	19.4
PTEN $(A)_6$, $(A)_6$	tumor suppressor	19.4

An example of a frameshift mutation is shown in Figure 2, and the frequencies of mutations of various genes are listed in Table 4. The TGFßRII gene is a component of the TGF-ß signaling pathway, including Smad2, Smad3 and Smad4, and this pathway functions as a growth suppressor of epithelial cells. A frameshift mutation at the $(A)_{10}$ region in the TGFßRII gene forms a truncated protein, and mutations in both alleles cause inactivation of this gene, resulting in a disappearance of the growth suppression activity. Mutations of the TGFßRII gene were frequently (77%) detected in HNPCC colorectal cancers even at the early stage. The BAX gene product, a proapoptotic factor, is directly transactivated by p53. The $(G)_8$ region of the BAX gene was mutated at 29% in the early stage of colorectal cancer and at 65% in the advanced stage. Since the p53 mutation is infrequent in HNPCC colorectal cancer [19], the alteration of the BAX gene probably plays a more important role than p53 gene mutations in both the development and progression of HNPCC cancer. The IGFIIR gene has been proposed as being a growth suppression gene in colorectal cancer cells [21], and the PTEN gene as a tumor suppressor [25]. No mutations of these two genes were detected in the early stage, whereas 35% of advanced cancer had mutations in these genes. This suggests that inactivation of IGFIIR and PTEN genes plays a role in cancer progression in HNPCC colorectal carcinogenesis. CASP5 cleaves pro-caspase-3 resulting in caspase-3, which is involved in apoptotic cell death. Alteration of the $(A)_{10}$ repeat in CASP5 occurred in 52% of the cancers, suggesting that alteration of CASP5 may convey a growth advantage to cancer cells. The $(A)_{10}$ tract of the MBD4 and $(A)_9$ tract of the RAD50, which are DNA repair genes, mutated in 45% of HNPCC cancers, suggesting that genomic instability may be increased in these cancers. Frameshift mutations were detected at $(A)_8$ of the hMSH3 gene in 55% of the cancers, and $(C)_8$ of the hMSH6 gene in 36% of cancers. Alteration of these genes, which are components of the mismatch repair complex [23], may cause more severe replication errors in HNPCC cancers, although these alterations contribute indirectly in tumorigenesis.

Mean numbers of altered genes within the 11 genes were estimated as 3.6 for Dukes A, 5.3 for Dukes B and 5.7 for Dukes C cancers. These data suggest that it is possible to observe the gradual development of HNPCC colorectal cancers by the gradual accumulation of the number of altered genes with repeated sequences.

Somatic Mutations of ß-catenin and APC Genes

We have observed that the frequency of APC gene mutations was low (nearly 20%) in HNPCC tumors compared to the high frequency (more than 70%) in non-HNPCC tumors [19]. It is known that wild-type APC protein forms a complex with ß-catenin and GSK3ß, leading to a degradation of ß-catenin in normal cells, whereas mutant APC protein in tumor cells lacks the ability for a complex formation and ß-catenin accumulates in the nuclei. This causes an interaction of ß-catenin with the nuclear transcription factor (Lef/Tcf) family, resulting in the activation of target genes, including cyclin D1 and c-myc. A similar accumulation of ß-catenin has been demonstrated in colorectal cancer cell lines without APC mutations but with mutations in the regulatory domain (codons 29 to 48) of the ß-catenin gene, suggesting that activation of the ß-catenin-Tcf signaling pathway by mutation in either the APC or ß-catenin gene contributes to colorectal carcinogenesis [44]. To assess the possible contribution of this signaling pathway in HNPCC carcinogenesis, we analyzed ß-catenin mutations in colorectal tumors from HNPCC patients.

Table 5. Mutations of ß-catenin and APC genes in HNPCC colorectal tumors

Tumor	ß-catenin mutation Codon	DNA change	APC mutation Codon	DNA change
HNP10 CoAd1	-			-
HNP10 CoAd2	32	GAC to GGC		-
HNP14 CoAd	-		1338	CAG to TAG
HNP6 CoCa	-			-
HNP10 CoCa1	45	TCT to TTT		-
HNP1 CoCa1	-			-
HNP3 CoCa	-			-
HNP4 CoCa	34	GGA to GAA		-
HNP5 CoCa1	-			-
HNP5 CoCa2		-	901-902	CAGGAA to CAGAA
			1554-1556	GAAAAACT to GAAAAAACT
HNP5 CoCa3	-			-
HNP5 CoCa4	-		874	TCA to TAA
HNP7 CoCa1	-		1466	GGA to GGGA
HNP8 CoCa1	41	ACC to GCC		-
HNP10 CoCa2	45	TCT to TTT		-
HNP12 CoCa	45	TCT to TTT		-
HNP13 CoCa	-			-
HNP14 CoCa2	-		1462-1465	AAGAGAGAGAGT to AAGAGAGAGAGAGT
HNP14 CoCa3	-			-
HNP15 CoCa	45	TCT to CCT		
	43	GCT deletion		
HNP16 CoCa1	45	TCT to TGT		-
HNP16 CoCa2	32	GAC to TAC		-
HNP16 CoCa3	-		1492	GCC to GC
HNP16 CoCa4	34	GGA to GAA		-
HNP17 CoCa	41	ACC to GCC		-
HNP18 CoCa	37	TCT to TGT		-
HNP19 CoCa1	-			-
HNP19 CoCa2	-			-

CoAd, colorectal adenoma; CoCa, colorectal cancer; -, mutation was not detected; HNP5 CoCa2 had two APC mutations. HNP15 CoCa had two ß-catenin mutations.

Somatic ß-catenin gene mutations were detected in 12 HNPCC colorectal tumors, including 11 cancers and 1 adenoma, in which no APC gene mutations were detected [32]

(Table 5). These mutations were single-base substitutions that were located within the NH$_2$-terminal regulatory domain of ß-catenin (codons 29 to 48): TCT(Ser) to TTT(Phe), CCT(Pro) or TGT(Cys) at codon 45; ACC(Thr) to GCC(Ala) at codon 41; TCT(Ser) to TGT(Cys) at codon 37; GGA(Gly) to GAA(Glu) at codon 34; GAC(Asp) to GGC(Gly) or TAC(Tyr) at codon 32; and a 3-bp deletion at codon 43. Such single-base substitutions are assumed to be caused by defects of DNA mismatch repair in HNPCC tumors. Immunohistochemical staining of HNPCC cancers with a ß-catenin mutation showed a high level of ß-catenin protein in both cytoplasm and nuclei, with stronger staining in the nuclei [32], although in normal epithelial cells of the colon ß-catenin protein was localized in the membrane but not in nuclei. ß-Catenin mutations were not detected in HNPCC tumors with APC mutations, indicating an alternative exclusion between ß-catenin mutations and APC mutations. However, the coexistence of mutations of TGFßRII and APC, and TGFßRII and ß-catenin was observed, which suggests that the TGFßRII mutation does not substitute for the activated ß-catenin-Tcf signaling pathway. The activation of the ß-catenin-Tcf signaling pathway, through either ß-catenin mutations (43%) or APC mutations (21%) may significantly contribute to HNPCC colorectal carcinogenesis. Because mutations in either APC or ß-catenin have been known to be associated with adenoma formation, the present observation may imply that more than half (64%) of HNPCC colorectal cancers develop via adenoma.

Somatic Mutations of the p53 gene

p53 gene mutations were detected in 2 of 15 colorectal cancers from HNPCC patients [19]. These included CGT to TGT at codon 110 and CGT to TGT at codon 273. The mutation frequency (13%) was lower than in non-HNPCC cancers (more than 50%), suggesting that colorectal cancer in HNPCC involves a more distinct pathogenic mechanism than in non-HNPCC cancer. Instead of p53 gene mutations, frequent frameshift mutations in the BAX gene appear to contribute to colorectal carcinogenesis in HNPCC patients.

Somatic mutations of K-ras and BRAF Genes

K-ras gene mutations have been demonstrated to generally occur at 30% to 40% in non-HNPCC colorectal cancers [45]. K-ras is a member of the RAS family which participates in the RAS-RAF signaling pathway, which mediates cellular responses to growth signals. BRAF is a member of the RAF family which is regulated by RAS and also mediates growth signals. It has recently been found that activation of RAS-RAF signaling is caused not only by K-ras gene mutations, but also by BRAF gene mutations in various human cancers [36], and a significantly high frequency of BRAF mutations has been observed in mismatch repair-deficient sporadic colorectal cancers compared to mismatch repair-proficient cancers [46]. HNPCC cancers are typical mismatch repair-deficient cancers. To clarify wether HNPCC colorectal cancers exhibit a high frequency of BRAF mutations similar to the mismatch repair-deficient sporadic cancers, we analyzed BRAF mutations in colorectal cancers from HNPCC patients. We also analyzed K-ras mutations in these cancers. We observed a low frequency of K-ras mutations (less than 18%) and no BRAF mutations in HNPCC colorectal cancers [33]. An obvious difference in the BRAF mutation frequency between mismatch repair-deficient sporadic (31%) and HNPCC (0%) cancers suggests a difference in the mechanisms of colorectal carcinogenesis between mismatch repair-deficient sporadic cancers and HNPCC cancers.

Loss of Heterozygosity

Colorectal cancers from FAP patients and the majority of sporadic colorectal cancers develop via an adenoma-carcinoma sequence through the accumulation of inactivations of tumor suppressor genes. High frequencies (40% to 70%) of LOH have been detected in FAP and sporadic colorectal cancers at tumor suppressor regions, including chromosomes 5q, 8p, 17p, 18q and 22q [13]. However, these LOH were not detected in colorectal cancers from HNPCC patients [19]. The absence of chromosomal instability is one aspect of the remarkable nature of HNPCC tumors, which is assumed to be related to the observation that HNPCC-associated tumors have generally diploid or near-diploid DNA.

CONCLUSION

Hereditary nonpolyposis colorectal cancer (HNPCC) is one of the most commom hereditary colon cancer syndromes with an autosomal dominant inheritance. The causative genes are germline mutations of DNA mismatch repair genes including hMSH2, hMLH1 and hMSH6. HNPCC also develops into extracolonic cancers such as cancer of the endometrium and other extracolonic organs. Inactivation of DNA mismatch repair genes through germline and somatic mutations leads to microsatellite instability, as well as frameshift mutations of repeated sequences in coding regions of various tumor-related genes. Frameshift mutations occurred in TGFßRII, IGFIIR, BAX, CASP5, RIZ, RAD50, MBD4, BLM, hMSH3, hMSH6 and PTEN genes. These genes include members of growth factor receptors, proapoptotic factors, DNA repair genes, components of the mismatch repair system, and tumor suppressor genes. Inactivation of these genes appears to cause the development and progression of HNPCC colorectal cancers. The gradual increase in the number of frameshift mutations during the progression from Dukes A to Dukes B and C cancers suggests the gradual progression of HNPCC colorectal cancers by the accumulation of mutations of genes with coding repeats. Mutations of ß-catenin and APC genes were also high in HNPCC colorectal tumors, which suggests that the majority of HNPCC colorectal cancers develop via adenomas.

The present data revealed that disruption of the WNT signaling pathway by mutations of ß-catenin and APC genes and disruption of the TGF-ß signaling pathway by mutation of the TGFßRII gene largely contribute to the development of HNPCC colorectal cancer. Moreover, it was suggested that mutations of apoptosis-related genes, such as the BAX, CASP5 and RIZ genes, contribute to the development, and inactivation of the IGFIIR and PTEN genes play a role in the progression of HNPCC colorectal cancer.

REFERENCES

[1] Lynch, H.T. & de la Chapelle, A. (2003). Hereditary colorectal cancer. *New Engl. J. Med.*, *348*, 919-932.

[2] Fishel, R., Lescoe, M.K., Rao, M.RS., Copeland, N.G., Jenkins, N.A., Garber, J., Kane, M. & Kolodner, R. (1993). The human mutator homolog MSH2 and its association with hereditary nonpolyposis colon cancer. *Cell*, *75*, 1028-1038.

[3] Leach, F.S., Nicolaides, N.C., Papadopoulos, N., Liu. B., Jen, J., Parsons, R., Peltomaki, P., Sistonen, P., Aaltonen, L.A., Nystrom-Lahti, M., Guan, X.-Y., Zang, J., Meltzer, P.S., Yu, J.-W., Kao, F.-T., Chen, D.J., Cerosaletti, K.M., Fournier, R.E.K., Todd, S., Lewis, T., Leach, R.J., Naylor, S.L., Weissenbach, J., Mecklin, J.-P., Jarvinen, H., Petersen, G.M., Hamilton, S.R., Green, J., Jass. J., Watson, P., Lynch, H.T., Trent, J.M., de la Chapelle, A., Kinzler, K.W. & Vogelstein, B. (1993). Mutations of a mutS homolog in hereditary nonpolyposis colorectal cancer. *Cell*, *75*, 1215-1225.

[4] Bronner, C.E., Baker, S.M., Morrison, P.T., Warren, G., Smith, L.G., Lescoe, M.K., Kane, M., Earabino, C., Lipfold, J., Lindblom, A., Tannergard, P., Bollag, R.J., Godwin, A.R., Ward, D.C., Nordenskjold, M., Fishel, R., Kolodner. R & Liskay, R.M. (1994). Mutation in the DNA mismatch repair gene homologue hMLH1 is associated with hereditary non-polyposis colon cancer. *Nature*, *368*, 258-261.

[5] Papadopoulos, N., Nicolaides, N.C., Wei, Y.-F., Ruben, S.M., Carter, K.C., Rosen, C.A., Haseltine, W., Fleischmann, R.D., Fraser, C.M., Adams, M.K., Venter, J.C., Hamilton, S.R., Petersen, G.M., Watson, P., Lynch, H.T., Peltomaki, P., Mecklin, J.-P., de la Chapelle, A., Kinzler, K.W. & Vogelstein, B. (1994). Mutation of a mutL homolog in hereditary colon cancer. *Science*, *263*, 1625-1629.

[6] Miyaki, M., Konishi, M., Tanaka, K., Kikuchi-Yanoshita, R., Muraoka, M., Yasuno, M., Igari, T., Koike, M., Chiba, M. & Mori, T. (1997). Germline mutation of MSH6 as the cause of hereditary nonpolyposis colorectal cancer. *Nature Genet.*, *17*, 271-272.

[7] Akiyama, Y., Sato, H., Yamada, T., Nagasaki, H., Tsuchiya, A., Abe, R. & Yuasa, Y. Germ-line mutation of the hMSH6/GTBP gene in an atypical hereditary nonpolyposis colorectal cancer kindred. (1997). *Cancer Res.*, *57*, 3920-3923.

[8] Nicolaides, N.C., Papadopoulos, N., Liu, B., Wei, Y.-F., Carter, K.C., Ruben, S.M., Rosen, C.A., Haseltine, W.A., Fleischmann, R.D., Fraser, C.M., Adams, M.D., Venter, J.C., Dunlop, M.G., Hamilton, S.R., Petersen, G.M., de la Chapelle, A., Vogelstein, B. & Kinzler, K.W. (1994). Mutation of two PMS homologues in hereditary nonpolyposis colon cancer. *Nature*, *371*, 75-80.

[9] Aaltonen, L.A., Peltomaki, P., Leach, F.S., Sistonen, P., Pylkkanen, L., Mecklin, J.-P., Jarvinen, H., Powell, S.M., Jen, J., Hamilton, S.R., Petersen, G.M., Kinzler, K.W., Vogelstein, B. & de la Chapelle, A. (1993). Clues to the pathogenesis of familial colorectal cancer. *Science*, *260*, 812-816.

[10] Ionov, Y., Peinads, M.A., Malkosyan, S., Shibata, D. & Perucho, M. (1993). Ubiquitous somatic mutations in simple repeated sequences reveal a new mechanisms for colonic carcinogenesis. *Nature*, *363*, 558-561.

[11] Markowitz, S., Wang, J., Myeroff, L., Parsons, R., Sun, L., Lutterbaugh, J., Fan, R.S., Zborowska, E., Kinzler, K.W., Vogelstein, B., Brattain, M. & Willson, J.K.W. (1995).

Inactivation of the type II TGF-ß receptor in colon cancer cells with microsatellite instability. *Science, 268*, 1336-1338.

[12] Fearon, E.R. & Vogelstein, B. (1990). A genetic model for colorectal tumorigenesis. *Cell, 61*, 759-767.

[13] Miyaki, M., Tanaka, K., Kikuch-Yanoshita, R., Muraoka, M.& Konishi, M. (1995). Familial polyposis: recent advances. *Crit. Rev. Oncol. Hematol., 19*, 1-31.

[14] Vasen, H.F.A., Watson, P., Mecklin, J.-P. & Lynch, H.T. (1999). New clinical criteria for hereditary nonpolyposis colorectal cancer (HNPCC, Lynch syndrome) proposed by the International Collaborative Group on HNPCC. *Gastroenterology, 116*, 1453-1456.

[15] Liu, B., Parsons, R.E., Hamilton, S.R., Petersen, G.M., Lynch, H.T., Watson, P., Markowitz, S., Willson, J.K.V., Green, J., de la Chapelle, A., Kinzler, K.W. & Vogelstein, B. (1994). HMSH2 mutations in hereditary nonpolyposis colorectal cancer kindreds. *Cancer Res., 54*, 4590-4594.

[16] Kolodner, R.D., Hall, N.R., Lipford, J., Kane, M.F., Rao, M.R.S., Morson, P., Wirth, L., Finan, P.J., Burn, J., Chapman, P., Earabino, C., Merchant, E. & Bishop, D.T. (1994). Structure of the human MSH2 locus and analysis of two Muir-Torre kinders for msh2 mutations. *Genomics, 24*, 516-526.

[17] Acharya, S., Wilson, T., Gradia, S., Kane, M.F., Guerrette, S., Marsischky, G.T., Kolodner, R. & Fishel, R. (1996). HMSH2 forms specific mispair-binding complexes with hMSH3 and hMSH6. *Proc. Natl. Acad. Sci. USA, 93*, 13629-13634. Genbank [U73732-7].

[18] Miyaki, M., Iijima, T., Yamaguchi, T., Shirahama, S., Ito, T., Yasuno, M. & Mori, T. (2004). Novel germline hMSH2 genomic deletion and somatic hMSH2 mutations in a hereditary nonpolyposis colorectal cancer family. *Mutation Res., 548*, 19-25.

[19] Konishi, M., Kikuchi-Yanoshita, R., Tanaka, K., Muraoka, M., Onda, A., Okumura, Y., Kishi, N., Iwama, T., Mori, T., Koike, M., Ushio, K., Chiba, M., Nomizu, S., Konishi, F., Utsunomiya, J. & Miyaki, M. (1996). Molecular nature of colon tumors in hereditary nonpolyposis colon cancer, familial polyposis, and sporadic colon cancer. *Gastroenterology, 111*, 307-317.

[20] Boland, C.R., Tibodeau, S.N., Hamilton, S.R., Sidransky, D., Eshleman, J.R., Burt, R.W., Meltzer, S.J., Rodoriguez-Bigas, M.A., Fodde, R., Ranzani, G.N., & Srirastava, S. (1998). A National Cancer Institute workshop on microsatellite instability for cancer detection and familial predisposition: Development of international criteria for the determinations of microsatellite instability in colorectal cancer. *Cancer Res., 58*, 5248-5257.

[21] Souza, R.F., Appel, R., Yin, J., Wang, S., Smolinski, K.N., Abraham, J.M., Zou, T.T., Shi, Y.Q., Leu, J., Cottrell, J., Cymes, K., Bider, K., Simms, L., Leggett, B., Lynch, P.M., Frazier, M., Powell, S.M., Harpaz, N., Sugimura, H., Young, J. & Meltzer, S.J. (1996). Microsatellite instability in the insulin-like growth factor II receptor gene in gastrointestinal tumors. *Nature Genet., 14*, 255-257.

[22] Rampino, N., Yamamoto, H., Ionov, Y., Li, Y., Sawai, H., Reed, J.C. & Perucho, M. (1997). Somatic frameshift mutations in the BAX gene in colon cancers of the microsatellite mutator phenotype. *Science, 275*, 967-969.

[23] Malkhosyan, S., Rampino, N., Yamamoto, H. & Perucho, M. (1996). Frameshift mutator mutations. *Nature*, *382*, 499-500.

[24] Schwartz, S. Jr, Yamamoto, H., Navarro, M., Maestro, M., Reventos, J. & Perucho, M. (1999). Frameshift mutations at mononucleotide repeats in Caspase-5 and other target genes in endometrial and gastrointestinal cancer of the microsatellite mutator phenotype. *Cancer Res.*, *59*, 2995-3002.

[25] Guanti, G., Resta, N., Simone, C., Cariola, F., Demma, I., Fiorente, P. & Gentile, M. (2000). Involvement of PTEN mutations in the genetic pathway of colorectal carcinogenesis. *Hum. Mol. Genet.*, *9*, 283-287.

[26] Riccio, A., Aaltonen, L.A., Godwin, A.K., Loukola, A., Percesepe, A., Salovaara, R., Masciullo, V., Genuardi, M., Papavatou-Petsotas, M., Bassi, D.E., Ruggeri, B.A., Klein-Szanto, A.J., Testa, J.R., Neri, G. & Bellacosa, A. (1999). The DNA repair gene MBD4 (MED1) is mutated in human carcinomas with microsatellite instability. *Nature Genet.*, *23*, 266-268.

[27] Chadwick, R.B., Jiang, G.L., Bennington, G.A., Yuan, B., Johnson, C.K., Stevens, M.W., Niemann, T.H., Peltomaki, P., Huang, S. & de la Chapelle, A. (2000). Candidate tumor suppressor RIZ is frequently involved in colorectal carcinogenesis. *Proc. Natl. Acad. Sci. USA*, *97*, 2662-2667.

[28] Calin, G., Herlea, V., Barbanti-Brodano, G & Negrimi, M. (1998). The coding region of the Bloom syndrome BLM gene and of the CBL proto-oncogene is mutated in genetically unstable sporadic gastrointestinal tumors. *Cancer Res.*, *58*, 3777-3781.

[29] Kim, N.J., Choi, Y.R., Beak, M.J., Kim, Y.H., Kang, H., Kim, N.K., Min, J.S. & Kim, H. (2001). Frameshift mutations at coding mononucleotide repeats of the hRAD50 gene in gastrointestinal carcinomas with microsatellite instability. *Cancer Res.*, *61*, 36-38.

[30] Miyaki, M., Konishi, M., Kikuchi-Yanoshita, R., Enomoto, M., Igeri, T., Tanaka, K., Muraoka, M., Takahashi, H., Amada, Y., Fukayama, M., Maeda, Y., Iwama, T., Mishima, Y., Mori, T. & Koike, M. (1994). Characteristics of somatic mutation of the adenomatous polyposis coli gene in colorectal tumors. *Cancer Res.*, *54*, 3011-3020.

[31] Kikuch-Yanoshita, R., Konishi, M., Ito, S., Seki, M., Tanaka, K., Maeda, Y., Iino, H., Fukayama, M., Koike, M., Mori, T., Sakuraba, H., Fukunari, M., Iwama, T. & Miyaki, M. (1992). Genetic changes of both p53 alleles associated with the conversion from colorectal adenoma to early carcinoma in familial adenomatous polyposis and non-familial adenomatous polyposis patients. *Cancer Res.*, *52*, 3965-3971.

[32] Miyaki, M., Iijima, T., Kimura, J., Yasuno, M., Mori, T., Hayashi, Y., Koike, M., Shitara, N., Iwama, & Kuroki, T. (1999). Frequent mutations of ß-catenin and APC genes in primary colorectal tumors from patients with hereditary nonpolyposis colorectal cancer. *Cancer Res.*, *59*, 4506-4509.

[33] Miyaki, M., Iijima, T., Yamaguchi, T., Kadofuku, T., Funata, N. & Mori, T. (2004). Both BRAF and KRAS mutations are rare in colorectal carcinomas from patients with hereditary nonpolyposis colorectal cancer. *Cancer Lett.*, *211*, 105-109.

[34] Groden, J., Thliveris, A., Samowitz, W., Carlson, M., Gelbert, L., Albertsen, H., Joslyn, G., Stevens, J., Spirio, L., Robertson, M., Sargeant, L., Krapcho, K., Walff, E., Burt, R., Hunghes, J.P., Warrington, J., McPherson, J., Wasmuth, J., LePaslier, D., Abderrahim,

H., Cohen, D., Leppert, M. & White, R. (1991). Identification and characterization of the familial adenomatous polyposis coli gene. *Cell, 66*, 589-600.
[35] Voeller, H.J., Truica, C.I. & Gelmann, E.P. (1998). ß-Catenin mutation in human prostate cancer. *Cancer Res., 58*, 2520-2523.
[36] Davis, H., Bignell, G.R., Cox, C., Stephens, P., Edkins, S., Clegg, S., Teague, J., Woffendin, H., Garnett, M.J., Bottomley, W., Davis, N., Dicks, E., Ewing, R., Floyd, Y., Gray, K., Hall, S., Hawes, R., Hughes, J., Kosmidou, V., Menzies, A., Mould, C., Parker, A., Stevens, C., Watt, S., Hooper, S., Wilson, R., Jayatilake, H., Gusterson, B.A., Cooper, C., Shipley, J., Hargrave, D., Pritchard-Jones, K., Maltland, N., Chenevix-Trench, G., Riggs, G.J., Bigner, D.D., Palmleri, G., Cossu, A., Flanagan, A., Nicholson, A., Ho, J.W.C., Leung, S.Y., Weber, B.L., Selgler, H.F., Darrow, T., Paterson, H., Marals, R., Marshall, C.J., Wooster, R., Stratton, M. & Futreal, P.A. (2002). Mutations of the BRAF gene in human cancer. *Nature, 417*, 949-954.
[37] Miyaki, M., Seki, M., Okamoto, M., Yamanaka, A., Maeda, Y., Tanaka, K., Kikuchi, R., Iwama, T., Ikeuchi, T., Tonomura, A., Nakamura, Y., White, R., Miki, Y., Utsunomiya, J. & Koike, M. (1990). Genetic changes and histopathological types of colorectal tumors from patients with familial adenomatous polyposis. *Cancer Res., 50*, 7166-7173.
[38] Wijnen, J., van der Klift, H., Vasen, H., Meera Khan, P. & Fodde, R. (1998). MSH2 genomic deletions are a frequent cause of HNPCC. *Nature Genet., 20*, 326-328
[39] Chanbonnier, F., Olschwang, S., Wang, Q., Boisson, C., Martin, C., Buisine, M.-P., Puisieux, A. & Frebourg, T. (2002). MSH2 in contrast to MLH1 and MSH6 is frequently inactivated by exonic and promoter rearrangements in hereditary nonpolyposis colorectal cancer. *Cancer Res., 62*, 848-853.
[40] Miyaki, M., Konishi, M., Muraoka, M., Kikuchi-Yanoshita, R., Tanaka, K., Iwama, T., Mori, T., Koike, M., Ushio, K., Chiba, M., Nomizu, S. & Utsunomiya, J. (1995). Germ line mutations of hMSH2 and hMLH1 genes in Japanese families with hereditary nonpolyposis colorectal cancer (HNPCC): usefulness of DNA analysis for screening and diagnosis of HNPCC patients. *J. Mol. Med., 73*, 515-520.
[41] Wijnen, J., de Leeuw, W., Vasen, H., van der Klift, H., Moller, P., Stormorken, A., Meijers-Heijboer, H., Lindhout, D., Menko, F., Vossen, S., Moslein, G., Tops, C., Brocker-Vriends, A., Wu, Y., Hofstra, R., Sijmons, R., Cornelisse, C., Morreau, H. & Fodde, R. (1999). Familial endometrial cancer in female carriers of MSH6 germline mutations. *Nature Genet., 23*, 142-144.
[42] Rhyu, M.S. (1996). Molecular mechanisms underlying hereditary nonpolyposis colorectal carcinoma. *J. Natl. Cancer Inst., 88*, 240-251.
[43] Strand, M., Prolla, T.A., Liskay, R.M. & Petes, T.D. (1993). Destabilization of tracts of single repetitive DNA in yeast by mutation affecting DNA mismatch repair. *Nature, 365*, 274-276.
[44] Morin, P.J., Sparks, A.B., Korinek, V., Baker, N., Clevers, H., Vogelstein, B. & Kinzler, K.W. (1997). Activation of ß-catenin-Tcf signaling in colon cancer by mutation in ß-catenin or APC. *Science, 275*, 1787-1790.

[45] Bos, J.L., Fearon, E.R., Hamilton, S.R., Verlaan-de Vries, M., van Boom, J.H., van der Eb, A.J. & Vogelstein, B. (1987). Prevalence of ras gene mutations in human colorectal cancers. *Nature*, *327*, 293-297.

[46] Rajagopalan, H., Bardelli, A., Lengauer, C., Kinzler, K.W., Vogelstein, B. & Veculescu, V.E. (2002). RAF/RAS oncogenes and mismatch-repair status. *Nature*, *418*, 934.

In: Rectal Cancer: Etiology, Pathogenesis and Treatment
Editors: Paula Wells and Regina Halstead

ISBN 978-1-60692-563-8
© 2009 Nova Science Publishers, Inc.

Chapter IX

WOMEN AND COLORECTAL CANCER[*]

Samantha Hendren[†]

Department of Surgery, University of Rochester, USA.

ABSTRACT

Colorectal cancer deaths are equally distributed among women and men. Prevention is possible using risk-stratified screening strategies and healthy lifestyle. Good outcomes are possible if the disease is discovered and treated at an early stage. Quality of life can be preserved but in rectal cancer patients, sexual function and changes in body image occur.

INTRODUCTION

It is a common misconception that colorectal cancer is a "male disease". On the contrary, colorectal cancer cases and deaths are approximately equally distributed between men and women in North America [1]. For women in Ontario, colorectal cancer (CRC) is the second most common cancer diagnosis, after breast cancer [2]. In terms of cancer deaths, it is third after breast and lung cancers. One in 16 Canadian women will develop CRC in her lifetime, compared to 1 in 14 men [3].

Table 1 displays American statistics for digestive system cancers [1]. These data illustrate that CRC is by far the most common digestive system cancer. It is also one of the most curable, as evidenced by the relatively low ratio of deaths to new cases diagnosed.

---

[*] A version of this chapter was also published in *Women and Cancer*, edited by Laurie Elit, published by Nova Science Publishers, Inc. It was submitted for appropriate modifications in an effort to encourage wider dissemination of research.

[†] Correspondence concerning this article should be addressed to: Dr. S. Hendren, 601 Elmwood Avenue, Box SURG, Rochester, New York 14642, USA. Phone: (585)275-0606; Email: samantha_hendren@urmc.rochester.edu.

Canadian statistics show that in 2006, an estimated 20,000 Canadians will be diagnosed with CRC and 8,500 will die of it [3].

Colorectal cancer diagnosis rates decreased in the USA between 1998 and 2002, by approximately 1.8% per year [4]. This may be due to improved cancer screening and the removal of pre-cancerous polyps. Death rates from CRC are also decreasing, probably due to improvements in early detection and treatment [4]. In Canada CRC rates have been decreasing since the mid-1980's, particularly in women, and in the distal colon and rectum [5]. In Ontario, an increase in incidence was seen more recently, from the mid-1990's to the present; the reason for this is not clear [2]. It is possible that improved detection from screening is a factor.

Table 1. Digestive Cancer Statistics for the USA, 2004*

	Estimated New Cases			Estimated Deaths		
	Both Genders	Male	Female	Both Genders	Male	Female
All Digestive System Cancers	255,640	135,410	120,230	134,840	73,240	61,600
Esophagus	14,250	10,860	3,390	13,300	10,250	3,050
Stomach	22,710	13,640	9,070	11,780	6,900	4,880
Small Intestine	5,260	2,750	2,510	1,130	610	520
Colon	**106,370**	**50,400**	**55,970**	56730**	28320**	28410**
Rectum	**40,570**	**23,220**	**17,350**			
Anus	4,010	1,890	2,120	580	210	370
Liver and Extrahepatic Bile Duct	18,920	12,580	6,340	14,270	9,450	4,820
Gallbladder and Other Biliary	6,950	2,960	3,990	3,540	1,290	2,250
Pancreas	31,860	15,740	16,120	31,270	15,440	15,830
Other	4,740	1,370	3,370	2,240	770	1,470

*CA Cancer J Clin 2004; 54:8-29; **Estimated deaths combined for colon and rectum.

ANATOMY

As illustrated in Table 1, the vast majority of "bowel cancers" are colorectal cancers due to the low rates of small intestine and anal cancers. The majority of colorectal cancers are distal, in the sigmoid colon and rectum [2]. The rectum is the last 12-15 cm of the large bowel; it is defined by its pelvic anatomic location and its distinct muscular, lymphatic and vascular anatomy. Rectal cancers in the final 12 cm of the large bowel are treated somewhat differently from colon cancers, due to their location, the proximity of nerve and genitourinary structures, and more aggressive tumour behavior. However, rectosigmoid cancers are similar to sigmoid cancers, and the treatment is usually the same as for other colon cancers.

The term "colorectal cancer" refers to adenocarcinomas of the large bowel. These cancers arise from the glandular epithelial lining of the interior of the bowel. Other types of tumors of the bowel, such as lymphomas, carcinoid tumors, squamous cell cancers, melanomas and gastrointestinal stromal tumors are quite different, and are not discussed here.

RISK FACTORS AND PREVENTION

Risk factors for colorectal cancer include: increasing age; a personal history of colorectal cancer or adenomatous polyps; a family history of CRC, particularly when the cancer is in a first-degree relative and/or the cancer was diagnosed at a young age; a family history of adenomatous polyps; inherited colorectal cancer syndromes; and having inflammatory bowel disease, including ulcerative colitis and Crohn's disease [4] (Table 2). However, in more than 75% of CRC, no specific risk factor is found [2].

There are several modifiable factors that may contribute to CRC and adenoma risk. The most important of these is cigarette smoking. Multiple cohort and case-control studies have also shown that former or current cigarette smoking increases the risk of colorectal cancer by a factor of 1.5 to 2 [6,7]. Several other dietary, lifestyle and pharmacologic interventions have been suggested to decrease colorectal cancer risk, and the data for these are reviewed below.

Table 2. Risk Factors for Colorectal Cancer

Age Over 50
Inflammatory Bowel Disease (Crohn's Disease, Ulcerative Colitis)
Personal History of CRC or Adenomatous Polyps
Family History of CRC or Adenomatous Polyps in a 1st Degree Relative
Genetic Syndromes (Familial Polyposis (FAP), Hereditary NonPolyposis Colon Cancer (HNPCC))

DIET, VITAMINS AND EXERCISE

Large cohort studies of women, such as the Nurses' Health Study have suggested that diet has a significant impact on the risk of CRC. Possible risk factors include low fruit intake [8], low legume intake [8], obesity, low physical activity, low folate intake, high red meat intake, high processed meat intake and high alcohol intake [9].

A case-control study of the diets of women found to have colorectal adenomas suggested that higher intake of calories, total fat, saturated fat, and red meat were risk factors for adenomas, while fish and chicken, vitamin A, and total fiber were protective [10]. It is interesting to note that these authors failed to find the same relationships between diet and adenomas in males. Meat, fat and fiber intake were prospectively studied in 88,000 women with a 6-year follow-up [11]. After adjusting for total calorie intake, several factors were associated with a higher risk of CRC: animal fat (not vegetable fat); red meat; processed meat and liver; and low intake of fruits. Fish and skinless chicken were protective. The same cohort study failed to show a protective effect of dietary fiber against CRC or adenomas [12]. A smaller cohort study with a 7-year follow-up showed an inverse relationship between protein intake and CRC risk in women [13]. Fish and dairy were protective in this study, but no relationship with total calories or fat was seen.

Prospective cohort studies have shown varying results with respect to dietary fiber and CRC risk. The large European EPIC study showed a significant protective effect of fiber [14], while large American cohort studies have failed to show an effect [15]. Randomized trials of dietary fiber conducted to prevent recurrent adenomatous polyps in patients with prior polyps have had mixed results. A metaanalysis of randomized trials showed no effect of dietary fiber on polyp or cancer prevention [16], but studies had a relatively short follow-up of 2-4 years, and the possibility of a long-term benefit exists. Gender differences in the response to dietary fiber may exist, with a specific benefit for women [17].

Long-term (>15 years) multivitamin supplementation in women was associated with a decreased risk of colorectal cancer in the Nurses Health Study [18]. The pattern of benefit suggested that folate supplementation might be an important factor in the observed benefit. Antioxidant vitamins have also been studied in relatively short-term experimental studies, without a benefit observed [19,20]; however, these studies are limited by relatively short follow-up.

Calcium plus Vitamin D supplementation has been associated with lower risk of CRC in epidemiologic studies, and has been found to prevent adenomatous polyps [21,22]. In addition, dietary intake of milk and dairy foods has strong support from prospective cohort studies for a protective effect [23]. However a recent randomized trial of calcium plus Vitamin D supplementation in 36,000 post-menopausal women showed no effect on the risk of colorectal cancer in 7 years of follow-up [24]. It is possible that the long latency in the development of CRC and a very low-risk cohort may have led to this negative result, and longer follow-up is needed.

Physical exercise has been suggested to protect against the development of CRC [25]; however, the Physicians' Health Study failed to confirm this benefit after controlling for obesity and other risk factors [26]. Obesity may also predispose to CRC [9,25]. Finally, a pooled analysis of large, prospective cohort studies showed a moderate increase in CRC risk amongst people with high alcohol intake [27].

In summary, there is some evidence suggesting that multivitamins, calcium/Vitamin D supplementation, dairy intake, fruit intake, fish and lean chicken intake, dietary fiber, a lean body weight, physical activity and avoidance of red and processed meats and excessive alcohol may reduce the risk of CRC. The evidence is mixed for most of these interventions; however, they are unlikely to have a deleterious effect on health if recommended (Table 3).

CHEMOPROPHYLAXIS

Several medications have been shown to decrease the number of polyps in patients with familial adenomatous polyposis, the highest-risk individuals for polyp formation. The use of these agents in usual-risk persons has not been shown to be effective when rigorously tested. In high-risk individuals, chemoprevention may be considered, but risks of medications must be weighed against potential benefit. This issue was brought into focus with the recent finding of increased cardiovascular risk with COX-2 inhibitor medications.

Non-steroidal anti-inflammatory drugs and aspirin have been tested extensively for polyp- and cancer-prevention. A recent randomized trial of aspirin (100 mg) for the prevention of cancer in women contained 39,000 women, who were followed-up for 10 years. No reduction in colorectal cancer risk was demonstrated [28]. Therefore, low-dose aspirin does not appear to be useful for chemoprevention of CRC in healthy women, at least over a 10-year time frame. However, cohort studies have suggested a lower risk in healthy subjects who take aspirin, and both aspirin and NSAIDS are effective in decreasing the number of polyps in patients with FAP, although not sufficiently to avoid colectomy [29]. The most effective agents for use in the setting are sulindac and celecoxib [29].

Statins (HMG-CoA reductase inhibitors designed for cholesterol reduction) and ursodeoxycholic acid may reduce the risk of colorectal cancer [30]; however, studies have mixed results and further analysis is warranted. Hormone replacement therapy was associated with decreased risk of colorectal cancer in prospective cohort studies, but randomized trials have shown mixed results. HRT can not currently be recommended for chemoprophylaxis of CRC [29]. In summary, several medications may provide a protective effect against colorectal polyps and cancer. However their use in average-risk persons has not been shown to reduce risk in randomized trials, and use should only be considered in high risk people such as those with FAP or multiple prior polyps [4].

Table 3. Modifiable Factors in Colorectal Cancer Risk for Women

May Increase Risk of CRC	May Decrease Risk of CRC
Cigarette Smoking	Long-Term Multivitamin Supplementation
Obesity	
High Alcohol Intake	High Fiber Intake
High Intake of Animal, Saturated or Total Fat	High Fruit Intake
High Intake of Red or Processed Meat	Fish and Lean Chicken Intake
	Dairy Intake
	Calcium/Vitamin D Supplementation
	Folate Supplementation
	Physical Activity
Possible Chemoprevention for High-Risk Individuals	
Aspirin	
Calcium/Vitamin D	
Non-Steroidal Anti-Inflammatory Drugs	
Statins	
Hormone Replacement Therapy	
Ursodeoxycholic Acid	

SUMMARY RECOMMENDATIONS FOR CRC PREVENTION

For people at average risk, regular screening starting at age 50 combined with a healthy lifestyle will minimize the risk of developing colorectal cancer. Healthy lifestyle recommendations include: limiting fat and red meat; eating more fruits, vegetables and dairy; and increasing fiber and whole grains. A daily multivitamin containing folate, plus additional calcium and vitamin D should be considered. In addition, quitting smoking, physical exercise, avoiding excessive alcohol intake, and maintaining a healthy weight should be recommended.

INHERITED COLORECTAL CANCER SYNDROMES

About 80% of patients with CRC have no family history for the disease, but about 20% have a genetic syndrome or a familial predisposition to the disease [31]. Identifying those few patients with familial syndromes is important, because prophylactic surgery will be required to prevent premature cancer in affected family members. The two autosomal-dominant colorectal cancer syndromes are the hereditary non-polyposis colon cancer syndrome (HNPCC or Lynch syndrome) and familial polyposis (FAP). These syndromes account for less than 4 percent of CRC [32]. Other patients with a positive family history may have the recessively-inherited MYH mutation, or hereditary colorectal adenomas.

Even if there is no definable genetic syndrome in a family, a person with a first degree relative with colorectal cancer has a 2.25 relative risk of developing CRC [32]. It is important to take a detailed family history for patients with colorectal cancer or adenomas, in order to identify those patients who should be referred for genetic counseling, and whose family members should be screened and counseled.

Patients with twenty or more adenomas should definitely be referred for genetic testing, and first-degree relatives should be screened with colonoscopy, because a hereditary syndrome is likely. A strongly positive family history meeting the Amsterdam or Bethesda criteria should also have genetic testing and relatives must be screened. Furthermore, any patient under the age of 50 with colorectal cancer, or under age 40 with adenomatous polyps, should be considered for genetic counseling and testing [31]. At the very least, first degree relatives of such a patient must be counseled to undergo colonoscopy, beginning at an age 10 years earlier than the earliest age of diagnosis in the family.

SCREENING FOR COLORECTAL CANCER

The rationale for colorectal cancer screening derives from the knowledge that colorectal cancers begin as pre-malignant adenomatous polyps. Early detection and removal of adenomatous polyps prevents cancers. There is strong evidence from randomized controlled trials to show that the cancer cases and mortality are decreased by screening, followed by the removal of pre-cancerous polyps or early treatment of cancers [33]. For fecal occult blood testing (FOBT), screening results in an absolute risk reduction for colorectal cancer death of between 0.8 and 4.6 per 1000. Seen another way, between 217 and 1250 persons will need to be regularly screened to prevent one death from colorectal cancer [33].

Women and men at average risk for the development of colorectal cancer are currently recommended to begin screening at age 50. The "best" method for population screening for colorectal cancer is a matter of considerable debate [34]. Options for screening average-risk patients include: annual or biennial FOBT (with a home testing kit such as Hemoccult II); flexible sigmoidoscopy every 5 years; colonoscopy every 10 years; a combination of FOBT and sigmoidoscopy; or double-contrast barium enema every 5 years [4]. In addition to these well-established tests, new tests such as "virtual colonoscopy" (also called CT colonography) and stool-based molecular screening are becoming available. There are pros and cons to each of these screening strategies; and the main issues are risk, sensitivity, cost, patient compliance and resource availability.

At present, Cancer Care Ontario, Health Canada and the Canadian Task Force on Preventive Health Care recommend annual or biennial FOBT for all people over age 50 [2]. Positive tests must be followed-up by a full colon examination with colonoscopy (preferably) or double-contrast barium enema. Rates of screening for colorectal cancer are much poorer than cancer screening for cervical cancer or breast cancer; approximately 20% of eligible persons are screened in Ontario [35]. A concerted effort to improve this statistic is underway in Ontario [2]. A recent study in Alberta showed that only 7.7% of people aged 50-59, and 12.5% of people 60-69 had an FOBT test in the last 2 years. Amongst women in the study, having a recent Pap test or mammogram, being employed or having a higher educational level were associated with a greater likelihood of having colorectal cancer screening [36].

In the USA, colorectal cancer screening rates have increased in recent years, and 43.1% of eligible women were screened in 2003 [37]. Much of the increase is attributable to increased colonoscopy rates. Women were slightly less likely than men to be screened, perhaps due to the perception of women that CRC is a "male" disease. Factors associated with being more likely to be screened included: having a higher educational level, having health insurance, older age (>65 years), having a "usual source" for health care, being a former smoker, having recently talked with a general doctor, having a greater number of recent doctors' visits, having a recent Pap test or mammogram, and having a non-Hispanic gender [37]. Women's preference for female practitioners may be another barrier to screening [38].

The above recommendations for CRC screening apply to asymptomatic people at average risk for colorectal cancer. Symptomatic patients or patients at increased risk of colorectal cancer (Table 2) should undergo colonoscopy at more frequent intervals.

SYMPTOMS

Early colorectal cancers are usually asymptomatic, but may be detected by screening. Later signs and symptoms of colorectal cancer include rectal bleeding, a change in the bowel habits, abdominal pain and weight loss [4]. Microcytic anemia in an older person is colorectal cancer, until proven otherwise. Rectal cancers can cause rectal pain and bloody or mucus discharge. Symptoms may mimic hemorrhoids, but careful digital rectal examination will make the diagnosis clear in many cases.

STAGE AND PROGNOSIS

When a person is diagnosed with colorectal cancer, the first priorities are addressing immediate risks to the patient such as bowel obstruction or bleeding, and determining the stage of the cancer. Chest X-ray, CT scan of the Abdomen and pelvis, and CEA level are routinely obtained to estimate stage. In addition, full colonoscopy or barium enema is required to determine if synchronous polyps or tumors elsewhere in the colon will require treatment, unless significant obstruction is present. PET scan is a valuable tool for staging a patient with questionable findings by CT scanning, but is not routinely used. For rectal cancer 12 cm or less from the anal verge, a transanal ultrasound or pelvis MRI is recommended to assess the status of mesorectal lymph nodes and the depth of wall-penetration of the primary tumor, because these factors will determine who should have preoperative chemoradiotherapy. A colorectal surgeon, surgical oncologist or general surgeon is the primary practitioner who coordinates the care of a patient with curable colorectal cancer.

Stages I and II colorectal cancer represent lymph node-negative disease, while Stage III is lymph-node positive ("regional"). Stage IV means that distant metastases are present. The most common location for distant metastasis is the liver. The distribution of stage at diagnosis and 5-year survival by stage are shown in Figure 1 (USA data) [1].

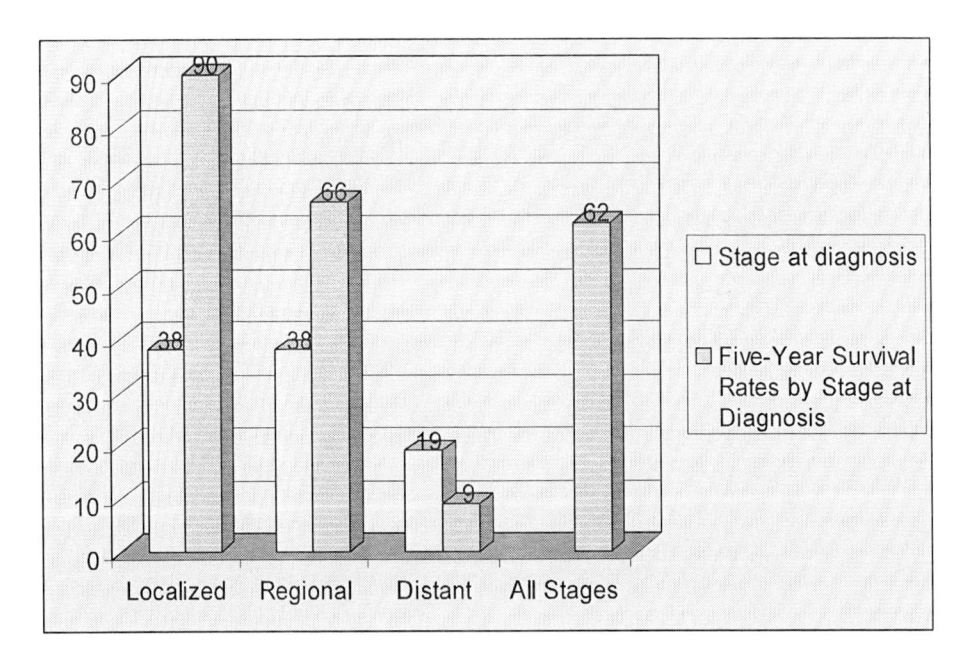

Figure 1. Stage at Diagnosis and Prognosis by Stage*.

TREATMENT

The primary treatment for curable colorectal cancer is surgery. The exact combination of therapies used depends on the Tumor-Node-Metastasis (TNM) Stage of the cancer (Table 4), the overall health status of the patient and the patient's preferences [39]. Stage I colorectal cancer is curatively treated by surgery alone. Stage II disease is treated by surgery with or without adjuvant chemotherapy. The use of adjuvant chemotherapy for stage II colorectal cancer is established for low rectal cancers, in which case it is combined with pelvic radiotherapy. For Stage II colon cancer, adjuvant chemotherapy was not felt to be beneficial until recent evidence showed a small benefit in Stage II colon cancer patients, particularly with high-risk features such as poor differentiation, lymphovascular invasion or T4 tumors. Because the survival advantage is modest amongst Stage II patients, adjuvant chemotherapy is currently used selectively in this situation [39].

There is great research interest in identifying molecular markers that will help to stratify patients, particularly with Stage II colon cancer, into high and low risk groups. This would allow better selection of people likely to benefit from chemotherapy or biologic therapies. Microsatellite instability (MSI) and loss of heterozygosity at chromosome 18q are possible markers under study in clinical trials.

The benefit of adjuvant chemotherapy for Stage III CRC is well-established [40]. Recent trials have confirmed the superiority of FOLFOX (5-fluorouracil/leukovorin and oxaliplatin) over 5-FU/leukovorin in the adjuvant setting, showing an approximate 5% improvement in disease-free survival over 5-FU/leukovorin [41]. As a result, FOLFOX is becoming the standard adjuvant treatment in Stage III and selected Stage II patients.

For Stage IV colorectal cancer, treatment is highly individualized. Surgical resection of the primary tumor is recommended if it is symptomatic and/or the life expectancy is long. Limited metastatic disease may be treated for cure in good-risk patients with single-sided liver or lung metastases, in whom staged or synchronous surgical resection is performed. In highly-selected patients with surgical resection of liver metastases, five-year survival of approximately 30% has been achieved [42]. Even the use of a combination of liver resection and radiofrequency ablation for bi-lobar liver metastatic disease may be considered in selected, healthy patients.

Table 4. Stage Definitions for Colorectal Cancer

AJCC Stage	TNM	Dukes Stage
I	T1/2, N0, M0	A
II	T3/4, N0, M0	B
III	Any T, N1/2, M0	C
IV	Any T, Any N, M1	

Whether or not the disease is resectable, chemotherapy clearly improves survival in Stage IV CRC [43-45]. Standard chemotherapy for Stage IV CRC is FOLFOX or FOLFIRI (5-FU/leukovorin plus irinotecan), often with the addition of bevacizumab or cetuximab biologic therapy. Median overall survival of 20 months has been achieved using these treatments for Stage IV CRC [44]. The timing of surgical intervention, radiation and medical treatments must be individualized, and presentation of these patients in a multidisciplinary tumor board is essential when aggressive treatment is warranted.

MANAGEMENT OF THE "MALIGNANT POLYP"

The finding of early invasive cancer (T1) within a completely-excised polyp is an area of controversy. If the polyp is completely excised as a single specimen, the margins are definitely negative, and the histologic features are uniformly favorable, selected patients can be observed, after marking the site with india ink on repeat endoscopy [46]. The rationale for this management strategy is that in such a situation the statistical likelihood of lymph node metastasis is very low. Specimens should be reviewed with the pathologist to confirm the histologic features.

ADVANCES IN CHEMOTHERAPY FOR COLORECTAL CANCER

Significant advances have been made in pharmacotherapy for colorectal cancer in recent years. Traditionally, 5-fluorouracil and leukovorin were used for adjuvant and palliative treatment of colorectal cancer. The most important new treatments are oxaliplatin and irinotecan as new chemotherapeutic agents, and the biologic agents bevacizumab (Avastin) and cetuximab. In addition, an oral form of fluorouracil, capecitabine (Xeloda), may have equivalent efficacy and allow for oral administration [44]. Increased sensory neurotoxicity with oxaliplatin had been dose-limiting in many patients, and neuroprotective treatments are under study.

Future directions in the treatment of colorectal cancer include: increased use of laparoscopic surgery; use of new biologic agents in the adjuvant setting; increased use of adjuvant therapy in Stage II disease; and increased surgical resection and/or ablation for stage IV disease.

SURGERY FOR COLON CANCER

Surgery for colon cancer involves removal of a segment of the intestine, with re-connection of the two ends. The extent of resection depends primarily on the vascular supply of the involved part of the large intestine, because removal of accompanying lymph nodes requires division of the mesenteric blood vessels near their origins. Practically speaking, tumors of the ascending colon require right hemicolectomy, tumors of the descending colon require left hemicolectomy, sigmoid tumors may be treated by sigmoid colectomy, and the resection for transverse colon cancers varies depending on the relationship of the individual tumor to associated mesenteric blood vessels. Randomized trials have proven that laparoscopic surgery provides equivalent 5-year colon cancer outcomes to open surgery, at least when performed by surgeons experienced in the technique of laparoscopic colon surgery [47]. Tumors excluded from the multi-institutional, North American COST trial included tumors invading other organs or structures (T4 tumors), transverse colon tumors, and rectal tumors [47], and these tumors should be approached via conventional surgery for most patients at present. A "learning curve" of laparoscopic colon surgery for benign diseases should be completed by a surgeon prior to offering laparoscopic surgery for colon cancer.

Short-term quality of life is improved by laparoscopic surgery, compared to open surgery [48,49]. Advantages include decreased postoperative pain, a smaller scar, slightly reduced length of hospitalization, and slightly lower complication rates [48]. It should be noted that all of the information of laparoscopic surgery for colon cancer comes from specialized centers and surgeons, and the translation of these benefits to the surgical community as a whole has not been proven.

Surgery for colon cancer carries a very low risk of death within 30 days of surgery, ranging from about 1% for elective surgery in a specialized center [47,50] to about 4-5% when emergent procedures and patients with serious comorbidities are added into the population mix [51]. Complication rates for elective surgery are about 20%, most of which are minor [47]. After surgery for colon cancer, most patients will have normal bowel function, as the remainder of the intestine compensates for the segment removed. A temporary or permanent ostomy is rarely required for treatment of colon cancer. One exception is the case of an obstructing, left-sided cancer, in which case a temporary colostomy or ileostomy is selectively used [52].

SURGERY FOR RECTAL CANCER

Surgery for rectal cancer differs from surgery for colon cancer, due to the pelvic location of the tumor, which places nerves and reproductive organs at risk for temporary or permanent injury. In addition, removing part of the rectum may have a significant impact on the bowel function or, rarely, require a permanent colostomy. Another major difference is the use of radiation therapy before or after surgery to reduce the risk of local recurrence and improve survival.

There are three broad categories of surgery for rectal cancer: anterior resection (AR), abdominoperineal resection (APR), and trans-anal excision (TAE). AR is the operation of choice in healthy patients with rectal cancers, in whom the tumor is at least 1 cm above the anal sphincters. If the tumor is in the upper rectum, AR carries a lower risk of nerve damage and significant bowel function changes compared to a "low AR", in which the anastomosis is in the low rectum. Quality of life and bowel function are improved with a "pouch" reconstruction of the rectum [53]. Many patients having a low AR operation will require a temporary ileostomy for several months.

APR is required when technical or tumor factors require removal of the anus to achieve an adequate margin around the tumor. In this case, a permanent colostomy is required and the patient has an incision on the perineum as well as the abdomen. Newer surgical techniques and preoperative radiation therapy have greatly decreased the frequency with which this operation is required. Transanal excision of rectal cancers is limited to small, low, early-stage

(T1) tumors with good histologic features. Even in these situations, transanal excision for rectal cancer has a higher recurrence rate than radical surgery, and radical surgery is the "gold standard" for treatment in good-risk patients [54]. This is a situation in which patients' preferences are important in the risk-benefit analysis.

Radiation therapy, usually combined with chemotherapy in North America, has become an important part of the treatment for low- and mid-rectal cancers with positive lymph nodes or full-thickness penetration through the rectal wall (T3/4). Preoperative (neoadjuvant) radiotherapy is preferred in cases where preoperative staging by transanal ultrasound, CT or MRI shows mesorectal lymphadenopathy or invasion of the tumor through the full-thickness of the muscular layer of the rectal wall [55-58]. In these situations, local recurrence rates and survival are both improved by neoadjuvant treatment [55-60]. Preoperative treatment may also improve the likelihood that an AR can be performed, rather than APR. If the stage is not clear, postoperative chemoradiotherapy can be given selectively based on the surgical pathology results [60].

Chemo-radiotherapy is clearly beneficial to selected patients with rectal cancer. However, the short-term and long-term toxicity of radiation treatment is significant, and patients should be well-informed.

POSTOPERATIVE RECOVERY

After surgery for colorectal cancer, most patients spend between 3 and 7 days in the hospital. An epidural analgesia catheter, a patient-controlled narcotic pump (PCA), or intermittently-dosed pain medicine may be used for pain control. Thoracic epidural analgesia may be superior to PCA in terms of pain control and postoperative ileus, although these are not routinely done in all hospitals [61]. Early ambulation is encouraged after surgery, and clear liquids are often allowed within 48 hours of surgery. It is common for patients to feel fatigued for 4-6 weeks after surgery, and most will require extra help at home during recovery.

BOWEL FUNCTION AFTER RECTAL CANCER TREATMENT

After colon cancer surgery, bowel changes are uncommon. However, rectal surgery frequently causes changes in the bowel function. The severity of these changes is determined by how low the anastomosis is, whether or not radiation treatment was given, the type of surgical reconstruction performed, and individual patient variation. With very low rectal anastomoses, median 24-hour bowel frequency is about 6.4 at 3 months and 3.5 at one year [62]. These numbers are improved to a median of 2 times per day at both time points if a pouch reconstruction is performed [62]. Other problems include nocturnal bowel movements, fecal urgency, incontinence or leakage of stool which requires wearing a pad, and a feeling of incomplete evacuation. Older patients and those with impaired continence preoperatively may have particular difficulty compensating for the bowel changes. Anti-diarrheal medication and fiber supplementation are frequently required, even one year postoperatively

[62,63]. Patients can be reassured by evidence showing that most individuals see improvement in bowel function up to one year after surgery.

OSTOMIES

Permanent or temporary ostomies are infrequently required in the modern treatment of CRC. However, having an ostomy causes a change in the body image, and may negatively impact on the quality of life, although this is controversial [64]. Fortunately, modern ostomy appliances are excellent, and a completely normal lifestyle is possible for patients with ostomies. The services of a WOCN-certified enterostomal nurse is extremely valuable for preoperative and postoperative care of the patient with a temporary or permanent ostomy. Many support groups are also available.

FEMALE SEXUAL AND URINARY FUNCTION

Female sexual function has seldom been measured after treatment for rectal cancer, while male sexual problems due to nerve damage from surgery and radiation were recognized long ago. Recent research has finally begun to shed some light on this under-recognized problem. Our recent study of 81 women, curatively treated for rectal cancer, showed that almost 30% of women felt that their treatment had a negative impact on their sexual function [65]. Sexual problems varied, and included dyspareunia (in almost half of the women), loss of libido, problems with arousal, lubrication, and orgasm. The ostomy had a negative impact for about one-third of those with an ostomy. Older age, radiation therapy, and having an APR made sexual dysfunction more likely. Our hypothesis is that scarring of the pelvis, nerve damage, stress surrounding the cancer diagnosis and changes in body image each has a role in these problems. Of note, only 9% of the women remembered any preoperative discussion of potential sexual effects of surgery [65]. Greater awareness of this issue is needed.

For women with rectal cancer who receive pelvic radiation therapy, sexual dysfunction is probably worse. Possible therapeutic interventions for women with sexual dysfunction after radiation therapy (mixed cancer diagnoses) was performed by the Cochrane Collaboration, but the quality of the evidence was found to be poor. Nevertheless, the use of topical estrogens and benzydamine to the vagina is supported by randomized trials, for the treatment of acute radiation toxicity [66].

QUALITY OF LIFE

After curative treatment for colorectal cancer, overall quality of life is excellent, particularly after 3 years, at which time full recovery from surgery and chemotherapy has been achieved. Most patients with long-term remission from colon cancer have a quality of life that is similar to age-matched controls [67]. Cancer recurrence is the most important factor impacting on the quality of life. For rectal cancer, numerous studies have confirmed that despite bowel and sexual changes, the overall quality of life is very high amongst survivors [65,68,89], including those with ostomies.

SURVEILLANCE

About 80% of curatively-treated patients who experience disease recurrence do so within the first 3 years [70]. Regular cancer surveillance (or "follow-up") is recommended for all patients with stage II/III disease, who are candidates for additional treatment, until 5 years. Stage I cancer patients have a very low risk of recurrence, and surveillance is not thought to improve outcome. Early-stage rectal cancer patients treated by transanal excision or whose tumors were pathologically down-staged by preoperative chemo-radiotherapy are exceptions, and should have intensive surveillance. The rationale for cancer surveillance is the early detection of recurrent CRC. While the majority of patients with disease recurrence will die of colorectal cancer, a minority can be treated for their recurrence with curative intent. It is these patients for whom surveillance is designed.

There is good evidence to show that "intensive" colorectal cancer surveillance improves overall survival for Stage II/III patients, and a 20-33% lower risk of death has been shown in metaanalyses [71,72]. However, the best surveillance regimen is not clear from existing evidence [72], and this is a controversial area. Surveillance should be performed by the surgeon or medical oncologist who is coordinating care. The American Society of Clinical Oncology currently recommends intensive surveillance for 3 years, and less intensive for 2 additional years [71]. For the first 3 years, CEA measurement is performed every 3 months, starting after completion of 5-FU-based chemotherapy, which can falsely elevate the CEA. History and physical examination are performed every 3-6 months for 3 years, then every 6 months for years 4-5. In addition, annual chest, abdomen and pelvis CT scan is performed for 3 years. Colonoscopy is recommended postoperatively if not complete preoperatively. If complete preoperatively it should be performed at 3 years, and then every 5 years if normal.

For rectal cancer patients, sigmoidoscopy should be performed about every 6 months, particularly if no radiation therapy was performed or if trans-anal excision was used as surgical therapy. Finally, all patients should be counseled to report symptoms or signs such as abdominal pain, bowel changes, anorexia, weight loss or a mass as soon as they occur. However, most patients who develop symptomatic recurrences are not curable.

CONCLUSION

Colorectal cancer is a significant public health concern for women. Prevention of CRC is possible with the use of a timely, risk-stratified screening strategy and a healthy lifestyle. High priority should be given to improving rates of CRC screening in North America. Women with CRC can expect a good outcome if the disease is discovered and treated at an early stage; and new advances in chemotherapy have improved the outlook even for women with advanced disease. Overall quality of life is preserved after curative treatment for colorectal cancer, but rectal cancer patients may experience sexual dysfunction and changes in body image. Recognition of these concerns and support for those affected is important.

REFERENCES

[1] Jemal A, Tiwari RC, Murray T, et al. Cancer statistics, 2004. *CA Cancer J Clin* 2004;54:8-29.
[2] Website CCO. *Cancer Incidence and Mortality in Ontario* 1964-2002, 2006.
[3] Society CC. *Colorectal Cancer Stats*, 2006.
[4] Society AC. *Cancer Facts and Figures* 2006. Atlanta: American Cancer Society, 2006.
[5] Gibbons L, Waters C, Mao Y, Ellison L. Trends in colorectal cancer incidence and mortality. *Health Rep* 2001;12:41-55.
[6] Sturmer T, Glynn RJ, Lee IM, Christen WG, Hennekens CH. Lifetime cigarette smoking and colorectal cancer incidence in the Physicians' Health Study I. *Journal of the National Cancer Institute* 2000;92:1178-81.
[7] Larsen IK, Grotmol T, Almendingen K, Hoff G. Lifestyle as a predictor for colonic neoplasia in asymptomatic individuals. *BMC Gastroenterology* 2006;6:5.
[8] Michels KB, Giovannucci E, Chan AT, Singhania R, Fuchs CS, Willett WC. Fruit and vegetable consumption and colorectal adenomas in the Nurses' Health Study. *Cancer Res* 2006;66:3942-53.
[9] Wei EK, Giovannucci E, Wu K, et al. Comparison of risk factors for colon and rectal cancer. *Int J Cancer* 2004;108:433-42.
[10] Neugut AI, Garbowski GC, Lee WC, et al. Dietary risk factors for the incidence and recurrence of colorectal adenomatous polyps. A case-control study. [see comment]. *Annals of Internal Medicine* 1993;118:91-5.
[11] Willett WC, Stampfer MJ, Colditz GA, Rosner BA, Speizer FE. Relation of meat, fat, and fiber intake to the risk of colon cancer in a prospective study among women.[see comment]. *New England Journal of Medicine* 1990;323:1664-72.
[12] Fuchs CS, Giovannucci EL, Colditz GA, et al. Dietary fiber and the risk of colorectal cancer and adenoma in women. *N Engl J Med* 1999;340:169-76.
[13] Kato I, Akhmedkhanov A, Koenig K, Toniolo PG, Shore RE, Riboli E. Prospective study of diet and female colorectal cancer: the New York University Women's Health Study. *Nutrition & Cancer* 1997;28:276-81.
[14] Bingham SA, Day NE, Luben R, et al. Dietary fibre in food and protection against colorectal cancer in the European Prospective Investigation into Cancer and Nutrition (EPIC): an observational study. *Lancet* 2003;361:1496-501.
[15] Michels KB, Fuchs CS, Giovannucci E, et al. Fiber intake and incidence of colorectal cancer among 76,947 women and 47,279 men. *Cancer Epidemiol Biomarkers Prev* 2005;14:842-9.
[16] Asano TK, McLeod RS. Dietary fibre for the prevention of colorectal adenomas and carcinomas [Systematic Review]: *Cochrane Database of Systematic Reviews* 2006;(3).
[17] McKeown-Eyssen GE, Bright-See E, Bruce WR, et al. A randomized trial of a low fat high fibre diet in the recurrence of colorectal polyps. Toronto Polyp Prevention Group.

[erratum appears in J Clin Epidemiol 1995 Feb;48(2):i]. *Journal of Clinical Epidemiology* 1994;47:525-36.
[18] Giovannucci E, Stampfer MJ, Colditz GA, et al. Multivitamin use, folate, and colon cancer in women in the Nurses' Health Study.[see comment]. *Annals of Internal Medicine* 1998;129:517-24.
[19] Greenberg ER, Baron JA, Tosteson TD, et al. A clinical trial of antioxidant vitamins to prevent colorectal adenoma. Polyp Prevention Study Group. [see comment]. *New England Journal of Medicine* 1994;331:141-7.
[20] Albanes D, Malila N, Taylor PR, et al. Effects of supplemental alpha-tocopherol and beta-carotene on colorectal cancer: results from a controlled trial (Finland) [see comment]. *Cancer Causes & Control* 2000;11:197-205.
[21] Weingarten MA, Zalmanovici A, Yaphe J. Dietary calcium supplementation for preventing colorectal cancer and adenomatous polyps. [update of Cochrane Database Syst Rev. 2004;(1):CD003548; PMID: 14974021]. *Cochrane Database of Systematic Reviews* 2005:CD003548.
[22] Shaukat A, Scouras N, Schunemann HJ. Role of supplemental calcium in the recurrence of colorectal adenomas: a metaanalysis of randomized controlled trials. [see comment]. *American Journal of Gastroenterology* 2005;100:390-4.
[23] Cho E, Smith-Warner SA, Spiegelman D, et al. Dairy foods, calcium, and colorectal cancer: a pooled analysis of 10 cohort studies. *J Natl Cancer Inst* 2004;96:1015-22.
[24] Wactawski-Wende J, Kotchen JM, Anderson GL, et al. Calcium plus vitamin D supplementation and the risk of colorectal cancer. [see comment]. *New England Journal of Medicine* 2006;354:684-96.
[25] Mao Y, Pan S, Wen SW, Johnson KC. Physical inactivity, energy intake, obesity and the risk of rectal cancer in Canada. *Int J Cancer* 2003;105:831-7.
[26] Lee IM, Manson JE, Ajani U, Paffenbarger RS, Jr., Hennekens CH, Buring JE. Physical activity and risk of colon cancer: the Physicians' Health Study (United States). *Cancer Causes & Control* 1997;8:568-74.
[27] Cho E, Smith-Warner SA, Ritz J, et al. Alcohol intake and colorectal cancer: a pooled analysis of 8 cohort studies. *Ann Intern Med* 2004;140:603-13.
[28] Cook NR, Lee IM, Gaziano JM, et al. Low-dose aspirin in the primary prevention of cancer: the Women's Health Study: a randomized controlled trial. *Jama* 2005;294:47-55.
[29] Raju R, Cruz-Correa M. Chemoprevention of colorectal cancer. *Dis Colon Rectum* 2006;49:113-24; discussion 124-5.
[30] Poynter JN, Gruber SB, Higgins PD, et al. Statins and the risk of colorectal cancer. *N Engl J Med* 2005;352:2184-92.
[31] American Gastroenterological Association medical position statement: hereditary colorectal cancer and genetic testing. *Gastroenterology* 2001;121:195-7.
[32] Church JM. A scoring system for the strength of a family history of colorectal cancer. *Dis Colon Rectum* 2005;48:889-96.
[33] Walsh JME, Terdiman JP. Colorectal cancer screening: scientific review. [see comment]. *JAMA* 2003;289:1288-96.

[34] McLeod RS, Canadian Task Force on Preventive Health C. Screening strategies for colorectal cancer: a systematic review of the evidence.[see comment]. *Canadian Journal of Gastroenterology* 2001;15:647-60.

[35] Rabeneck L, Paszat LF. A population-based estimate of the extent of colorectal cancer screening in Ontario. *American Journal of Gastroenterology* 2004;99:1141-4.

[36] McGregor SE, Bryant HE. Predictors of colorectal cancer screening: a comparison of men and women. *Can J Gastroenterol* 2005;19:343-9.

[37] Meissner HI, Breen N, Klabunde CN, Vernon SW. Patterns of colorectal cancer screening uptake among men and women in the United States. *Cancer Epidemiol Biomarkers Prev* 2006;15:389-94.

[38] Menees SB, Inadomi JM, Korsnes S, Elta GH. Women patients' preference for women physicians is a barrier to colon cancer screening. *Gastrointestinal Endoscopy* 2005;62:219-23.

[39] NCCN Practice Guidelines in Oncology v.2.2006: Colon Cancer. *NCCN Practice Guidelines in Oncology v.2*.2006, 2006.

[40] Gill S, Loprinzi CL, Sargent DJ, et al. Pooled analysis of fluorouracil-based adjuvant therapy for stage II and III colon cancer: who benefits and by how much? *J Clin Oncol* 2004;22:1797-806.

[41] Andre T, Boni C, Mounedji-Boudiaf L, et al. Oxaliplatin, fluorouracil, and leucovorin as adjuvant treatment for colon cancer. *N Engl J Med* 2004;350:2343-51.

[42] Simmonds PC, Primrose JN, Colquitt JL, Garden OJ, Poston GJ, Rees M. Surgical resection of hepatic metastases from colorectal cancer: a systematic review of published studies. *British Journal of Cancer* 2006;94:982-99.

[43] Jonker DJ, Maroun JA, Kocha W. Survival benefit of chemotherapy in metastatic colorectal cancer: a meta-analysis of randomized controlled trials. *British Journal of Cancer* 2000;82:1789-94.

[44] Meyerhardt JA, Mayer RJ. Systemic therapy for colorectal cancer. *N Engl J Med* 2005;352:476-87.

[45] Palliative chemotherapy for advanced or metastatic colorectal cancer. Colorectal Meta-analysis Collaboration. *Cochrane Database of Systematic Reviews* 2000:CD001545.

[46] Bond JH. Polyp guideline: diagnosis, treatment, and surveillance for patients with colorectal polyps. Practice Parameters Committee of the American College of Gastroenterology. *Am J Gastroenterol* 2000;95:3053-63.

[47] A comparison of laparoscopically assisted and open colectomy for colon cancer. *N Engl J Med* 2004;350:2050-9.

[48] Schwenk W, Haase O, Neudecker J, Muller JM. Short term benefits for laparoscopic colorectal resection. *Cochrane Database Syst Rev* 2005:CD003145.

[49] Abraham NS, Young JM, Solomon MJ. Meta-analysis of short-term outcomes after laparoscopic resection for colorectal cancer. [see comment]. *British Journal of Surgery* 2004;91:1111-24.

[50] Ko CY, Chang JT, Chaudhry S, Kominski G. Are high-volume surgeons and hospitals the most important predictors of in-hospital outcome for colon cancer resection? *Surgery* 2002;132:268-73.

[51] Schrag D, Panageas KS, Riedel E, et al. Surgeon volume compared to hospital volume as a predictor of outcome following primary colon cancer resection. *J Surg Oncol* 2003;83:68-78; discussion 78-9.

[52] De Salvo GL, Gava C, Pucciarelli S, Lise M. Curative surgery for obstruction from primary left colorectal carcinoma: primary or staged resection?[update of Cochrane Database Syst Rev. 2002;(1):CD002101; PMID: 11869622]. *Cochrane Database of Systematic Reviews* 2004:CD002101.

[53] Sailer M, Fuchs KH, Fein M, Thiede A. Randomized clinical trial comparing quality of life after straight and pouch coloanal reconstruction. [see comment]. *British Journal of Surgery* 2002;89:1108-17.

[54] Bentrem DJ, Okabe S, Wong WD, et al. T1 adenocarcinoma of the rectum: transanal excision or radical surgery? *Ann Surg* 2005;242:472-7; discussion 477-9.

[55] Mohiuddin M, Winter K, Mitchell E, et al. Randomized phase II study of neoadjuvant combined-modality chemoradiation for distal rectal cancer: Radiation Therapy Oncology Group Trial 0012. *Journal of Clinical Oncology* 2006;24:650-5.

[56] Allal AS, Bieri S, Pelloni A, et al. Sphincter-sparing surgery after preoperative radiotherapy for low rectal cancers: feasibility, oncologic results and quality of life outcomes. *British Journal of Cancer* 2000;82:1131-7.

[57] Improved survival with preoperative radiotherapy in resectable rectal cancer. Swedish Rectal Cancer Trial.[see comment][erratum appears in *N Engl J Med* 1997 May 22;336(21):1539]. *New England Journal of Medicine* 1997;336:980-7.

[58] Sauer R, Becker H, Hohenberger W, et al. Preoperative versus postoperative chemoradiotherapy for rectal cancer. *N Engl J Med* 2004;351:1731-40.

[59] Camma C, Giunta M, Fiorica F, Pagliaro L, Craxi A, Cottone M. Preoperative radiotherapy for resectable rectal cancer: A meta-analysis. *JAMA* 2000;284:1008-15.

[60] Glimelius B, Gronberg H, Jarhult J, Wallgren A, Cavallin-Stahl E. A systematic overview of radiation therapy effects in rectal cancer. *Acta Oncologica* 2003;42:476-92.

[61] Carli F, Trudel JL, Belliveau P. The effect of intraoperative thoracic epidural anesthesia and postoperative analgesia on bowel function after colorectal surgery: a prospective, randomized trial. *Diseases of the Colon & Rectum* 2001;44:1083-9.

[62] Hallbook O, Pahlman L, Krog M, Wexner SD, Sjodahl R. Randomized comparison of straight and colonic J pouch anastomosis after low anterior resection. *Ann Surg* 1996;224:58-65.

[63] Ho YH, Tan M, Seow-Choen F. Prospective randomized controlled study of clinical function and anorectal physiology after low anterior resection: comparison of straight and colonic J pouch anastomoses. *Br J Surg* 1996;83:978-80.

[64] Pachler J, Wille-Jorgensen P. Quality of life after rectal resection for cancer, with or without permanent colostomy. [update of Cochrane Database Syst Rev. 2004;(3):CD004323; PMID: 15266529]. *Cochrane Database of Systematic Reviews* 2005:CD004323.

[65] Hendren SK, O'Connor BI, Liu M, et al. Prevalence of male and female sexual dysfunction is high following surgery for rectal cancer. *Ann Surg* 2005;242:212-23.

[66] Denton AS, Maher EJ. Interventions for the physical aspects of sexual dysfunction in women following pelvic radiotherapy [Systematic Review]: *Cochrane Database of Systematic Reviews* 2006;(3).

[67] Ramsey SD, Andersen MR, Etzioni R, et al. Quality of life in survivors of colorectal carcinoma. *Cancer* 2000;88:1294-303.

[68] Camilleri-Brennan J, Steele RJ. Quality of life after treatment for rectal cancer. *Br J Surg* 1998;85:1036-43.

[69] Camilleri-Brennan J, Steele RJ. Prospective analysis of quality of life and survival following mesorectal excision for rectal cancer. *Br J Surg* 2001;88:1617-22.

[70] Sargent DJ, Wieand HS, Haller DG, et al. Disease-free survival versus overall survival as a primary end point for adjuvant colon cancer studies: individual patient data from 20,898 patients on 18 randomized trials. *J Clin Oncol* 2005;23:8664-70.

[71] Desch CE, Benson AB, 3rd, Somerfield MR, et al. Colorectal cancer surveillance: 2005 update of an American Society of Clinical Oncology practice guideline. *J Clin Oncol* 2005;23:8512-9.

[72] Jeffery GM, Hickey BE, Hider P. Follow-up strategies for patients treated for non-metastatic colorectal cancer [Systematic Review]: *Cochrane Database of Systematic Reviews* 2006;(3).

In: Rectal Cancer: Etiology, Pathogenesis and Treatment
Editors: Paula Wells and Regina Halstead

ISBN 978-1-60692-563-8
© 2009 Nova Science Publishers, Inc.

Chapter X

DIETARY FATTY ACIDS AND ACYL-COA SYNTHETASES IN THE MODIFIER CONCEPT OF COLORECTAL CARCINOGENESIS[*]

Nikolaus Gassler[1,†], Elke Kaemmerer[2], Christina Klaus[1] and Andrea Reinartz[1,3]

[1]Institute of Pathology, RWTH Aachen University, Aachen, Germany;
[2]Department of Pediatrics, RWTH Aachen University, Aachen, Germany;
[3]School of Biology and Petit Institute for Bioengineering and Bioscience, Georgia Institute of Technology, Atlanta, USA

ABSTRACT

Epidemiological studies confirm a strong association between intake of saturated fatty acids and colon cancer risk. Fatty acids have been especially shown to be involved in gene expression and cellular reactivity mediated by several signaling cascades. However, the molecular pathways determining this phenomenon are not well elucidated. Here we discuss a putative pathway by which fatty acids could be able to modify the behaviour of intestinal epithelia via acyl-CoA synthetase isoform 5 (ACSL5), a mitochondrial located enzyme preferentially catalyzing the synthesis of long chain acyl-CoA derivatives. In enterocytes, strong association of ACSL5 over-expression and susceptibility for apoptosis has been shown. This physiological mechanism probably facilitates maturation and shedding of enterocytes along the crypt-plateau axis in normal

---

[*] A version of this chapter was also published in *Nutrition for Middle Aged and Elderly*, edited by Nancy E. Bernhardt and Artur M. Kasko, published by Nova Science Publishers, Inc. It was submitted for appropriate modifications in an effort to encourage wider dissemination of research.

[†] Correspondence concerning this article should be addressed to: Prof. Dr. med. N. Gassler (M.A.), Institute of Pathology, RWTH Aachen University, Pauwelsstrasse 30, 52074 Aachen, Germany. E-mail: ngassler@ukaachen.de; Phone: +49 241 8088897; Fax: +49 241 8082439.

intestinal mucosa. On the molecular level, ACSL5 synthesized acyl-CoA derivatives might interfere with ceramide synthesis, membrane composition, protein lipidation, activity of intramitochondrial enzymes, and finally gene transcription. Disturbances in this complex system are suggested to modify enterocyte behaviour promoting intestinal carcinogenesis.

INTRODUCTION

Colorectal cancer (CRC) is one of the most frequent malignancies in the world (Saunders and Iveson, 2006). Its development is based on a sequence of molecular events including gene mutations, epigenetic modifications, aberrant signaling in several pathways, and execution of modifier genes. From the *APC* mice evidence is given that the power of modifier gene activity depends on the individual genetic background of a susceptible person (Taketo and Edelmann, 2009). The molecular injuries determining CRCs are associated with the development of histomorphological lesions comprising intraepithelial neoplasia, i.e. aberrant crypt foci (ACF) or adenomas, and mucosa-invasive (early) colorectal cancer. Moreover, the differences in cellular morphology of such lesions are summarized in the tumour-grading which is suggested as a well-suitable indicator for tumour prognosis and molecular changes behind tumour growth. The sentinel molecular events occurring early in progression from adenoma to carcinoma have been integrated into a coherent adenoma-carcinoma sequence by molecular research (Fearon and Vogelstein, 1990). This sequence is a time-consuming process. It is assumed that the great number of CRCs has a natural history of transition from precursor to malignant lesions that spans approx. 15 – 20 years (Dvory-Sobol and Arber, 2007).

CRCs comprise a heterogeneous group of malignancies including hereditary forms and so-called sporadic tumours (Jass et al., 2002; Worthley et al., 2007). At present, the autosomal dominant condition, familial adenomatous polyposis (FAP) has been characterized as the counterpart of sporadic CRCs. Mutations in the *APC* gene are founder lesions in CRCs of FAP-type. In hereditary nonpolyposis colorectal cancer (HNPCC), the stepwise progression of tumours following the step of initiation is accelerated by an injured expression of mismatch repair genes. Consequently, HNPCC is not a hereditary form of CRC by its own (Jass et al., 2002). By defining subsets of colorectal cancer, it should be possible to characterize additional founder or modifying pathways and to develop more targeted approaches to tumour prevention and treatment.

In the last years, nutrition has been suggested as a fundamental factor in modifying initiation and progression of CRCs (Lipkin et al., 1999). Epidemiological data are indicating a link between the intake of dietary lipids and development of (sporadic) CRCs (Granados et al., 2006; Yeh et al., 2006). Among dietary lipids fatty acids are assumed to be the main component interfering with the development of intestinal neoplasia. However, pathways of fatty acid metabolism intervening in the adenoma-carcinoma sequence are not well elucidated so far (Kuniyasu, 2008). The association of fatty acids like n-3 polyunsaturated fatty acids or long-chain saturated fatty acids and inhibition or promotion of colorectal carcinogenesis is in discussion (Balk et al., 2007; Chapkin et al., 2007). Despite this discrepancy, development of a diet that provides adequate nutrition and effective cancer prevention is an important goal in nutrition and cancer research.

Here we provide a short overview about the putative modifier role of free fatty acids activated by acyl-CoA synthetases in the development of colorectal carcinoma. The focus is given on the acyl-CoA synthetase family member acyl-CoA synthetase 5.

ACSL5 AND ACYL-COA-DEPENDENT METABOLISM

Lipids comprise a heterogeneous group of chemical substances broadly defined as any hydrophobic, fat-soluble molecule. Fatty acids and their derivatives, e.g. glycerides and phospholipids as well as sterol-derivatives are important subgroups of lipids involved in diverse cellular pathways and functions. Evidence is given that fatty acids affect the behaviour of different cell types, e.g. enterocytes. Various molecular mechanisms including changes in membrane composition, intracellular calcium levels, and second messenger synthesis as well as protein lipidation and direct interaction with coding gene sequences in the nucleus are recorded (Sampath and Ntambi, 2005; Resh, 2006). Experimental evidence is given that dietary fatty acids and sphingoid bases are physiologically metabolized by enterocytes generating a multitude of cellular functions.

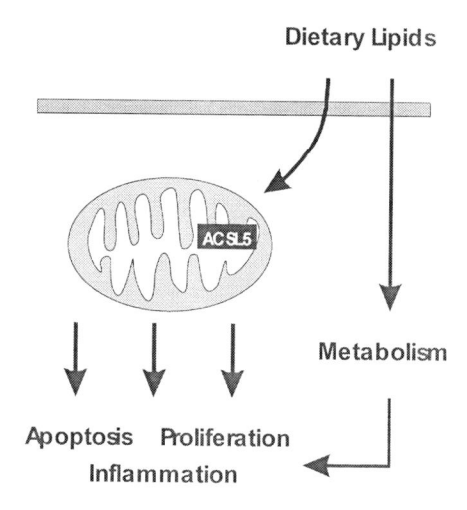

Figure 1. Putative pathways of dietary long chain fatty acid metabolism in enterocytes involving acyl-CoA synthetase 5. Dietary triglycerides are digested in free fatty acids and glycerol. The constituents are absorbed by enterocytes. Activation of free fatty acids to acyl-CoA derivatives is performed by several enzymes including acyl-CoA synthetases (ACSL) localized in endoplasmic reticulum (ER), mitochondria (M), and cytoplasm. ACSL5 catalyzed acyl-CoA derivatives are probably used in several biochemical pathways modifying cellular reagibility in apoptosis, proliferation, and inflammation.

Such activated lipid intermediates are precursor molecules in the formation of complex lipids and are involved in signal transduction, transcriptional activation, and modulation of a variety of cellular functions including membrane fusion, ion transportation, and cellular survival. Main pathways of dietary, apically incorporated fatty acids are illustrated in Figure

1. It is assumed that basolateral incorporated lipids initiate functions different from the dietary-induced phenomena (Murota and Storch, 2005). However, this issue is not well elucidated as yet and at present, dietary – not endogenous – fatty acids are assumed being critical in colorectal carcinogenesis (Granados et al., 2006). Recently, vectorial acylation has been characterized as to be important in the modification of cellular behaviour by fatty acids (Black and DiRusso, 2007). This molecular process involves a transport protein and activating protein, i.e. acyl-CoA synthetase, typically forming a physical complex.

An important step in the activation of long chain fatty acids is the synthesis of thioester derivatives by addition of coenzyme-A (CoA). This biochemical two-step synthesis is preferentially catalyzed by ATP-consuming enzymes of the acyl-CoA synthetase family (ACSL) (Mashek et al., 2004). The acyl-CoA derivatives are soluble in hydrophilic milieu which is one important difference to free fatty acids. Importantly, acyl-CoA derivatives are used in several biochemical pathways including the *de novo* synthesis of ceramides (Figure 2). Ceramides are central metabolites of bioactive sphingolipids which can be synthesized either in response to the activation of sphingomyelinases or *de novo*.

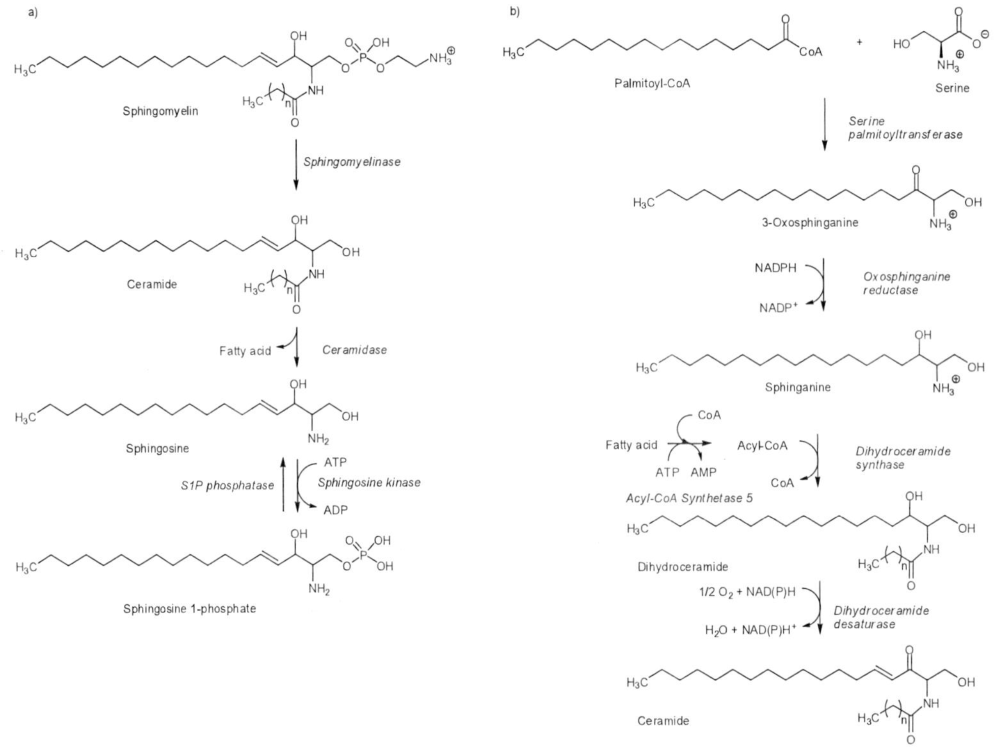

Figure 2. Sphingolipid metabolism. a) Central role of ceramide in sphingosine 1-phosphate metabolism and its synthesis by activation of sphingomyelinases. The amount of ceramide is further balanced by the *de novo* synthesis shown in more detail right hand. b) Ceramide *de novo* synthesis. In the scheme, the important role of acyl-CoA generating enzymes like acyl-CoA synthetase 5 (ACSL5) is addressed. Especially palmitoyl-CoA is used for the synthesis of the ceramide precursor 3-oxosphinganine, whereas several acyl-CoA derivatives are enzymatically added to sphinganine forming dihydroceramide. The acyl-CoA-forming enzyme ACSL5 is also located in mitochondrial membranes where ceramide synthesis is assumed to be highly important for the initiation of apoptosis.

Fatty acids activated by ACSLs are necessary in the *de novo* ceramide synthesis. Here, sphinganine is modified by the enzyme dihydroceramide synthase catalyzing the N-acylation of dihydrosphingosine to dihydroceramide. Finally, dihydroceramide desaturase catalyses the subsequent introduction of a *trans* double bond at C4-C5 to generate ceramide. Several inhibitors of the *de novo* ceramide synthesis have been identified including L-cycloserine, myriocin, fumonisin, D-*threo*-1-phenyl-2-palmitoylamino-3-morpholino-1-propanol (PPMP), and D-*threo*-1-phenyl-2-decanoylamino-3-morpholino-1-propanol (PDMP) (Pyne and Pyne, 2000; Ruvolo, 2003; Marasas et al., 2004).

The metabolic conversion of ceramide into sphingosine 1-phosphate is assumed to switch cells from an apoptotic state to a proliferative one. Ceramidases catalyze the deacylation of ceramide to produce non-esterified fatty acid and sphingosin (Bernardo et al., 1995). Condensation of serine and palmitoyl-CoA producing 3-oxosphinganine is the initial step in the intracellular *de novo* ceramide synthesis (Pyne and Pyne, 2000). Intracellular sphinganine (dihydrosphingosine) is generated from 3-oxosphinganine by rapid reduction catalyzed by a NAD(P)H reductase stereospecific for the D-isomer. Evidence is given that dietary sphinganine is absorbed by cellular systems and is able to interfere with the metabolism of sphingolipids (Ahn and Schroeder, 2002; Sugawara et al., 2003; Sugawara et al., 2004).

Strong evidence is given that the sphingosine-based lipid ceramide is involved in apoptosis of tumour as well as non-tumour cells by different pathways (Ruvolo, 2003; Ahn and Schroeder, 2006).

The release of ceramide from sphingomyelin by stress stimuli like irradiation or heat shock is mediated by the acid sphingomyelinase which is expressed in the cell surface membrane after stimulation with apoptotic triggers (Gulbins, 2003). Several apoptotic stimuli have been shown to induce apoptosis *via* an increase in mitochondrial ceramide levels probably mediated by both, release from sphingomyelin as well as *de novo* ceramide synthesis (Bionda et al., 2004; Birbes et al., 2001; Siskind, 2005). ACSL5 is assumed to be important in catalyzing intramitochondrial acyl-CoA for the ceramid *de novo* synthesis. This pathway could be of high interest to transfer pro-apoptotic ACSL5 activity. Some ceramide species are able to form large channels permeable for protein, especially in mitochondria outer membranes which are important in apoptosis execution (Siskind et al., 2006). It is assumed that the molecular basis of channel forming by ceramide is determined by the molecular structure of the ceramide backbone, especially the presence of the C4-C5 *trans* double-bound (Brockman et al., 2004). Given the interference of dietary sphinganine and sphinganine derivatives with intracellular ceramide *de novo* synthesis and ACSL5 activity, this class of molecules provides numerous opportunities for indirect modulation of channel formation by ceramide.

In small intestinal mucosa, where fatty acids are preferentially absorbed, isoform 5 of the ACSL family is abundantly expressed by enterocytes (Yamashita et al., 2000, Gassler et al., 2004). ACSL5 is found in a spatial distribution with high amounts of ACSL5 mRNA and protein in villus or plateau-lining epithelia when compared with crypts. Consequently, expression of ACSL5 is stronger in small than large intestinal mucosa reflecting the differences in cellular lipid metabolism. ACSL isoforms other than ACSL5 are additionally found in intestinal surface epithelia; their function in physiological as well as pathophysiological pathways has been investigated (Cao et al., 2001). Using an inducible cell expression system, prevention of apoptosis is found after over-expression of ACSL4 probably due to reduction of free arachidonic acid signaling apoptosis (Cao et al., 2000). In the majority of CRCs, ACSL4 and cyclooxygenase-2 (COX-2) are up-regulated and interference with arachidonic acid metabolism is suggested (Cao et al., 2001). The additive effect of the enzymes in lowering free arachidonic acid levels is suggested as an important modifying mechanism in prevention of cellular apoptosis and driving tumour progression.

However, it is suggested that in addition to ACSL4 ACSL isoform 5 plays a central role in intestinal lipid metabolism and probably in cellular differentiation (Yeh et al., 2006). This hypothesis is initiated by spatial distribution of ACSL5 along the crypt-villus axis in human small intestine and the crypt-plateau axis in human large intestine, cloning of two ACSL5 variants from human intestinal mucosa (accession no. AB033899; AM262166), and a functional link of ACSL5 activity to apoptosis.

The ACSL5 variants identified differ in a 72 bp region corresponding to exon 20 of the *ACSL5* gene (10q25.1-q25.2). Biochemical analysis of both recombinant proteins, ACSL5-fl and ACSL5-Δ20, shows a significant shift in pH dependency of enzyme activities. Whereas ACSL5-fl is active in a strong bimodal dependency at pH 7.5 and pH 9.5, ACSL5-Δ20 shows a more uniform performance over a broad pH spectrum with minor peaks at pH 7.5 and 8.5. The phenomenon is determined by molecular differences in organization of the fatty acid activation 1 domain (FAA1) encoded by exon 20.

It has been suggested that the ACSL5-fl/ ACSL5-Δ20 ratio has some input to the execution of apoptosis/ senescence of enterocytes involving mitochondria, because over-expression of ACSL5-fl sensitizes enterocytes to TRAIL-mediated apoptosis accompanied by surface expression of TRAIL-receptors and increased caspase 3-like activity (Gassler et al., 2007). In such TRAIL-sensitive cells, expression of the FLICE-inhibitory protein (FLIP) is substantially decreased. However, treatment of ACSL5-fl transfectants with fumonisin B1, a specific inhibitor of the ceramide synthase, restores FLIP-expression levels.

ACSL5 IN THE MODIFIER CONCEPT OF CRC DEVELOPMENT

It is assumed that the search for key modifier genes underlying carcinogenesis has not been highly successful because alleles of modifier genes have a moderate-to-high population frequency with a low penetrance (Samuelson et al., 2007). However, the use of whole-genome linkage studies in inbred animal cancer models in addition to functional studies is suggested as a modern approach to define potential cancer susceptibility genes. Consequently, an increasing number of studies focussed on gene – environment interactions and cancer predisposition has led to the identification of so-called tumour modifiers (Dragani and Manenti, 1997; Papanikolaou et al., 2000). In the last decades a plenty of mouse models of colon cancer have been used as powerful tools (Taketo and Edelmann, 2009). For example, important modifier genes identified in intestinal and colorectal carcinogenesis are DNA methyltransferase (*Dnmt*), *COX-2*, and the modifier of Min1 (*Mom1*) that decreases the number of tumour nodules in the *Min* (*Multiple Intestinal Neoplasia*) – mouse model (Dietrich et al., 1993; Laird et al., 1995; Oshima et al., 1996). *Min* mice develop numerous tumour nodules, predominantly in the small intestine, and die by about 5 months of age with anemia and intestinal obstruction from polyps and tumours. It was shown that tumour progress and tumour multiplicity in mice depend on the inbred strain in which the *Min* mutation was analyzed (McCart et al., 2008). This observation is paralleled by findings in humans. Patients carrying the same mutation in the *APC* gene [human ortholog of *Min* (Shoemaker et al., 1997)] can have dramatic differences in disease expression (Crabtree et al., 2002). However, the genes responsible for this variable expression of the FAP phenotype are widely unknown.

In the *Min* – *Mom1* scenario secretory phospholipase A2 was discussed as a molecule involved in modifying tumour progression as its expression was induced by the carcinogen azoxymethane (Papanikolaou et al., 2000). However, functional variants of phospholipase A2 have not been isolated so far, suggesting that other genetic loci might act as modifiers of the phenotype observed in CRC. From the data it is assumed that the number of so-called modifier genes is much higher, and that alleles acting in this manner comprise the majority of genetic risk for many common diseases including CRC (Reich and Lander, 2001). Moreover, it is speculated that inter-individual differences in susceptibility for colorectal tumours and modification in well-characterized pathways of colorectal carcinogenesis like the APC- or the so-called 'serrated-type' pathway is determined by the genetic polymorphism of modifiers in the epithelial and/or mesenchymal compartment.

In addition to *APC* and phospholipase A2, which are expressed by epithelial cells, *Foxl1* was identified as the first mesenchymal modifier gene of *Min* (Perreault et al., 2005). *Foxl1* encodes a winged helix transcription factor expressed in the mesenchyme of the gastrointestinal tract. The factor is an important regulator of the Wnt/APC/beta-catenin pathway influencing accumulation of nuclear beta-catenin. Loss of *Foxl1* was shown to increase tumour multiplicity in *Min* mice caused by accelerated loss of heterozygosity at the *Min* locus (Perreault et al., 2005). The data underline the important hypothesis that other genes, or even environmental conditions, that favour increased turnover of intestinal epithelial cells will likewise accelerate tumour initiation and tumour progression.

At present, regulation of modifier gene expression by environmental conditions, especially dietary components, is suggested (Perreault et al., 2005). This point of view is for example favoured by the coincidence of CRCs and an increased alimentary supply of fatty acids or *COX-2* expression as discussed above. Concerning putative modifiers, dietary-induced changes in the expression of ACSL isoforms have been recorded so far for rat liver (Lewin et al., 2001). In high alimentary feeding both ACSL1 and ACSL4 expression increased, whereas ACSL5 expression decreased. The opposite constellation was found in fasting animals. In a more subtle study, however, induction of ACSL5 expression in rat hepatocytes was found after feeding with a diet enriched with sucrose, whereas a fatty acid diet did not induce any change in ACSL5 expression (Oikawa et al., 1998). In contrary to a fatty acid enriched diet, ACSL5 expression was lowered by both, a cholesterol-enriched diet as well as fasting. The strong inductive effect of carbohydrate re-feeding on ACSL5 expression in rat hepatocytes recorded by Oikawa and colleagues was corroborated recently by another study (Achouri et al., 2005). In these experiments regulation of ACLS5 expression by dietary components was shown in cultured hepatocytes as well as in rats. The minor dietary effects of intestinal ACSL5 expression recorded in the Oikawa-study are probably due to the analysis of total bowel tissue preparations instead of dissected enterocytes. Therefore regulation of intestinal ACSL isoforms, especially ACSL5 variants, is not really investigated as yet. Our preliminary data indicate that ACSL5 is up-regulated by different fatty acids in enterocytes cultured as permanent cell lines or cultured as mucosal tissue biopsies. At present, this phenomenon is not systematically analyzed in cultured CRC biopsies.

Protein lipidation, especially protein palmitoylation, could be one important molecular mechanism of ACSL5 to act as potential modifier in CRC carcinogenesis. Accumulating evidence is given that protein palmitoylation is of high importance to modify a plenty of cellular signalling mechanism and pathways (Resh, 2006). Interestingly, palmitoylation of the CD95 on cysteine 199 was described recently as an early event that initiates apoptosis signalling (Feig et al., 2007). In mitochondria, protein lipidation following the regular biochemical pathway using acyl-CoA derivatives as precursors for covalent attachment to susceptible proteins (palmitoylation and myristoylation) is additionally found (Kostiuk et al., 2008). Several data indicate that ACSL5 could be of high importance in this scenario to modify cellular behaviour. Putative ACSL5 – associated pathways are summarized in Fig. 3.

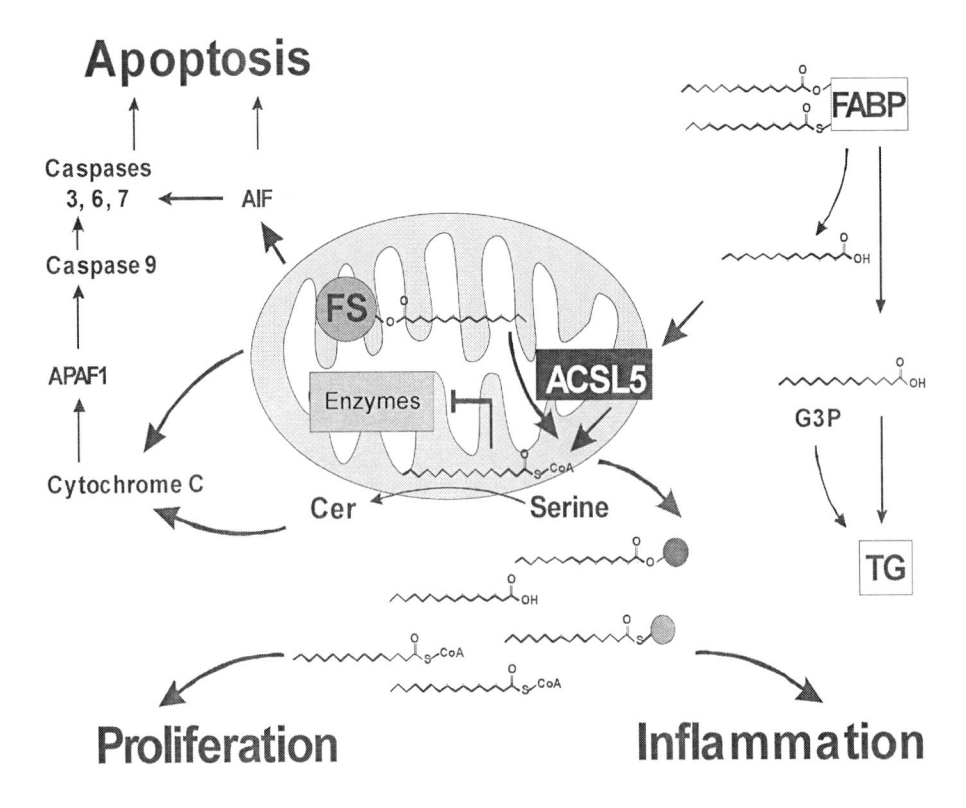

Figure 3. Main aspects of the putative ACSL5 pathways in enterocytes. Dietary fatty acids are provided by fatty acid binding proteins (FABP) probably for both intramitochondrial ACSL5 – dependent metabolism and intracytoplasmatic synthesis of triglycerides (TG) using glycerol-3-phosphate (G3P). *De novo* fatty acid synthesis (FS) is probably one additional source for intramitochondrial fatty acids utilized by ACSL5. Some pathways probably using ACLS5 catalyzed acyl-CoA derivatives are illustrated: (1) acyl-CoA dependent inhibition of intramitochondrial enzymes; (2) *de novo* synthesis of ceramide (Cer); (3) activation of caspases; (4) modification of cellular proliferation and inflammatory behaviour by lipidation.

Because ACSL5 expression is associated with susceptibility to apoptosis in enterocytes, disturbances of this ACSL5 - dependent system are assumed to be critical in modifying colorectal carcinogenesis. To further elucidate the putative molecular link of dietary-induced changes of the putative modifier gene ACSL5 additional functional studies, preferentially in mouse models, are necessary.

ACKNOWLEDGMENTS

The authors are grateful to P. Akens for typing and proofreading the manuscript.

REFERENCES

Achouri Y, Hegarty BD, Allanic D, Bécard D, Hainault I, Ferré P, Foufelle F. Long chain fatty acyl-CoA synthetase 5 expression is induced by insulin and glucose: involvement of sterol regulatory element-binding protein-1c. *Biochimie 87*:1149-1155;2005.

Ahn EH, Schroeder JJ. Sphinganine causes early activation of JNK and p38 MAPK and inhibition of AKT activation in HT-29 human colon cancer cells. *Anticancer. Res. 26*:121-127;2006.

Ahn EH, Schroeder JJ. Sphingoid bases and ceramide induce apoptosis in HT-29 and HCT-116 human colon cancer cells. *Exp. Biol. Med. 227*:345-353;2002.

Balk EM, Horsley TA, Newberry SJ, Lichtenstein AH, Yetley EA, Schachter HM, Moher D, MacLean CH, Lau J. A collaborative effort to apply the evidence-based review process to the field of nutrition: challenges, benefits, and lessons learned. *Am. J. Clin. Nutr. 85*:1448-1456;2007.

Bernardo K, Hurwitz R, Zenk T, Desnick RJ, Ferlinz K, Schuchman EH, Sandhoff K. Purification, characterization, and biosynthesis of human acid ceramidase. *J. Biol. Chem. 270*:11098-11102;1995.

Bionda C, Portoukalian J, Schmitt D, Rodriguez-Lafrasse C, Ardail D. Subcellular compartmentalization of ceramide metabolism: MAM (mitochondria-associated membrane) and/or mitochondria? *Biochem. J. 382*:527-533;2004.

Birbes H, El Bawab S, Hannun YA, Obeid LM. Selective hydrolysis of a mitochondrial pool of sphingomyelin induces apoptosis. *Fed. Am. Soc. Exp. Biol. J. 15*:2669-2679;2001.

Black PN, DiRusso CC. Yeast acyl-CoA synthetases at the crossroad of fatty acid metabolism and regulation. *Biochim. Biophys. Acta 1771*:286-298;2007.

Brockman HL, Momsen MM, Brown RE, He L, Chun J, Byun HS, Bittman R. The 4,5-double bond of ceramide regulates its dipole potential, elastic properties, and packing behavior. *Biophys. J. 87*:1722-1731;2004.

Cao Y, Dave KB, Doan TP, Prescott SM. Fatty acid CoA ligase 4 is up-regulated in colon adenocarcinoma. *Cancer Res. 61*:8429-8434;2001.

Cao Y, Pearman AT, Zimmerman GA, McIntyre TM, Prescott SM. Intracellular unesterified arachidonic acid signals apoptosis. *Proc. Natl. Acad. Sci. USA 97*:11280-11285;2000.

Chapkin RS, McMurray DN, Lupton JR. Colon cancer, fatty acids and anti-inflammatory compounds. *Curr. Opin. Gastroenterol. 23*:48-54; 2007.

Crabtree MD, Tomlinson IP, Hodgson SV, Neale K, Phillips RK, Houlston RS. Explaining variation in familial adenomatous polyposis: relationship between genotype and phenotype and evidence for modifier genes. *Gut 51*:420-423;2002.

Dietrich WF, Lander ES, Smith JS, Moser AR, Gould KA, Luongo C, Borenstein N, Dove W. Genetic identification of Mom-1, a major modifier locus affecting Min-induced intestinal multiple neoplasia in the mouse. *Cell 75*:631-639;1993.

Dragani TA, Manenti G. Mom1 leads the pack. *Nature Genet. 17*:7-8;1997.

Dvory-Sobol H, Arber N. Cyclooxygenase-2 as target for chemopreventive interventions: new approaches. *Cancer Biomark. 3*:153-161;2007.

Fearon ER, Vogelstein B. A genetic model for colorectal tumorigenesis. *Cell 61*:759-767;1990.

Feig C, Tchikov V, Schutze S, Peter ME. Palmitoylation of CD95 facilitates formation of SDS-stable receptor aggregates that initiate apoptosis signaling. *EMBO J. 26*:221-231;2007.

Gassler N, Kopitz J, Tehrani A, Ottenwälder B, Schnölzer M, Kartenbeck J, Lyer S, Autschbach F, Poustka A, Otto HF, Mollenhauer J. Expression of acyl-CoA synthetase 5 reflects the state of villus architecture in human small intestine. *J. Pathol. 202*:188-196;2004.

Gassler N, Roth W, Funke B, Schneider A, Herzog F, Tischendorf JJ, Grund K, Penzel R, Bravo IG, Mariadason J, Ehemann V, Sykora J, Haas TL, Walczak H, Ganten T, Zentgraf H, Erb P, Alonso A, Autschbach F, Schirmacher P, Knüchel R, Kopitz J. Regulation of enterocyte apoptosis by acyl-CoA synthetase 5 splicing. *Gastroenterology 133*:587-598;2007.

Granados S, Quiles JL, Gil A, Ramirez-Tortosa MC. Dietary lipids and cancer. *Nutr. Hosp. 2*:42-52, 44-54;2006.

Gulbins E. Regulation of death receptor signaling and apoptosis by ceramide. *Pharmacol. Res. 47*:393-399;2003.

Jass JR, Whitehall VL, Young J, Leggett BA. Emerging concepts in colorectal neoplasia. *Gastroenterology 123*:862-876;2002.

Kostiuk MA, Corvi MM, Keller BO, Plummer G, Prescher JA, Hangauer MJ, Bertozzi CR, Rajaiah G, Falck JR, Berthiaume LG. Identification of palmitoylated mitochondrial proteins using a bio-orthogonal azido-palmitate analogue. *FASEB J. 22*:721-732;2008.

Kuniyasu H. The roles of dietary PPARgamma ligands for metastasis in colorectal cancer. *PPAR Research.* Article ID 529720;2008.

Laird PW, Jackson-Grusby L, Fazeli A, Dickinson SL, Jung WE, Li E, Weinberg RA, Jaenisch R. Suppression of intestinal neoplasia by DNA hypomethylation. *Cell 81*:197-205;1995.

Lewin TM, Kim JH, Granger DA, Vance JE, Coleman RA. Acyl-CoA synthetase isoforms 1, 4, and 5 are present in different subcellular membranes in rat liver and can be inhibited independently. *J. Biol. Chem. 276*:24674-24679;2001.

Lipkin M, Reddy B, Newmark H and Lamprecht SA. Dietary factors in human colorectal cancer. *Annu Rev Nutr 19*:545-586;1999

Marasas WF, Riley RT, Hendricks KA, Stevens VL, Sadler TW, Gelineau-van Waes J, Missmer SA, Cabrera J, Torres O, Gelderblom WC, Allegood J, Martinez C, Maddox J, Miller JD, Starr L, Sullards MC, Roman AV, Voss KA, Wang E, Merrill AH Jr. Fumonisins disrupt sphingolipid metabolism, folate transport, and neural tube development in embryo culture and in vivo: a potential risk factor for human neural tube defects among populations consuming fumonisin-contaminated maize. *J. Nutr. 134*:711-716;2004.

Mashek DG, Bornfeldt KE, Coleman RA, Berger J, Bernlohr DA, Black P, DiRusso CC, Farber SA, Guo W, Hashimoto N, Khodiyar V, Kuypers FA, Maltais LJ, Nebert DW, Renieri A, Schaffer JE, Stahl A, Watkins PA, Vasiliou V, Yamamoto TT. Revised nomenclature for the mammalian long-chain acyl-CoA synthetase gene family. *J. Lipid. Res. 45*:1958-1961;2004.

McCart AE, Vickaryous NK, Silver A. Apc mice: models, modifiers and mutants. *Pathol. Res. Prac. 204*:479-490;2008.

Murota K, Storch J. Uptake of micellar long-chain fatty acid and sn-2-monoacylglycerol into human intestinal Caco-2 cells exhibits characteristics of protein-mediated transport. *J. Nutr. 135*:1626-1630;2005.

Oikawa E, Iijima H, Suzuki T, Sasano H, Sato H, Kamataki A, Nagura H, Kang MJ, Fujino TT, Suzuki H, Yamamoto TT. A novel acyl-CoA synthetase, ACS5, expressed in intestinal epithelial cells and proliferating preadipocytes. *J. Biochem. 124*:679-685;1998.

Oshima M, Dinchuk JE, Kargman SL, Oshima H, Hancock B, Kwong E, Trzaskos JM, Evans JF, Taketo MM. Suppression of intestinal polyposis in Apc delta716 knockout mice by inhibition of cyclooxygenase 2 (COX-2). *Cell 87*:803-809;1996.

Papanikolaou A, Wang QS, Mulherkar R, Bolt A, Rosenberg DW. Expression analysis of the group IIA secretory phospholipase A2) in mice with differential susceptibility to azoxymethane-induced colon tumorigenesis. *Carcinogenesis 21*:133-138;2000.

Perreault N, Sackett SD, Katz JP, Furth EE, Kaestner KH. Foxl1 is a mesenchymal modifier of Min in carcinogenesis of stomach and colon. *Genes Dev. 19*:311-315;2005.

Pyne S, Pyne NJ. Sphingosine 1-phosphate signalling in mammalian cells. *Biochem. J. 349*:385-402;2000.

Reich DE, Lander ES. On the allelic spectrum of human disease. *Trends Genet 17*:502-510;2001.

Resh D. Palmitoylation of ligands, receptors, and intracellular signaling molecules. *Sci. STKE. 359*:re14;2006

Ruvolo PP. Intracellular signal transduction pathways activated by ceramide and its metabolites. *Pharmacol. Res. 47*:383-392;2003.

Sampath H, Ntambi JM. The fate and intermediary metabolism of stearic acid. *Lipids 40*:1187-1191;2005.

Samuelson DJ, Hesselson SE, Aperavich BA, Zan Y, Haag JD, Trentham-Dietz A, Hampton JM, Mau B, Chen KS, Baynes C, Khaw KT, Luben R, Perkins B, Shah M, Pharoah PD, Dunning AM, Easton DF, Ponder BA, Gould MN. Rat Mcs5a is a compound quantitative trait locus with orthologous human loci that associate with breast cancer risk. *Proc. Natl. Acad. Sci. USA 104*:6299-6304;2007.

Saunders M, Iveson T. Management of advanced colorectal cancer: state of the art. *Br. J. Cancer 95*:131-138;2006

Shoemaker AR, Gould KA, Luongo C, Moser AR, Dove WF. Studies of neoplasia in the Min mouse. *Biochim. Biophys. Acta 1332*:F25-F48;1997.

Siskind LJ, Kolesnick RN, Colombini M. Ceramide forms channels in mitochondrial outer membranes at physiologically relevant concentrations. *Mitochondrion 6*:118-125;2006.

Siskind LJ. Mitochondrial ceramide and the induction of apoptosis. *J. Bioenerg. Biomembr. 37*:143-153;2005.

Sugawara T, Kinoshita M, Ohnishi M, Nagata J, Saito M. Digestion of maize sphingolipids in rats and uptake of sphingadienine by Caco-2 cells. *J. Nutr. 133*:2777-2782;2003.

Sugawara T, Kinoshita M, Ohnishi M, Tsuzuki T, Miyazawa T, Nagata J, Hirata T, Saito M. Efflux of sphingoid bases by P-glycoprotein in human intestinal Caco-2 cells. *Biosci. Biotechnol. Biochem. 68*:2541-2546;2004.

Taketo MM, Edelmann W. Mouse models of colon cancer. *Gastroenterology 136*:780-798;2009.

Worthley DL, Whitehall VL, Spring KJ and Leggett BA. Colorectal carcinogenesis: road maps to cancer. *World J. Gastroenterol. 13*:3784-3791;2007.

Yamashita Y, Kumabe T, Cho YY, Watanabe M, Kawagishi J, Yoshimoto T, Fujino T, Kang MJ, Yamamoto TT. Fatty acid induced glioma cell growth is mediated by the acyl-CoA synthetase 5 gene located on chromosome 10q25.1-q25.2, a region frequently deleted in malignant gliomas. *Oncogene 19*:5919-5925; 2000.

Yeh CS, Wang JW, Cheng TL, Juan CH, Wu CH, Lin SR. Fatty acid metabolism pathway play an important role in carcinogenesis of human colorectal cancers by microarray-bioinformatics analysis. *Cancer Let. 233*:297-308;2006.

In: Rectal Cancer: Etiology, Pathogenesis and Treatment
Editors: Paula Wells and Regina Halstead

ISBN 978-1-60692-563-8
© 2009 Nova Science Publishers, Inc.

Short Communication A

RISK FACTORS OF LOCAL RECURRENCE AFTER CURATIVE RESECTION IN PATIENTS WITH MIDDLE AND LOWER RECTAL CARCINOMA

Wu Ze-yu[1,], Wan Jin[1], Zhao Gang[1], Peng Lin[1], Du Jia-lin[1], Yao Yuan[1], Liu Quan-fang[1], Wang Zhi-du[1], Huang Zhi-ming[1] and Lin Hua-huan[2]*

[1]Department of General Surgery, Guangdong Provincial People's Hospital, Guangzhou 510080, China
[2]Department of Pathology, Guangdong Provincial People's Hospital, Guangzhou 510080, China

ABSTRACT

AIM: To explore the risk factors of local recurrence after curative resection in patients with middle and lower rectal carcinoma.

Materials and Methods: Cancer specimens from 56 patients with middle and lower rectal carcinoma who received total mesorectal excision at the Department of General Surgery of Guangdong Provincial People's Hospital were studied. A large slice technique was used to detect mesorectal metastasis and evaluate circumferential resection margin status. The relationships between mesorectal metastasis and local recurrence and the possible correlations between circumferential resection margin status and local recurrence were identified. The relationships between local recurrence and clinicopathologic characteristics of middle and lower rectal carcinoma were also evaluated.

Results: Local recurrence after curative resection occurred in 12.5 percent (7 of 56 cases) of patients with middle and lower rectal carcinoma. Local recurrence was

---

[*] Correspondence concerning this article should be addressed to: Dr. Wu Ze-yu, Department of General Surgery, Guangdong Provincial People's Hospital, Guangzhou 510080, Guangdong Province, China. E-mail: rainy1977@21cn.com; Telephone: +86-20-83827812 Ext 60821; Fax: +86-20-83827812.

significantly associated with family history ($P=0.047$), high CEA level ($P=0.026$), cancerous perforation ($P=0.004$), tumor differentiation ($P=0.009$) and vessel cancerous emboli ($P=0.001$). Conversely, No significant correlations were found between local recurrence and other variables such as age ($P=0.477$), gender ($P=0.0.749$), tumor diameter ($P=0.516$), diameter of tumor infiltration ($P=0.168$), Ming's classification ($P=0.727$), depth of tumor invasion ($P=0.101$), lymph node metastases ($P=0.055$) and TNM staging system ($P=0.152$). 21.4 per cent (12 of 56 cases) of patients with middle and lower rectal carcinoma had positive circumferential resection margin. Local recurrence rate of patients with positive circumferential resection margin was 33.3%(4/12), whereas it was 6.8%(3/44) in those with negative circumferential resection margin. The difference between these two groups was statistically significant ($P=0.014$). 64.3 per cent (36 of 56 cases) of patients with middle and lower rectal carcinoma were detected mesorectal metastasis. Local recurrence occurred in 16.7 per cent (6 of 36 cases) of patients with mesorectal metastasis, and in 5.0 per cent (1 of 20 cases) of patients without mesorectal metastasis. However, the difference between these two groups was not statistically significant ($P=0.206$).

Conclusion: Our results demonstrate that family history, high CEA level, cancerous perforation, tumor differentiation, vessel cancerous emboli and circumferential resection margin status are significant risk factors of local recurrence after curative resection in patients with middle and lower rectal carcinoma. Local recurrence may be more frequent in patients with mesorectal metastasis, compared with patients without mesorectal metastasis. Larger sample investigations are helpful to draw a further conclusion.

Keywords: Middle and lower rectal carcinoma; Local recurrence; Circumferential resection margin; Mesorectal metastasis.

It is well known that local recurrence is the most important prognostic factor of rectal carcinoma [1-3]. However, even after undergoing radical resection of primary tumors and lymph nodes, about 4~50 percent of patients with rectal carcinoma were reportedly with local recurrence [4-9]. Clinicopathologically, the risk factors of local recurrence remain unclear heretofore. Therefore, the aim of the current study was to explore the risk factors of local recurrence after curative resection in patients with middle and lower rectal carcinoma. Cancer specimens resected from 56 patients with middle and lower rectal carcinoma who received total mesorectal excision at the Department of General Surgery of Guangdong Provincial People's Hospital from November 2001 to July 2003 were studied. A large slice technique was used to detect mesorectal metastasis and evaluate circumferential resection margin status. The relationships between mesorectal metastasis and local recurrence and the possible correlations between circumferential resection margin status and local recurrence were identified. The relationships between local recurrence and clinicopathologic characteristics of middle and lower rectal carcinoma were also evaluated.

MATERIAL AND METHODS

Patients and Specimens

Cancer specimens resected from 56 patients with middle and lower rectal carcinoma who received total mesorectal excision at the Department of General Surgery of Guangdong Provincial People's Hospital from November 2001 to July 2003 were studied. There were 37 men and 19 women, ranging in age from 30 to 86 years, with a mean age of 60.5years. None of these patients had received preoperative chemotherapy or radiotherapy. There were 26 lower rectal carcinomas and 30 middle rectal carcinomas. Patients with tumor diameter≥5cm were in 18 cases, with tumor diameter＜5cm in 38 cases. Low anterior resection was performed in 40 patients, abdominal perineal resection in 16 patients. According to the Ming's criteria, 15 tumors were classified as expansive type carcinomas, 34 tumors classified as infiltrative type carcinomas, 7 tumors classified as mixed type carcinomas. TNM stage status: I stage in 5 patients, II stage in 22 patients, and III stage in 29 patients. There were 14 patients with poorly differentiated carcinoma, 37 patients with moderate differentiated carcinoma, 5 patients with well-differentiated carcinoma. A large slice technique was used to detect mesorectal metastasis and evaluate circumferential resection margin status. Two pathologists who had no knowledge of the clinicopathological data observed the specimens independently. If tumor cells were detected within 1 mm of the circumferential margin, the status was classified as positive circumferential resection margin [10-12].

Statistical Analysis

Statistical analysis was performed by the Pearson Chi-square test to examine the associations of local recurrence and circumferential resection margin status, mesorectal metastasis as well as clinicopathologic characteristics of patients with middle and lower rectal carcinoma. Statistical significance was defined as $P<0.05$.

RESULTS

Correlations between Local Recurrence and Clinicopathologic Characteristics of Patients with Middle and Lower Rectal Carcinoma

Local recurrence after curative resection occurred in 12.5 percent (7 of 56 cases) of patients with middle and lower rectal carcinoma. Local recurrence was significantly related with family history ($P=0.047$), high CEA level ($P=0.026$), cancerous perforation ($P=0.004$), tumor differentiation ($P=0.009$) and vessel cancerous emboli ($P=0.001$). Conversely, No significant correlations were found between local recurrence and other variables such as age ($P=0.477$), gender ($P=0.0.749$), tumor diameter ($P=0.516$), diameter of tumor infiltration

($P=0.168$), Ming's classification ($P=0.727$), depth of tumor invasion ($P=0.101$), lymph node metastases ($P=0.055$) and TNM staging system ($P=0.152$).

Correlations between Circumferential Resection Margin Status and Local Recurrence of Patients with Middle and Lower Rectal Carcinoma

21.4 per cent (12 of 56 cases) of patients with middle and lower rectal carcinoma had positive circumferential resection margin. Local recurrence occurred in 33.3 per cent (4 of 12 cases) of patients with positive circumferential resection margin, and in 6.8 per cent (3 of 44 cases) of patients with negative circumferential resection margin. The difference between these two groups was statistically significant ($P=0.014$).

Correlations between Mesorectal Metastasis and Local Recurrence of Patients with Middle and Lower Rectal Carcinoma

64.3 per cent (36 of 56 cases) of patients with middle and lower rectal carcinoma were detected mesorectal metastasis. Local recurrence rate of patients with mesorectal metastasis was 16.7 per cent (6 of 36 cases), whereas it was 5.0 per cent (1 of 20 cases) in those without mesorectal metastasis. However, the difference between these two groups was not statistically significant ($P=0.206$).

DISCUSSION

It is well known that middle and lower rectal carcinoma is of the most common carcinomas in China. Local recurrence after curative resection is followed by significant morbidity and mortality [4,13-16]. Local recurrence rate varies from less than 4% to greater than 50%. Since total mesorectal excision (TME) was adopted as the standard treatment of patients with rectal carcinoma, it has been reported that a significant decrease in local recurrence and a trend for improved relative survival in many centers [17-19]. In our sturdy, local recurrence occurred in 12.5 percent (7 of 56 cases) of in patients with middle and lower rectal carcinoma who underwent total mesorectal excision. The consequence indicates that implementation of TME for middle and lower rectal carcinomas can significantly reduce local recurrence rate.

The correlation between circumferential resection margin status and local recurrence of patients with rectal carcinoma is still controversial presently [11,12,20-22]. Wibe [11] et al. reported that positive circumferential resection margin had a significant and major prognostic impact on the rates of local recurrence of patients with rectal carcinoma who underwent total mesorectal excision. However, Luna-Perez [20] et al. reported that circumferential resection margin involvement was not correlated significantly with local recurrence of patients with rectal adenocarcinoma ($P=0.33$). Hall [12] et al. reported that local recurrence rate of patients with positive circumferential resection margin was 15%, whereas it was 11% in those with negative circumferential resection margin. The difference between these two groups was not statistically significant ($P=0.38$). Our result demonstrated that circumferential resection margin involvement had significant correlation with local recurrence of patients with middle and low rectal carcinoma. Local recurrence was more frequent in patients with positive circumferential resection margin (4 of 12 cases, 33.3%), compared with patients with negative circumferential resection margin (3 of 44 cases, 6.8%) ($P=0.014$). We conclude that the circumferential resection margin status is an important predictor of local recurrence of patients with middle and low rectal carcinoma. It has been also reported that residual mesorectal metastasis in rectal surgery may be the most important factor of local recurrence [23,24]. In the current study, local recurrence was more frequent in patients with mesorectal metastasis, compared with patients without mesorectal metastasis (16.7 per cent, 6 of 36 cases vs 5.0 per cent, 1 of 20 cases). However, the difference between these two groups was not statistically significant ($P=0.206$). The implementation of TME standard in surgery at our Department may be also the plausible explanation for the observation.

Sugihara [25] et al. investigated correlations between local recurrence and clinicopathologic characteristics of patients with rectal carcinoma. Multivariate analysis disclosed that lower rectal cancers, non-well-differentiated adenocarcinoma, T_3-T_4, lymph node metastasis, and positive lateral lymph nodes were significantly associated with an increased local recurrence. Das [26] et al. also reported that pathologic T and N stages significant predictors of local recurrence. In the present study, local recurrence rate of poorly differentiated carcinomas was 35.7 per cent (5 of 34 cases), while that of moderate and well-differentiated carcinomas were only 5.4% (2 of 37 cases) and 0% (0 of 6 cases) respectively. The difference between these three groups was statistically significant ($P=0.009$). The result showed that local recurrence was significantly related with tumor differentiation. We also found that local recurrence rate increased in accordance with the depth of tumor invasion. Local recurrence was more frequent in T_3 tumors (6 of 27 cases, 22.2%), compared with T_2 tumors (1 of 23 cases, 4.3%) and T_1 tumors (0 of 6cases, 0%). However, the difference between these three groups was not statistically significant ($P=0.101$). In 29 patients with lymph node metastases 6 (20.7%) occurred local recurrence, while in 27 patients without lymph node metastases only 1 (3.7%) occurred local recurrence. Similarly, the difference was not statistically significant ($P=0.055$). These observations may be explained by the fact that the cases in our study were comparatively few. To draw a further conclusion, larger sample investigations on middle and low rectal carcinoma are needed.

Park [27] et al. reported that the perioperative serum CEA change was a useful prognostic indicator to predict for recurrence and survival in stage III rectal cancer patients. Oh YT [28] et al. reported that the vascular invasion was significantly associated with local recurrence of rectal cancer. Our results also demonstrated that local recurrence had significant correlation with high CEA level ($P=0.026$) and vessel cancerous emboli ($P=0.001$). We also found that local recurrence was significant correlated with family history ($P=0.047$) and cancerous perforation ($P=0.004$). These observations indicate that extensive mesorectal excision and postoperative adjuvant chemotherapy should be followed in the management of patients with family history, cancerous perforation, high CEA level, vessel cancerous emboli.

Table 1. Correlations of local recurrence and circumferential resection margin status, mesorectal metastasis as well as clinicopathologic characteristics of patients with middle and lower rectal carcinoma

Clinicopathologic variable	Patients (n)	Local recurrence Positive (%)	Negative (%)	P value
Gender				
Male	37	5 (13.5)	32 (86.5)	
Female	19	2 (10.5)	17 (89.5)	P=0.749
Age				
<60 yrs	25	4 (16.0)	21 (84.0)	
≥60 yrs	31	3 (9.7)	28 (90.3)	P=0.477
Family history				
Yes	21	5 (23.8)	16 (76.2)	
No	35	2 (5.7)	33 (94.3)	P=0.047
CEA leve				
High	26	6 (23.1)	20 (76.9)	
Normal	30	1 (3.3)	29 (96.7)	P=0.026
Cancerous perforation				
Yes	3	2 (33.3)	1 (66.7)	
No	53	5 (9.4)	48 (90.6)	P=0.004
Superficial diameter				
<5 cm	38	4 (10.5)	34 (89.5)	
≥5 cm	18	3 (16.7)	15 (83.3)	P=0.516
Diameter of infiltration				
1/4	8	0 (0)	8 (100)	
1/2	16	1 (6.3)	15 (93.7)	
3/4	18	2 (11.1)	16 (88.9)	
4/4	14	4 (28.6)	10 (71.4)	P=0.168
Ming's classification				
Expansive	15	1 (6.7)	14 (93.3)	
Infiltrative	34	5 (14.7)	29 (85.3)	
Mixed	7	1 (14.3)	6 (85.7)	P=0.727
Depth of invasion				
T_1	6	0 (0)	6 (100)	
T_2	23	1 (4.3)	22 (95.7)	
T_3	27	6 (22.2)	21 (77.8)	P=0.101
Histologic differentiation				
Well	5	0 (0)	5 (100)	
Moderate	37	2 (5.4)	35 (94.6)	
Poorly	14	5 (35.7)	9 (64.3)	P=0.009
Lymph node metastasis				
Positive	29	6 (20.7)	23 (79.3)	
Negative	27	1 (3.7)	26 (96.3)	P=0.055
Vessel cancerous emboli				
Positive	12	5 (41.7)	7 (58.3)	
Negative	44	2 (4.5)	42 (95.5)	P=0.001
Circumferential resection margin				
Positive	12	4 (33.3)	8 (66.7)	
Negative	44	3 (6.8)	41 (93.2)	P=0.014
Mesorectal metastasis				
Positive	36	6 (16.7)	30 (83.3)	
Negative	20	1 (5.0)	19 (95.0)	P=0.206
TNM staging				
I	5	0 (0)	5 (100)	
II	22	1 (4.5)	21 (95.5)	
III	29	6 (20.7)	23 (79.3)	P=0.152

REFERENCES

[1] Noda K, Umekita N, Tanaka S, Ohkubo T, Inoue S, Kitamura M. A clinical study of therapy for local recurrent rectal cancer. *Gan To Kagaku Ryoho* 2006; 33(12):1830-1833.

[2] Bedrosian I, Giacco G, Pederson L, Rodriguez-Bigas MA, Feig B, Hunt KK, Ellis L, Curley SA, Vauthey JN, Delclos M, Crane CH, Janjan N, Skibber JM. Outcome after curative resection for locally recurrent rectal cancer. *Dis Colon Rectum* 2006; 49(2):175-182.

[3] Moriya Y, Akasu T, Fujita S, Yamamoto S. Total pelvic exenteration with distal sacrectomy for fixed recurrent rectal cancer. *Surg Oncol Clin N Am* 2005; 14(2):225-238.

[4] Radice E, Dozois RR. Locally recurrent rectal cancer. *Dig Surg* 2001; 18(5): 355-362.

[5] Piso P, Dahlke MH, Mirena P, Schmidt U, Aselmann H, Schlitt HJ, Raab R, Klempnauer J. Total mesorectal excision for middle and lower rectal cancer: a single institution experience with 337 consecutive patients. *J Surg Oncol* 2004; 86(3): 115-121.

[6] Maslekar S, Sharma A, Macdonald A, Gunn J, Monson JR, Hartley JE. Do supervised colorectal trainees differ from consultants in terms of quality of TME surgery? *Colorectal Dis* 2006; 8(9):790-794.

[7] Rengan R, Paty PB, Wong WD, Guillem JG, Weiser M, Temple L, Saltz L, Minsky BD. Ten-year results of preoperative radiation followed by sphincter preservation for rectal cancer: increased local failure rate in nonresponders. *Clin Colorectal Cancer* 2006; 5(6):413-421.

[8] Hohenberger W, Merkel S, Matzel K, Bittorf B, Papadopoulos T, Gohl J. The influence of abdomino-peranal (intersphincteric) resection of lower third rectal carcinoma on the rates of sphincter preservation and locoregional recurrence. *Colorectal Dis* 2006; 8(1):23-33.

[9] Lezoche E, Guerrieri M, De Sanctis A, Campagnacci R, Baldarelli M, Lezoche G, Paganini AM. Long-term results of laparoscopic versus open colorectal resections for cancer in 235 patients with a minimum follow-up of 5 years. *Surg Endosc* 2006; 20(4):546-553.

[10] Hermanek P, Junginger T. The circumferential resection margin in rectal carcinoma surgery. *Tech Coloproctol* 2005; 9(3): 193-199.

[11] Wibe A, Rendedal PR, Svensson E, Norstein J, Eide TJ, Myrvold HE, Soreide O. Prognostic significance of the circumferential resection margin following total mesorectal excision for rectal cancer. *Br J Surg* 2002; 89(3): 327-334.

[12] Hall NR, Finan PJ, al-Jaberi T, Tsang CS, Brown SR, Dixon MF, Quirke P. Circumferential margin involvement after mesorectal excision of rectal cancer with curative intent. Predictor of survival but not local recurrence? *Dis Colon Rectum* 1998; 41(8): 979-983.

[13] Okaro AC, Worthington T, Stebbing JF, Broughton M, Caffarey S, Marks CG. Curative resection for low rectal adenocarcinoma: abdomino-perineal vs anterior resection. *Colorectal Dis* 2006; 8(8):645-649.

[14] Chiappa A, Biffi R, Bertani E, Zbar AP, Pace U, Crotti C, Biella F, Viale G, Orecchia R, Pruneri G, Poldi D, Andreoni B. Surgical outcomes after total mesorectal excision for rectal cancer. *J Surg Oncol* 2006; 94(3):182-193.

[15] Martling AL, Holm T, Rutqvist LE, Moran BJ, Heald RJ, Cedemark B. Effect of a surgical training programme on outcome of rectal cancer in the County of Stockholm. Stockholm Colorectal Cancer Study Group, Basingstoke Bowel Cancer Research Project. *Lancet* 2000; 356(9224): 93-96.

[16] Temple WJ, Saettler EB. Locally recurrent rectal cancer: role of composite resection of extensive pelvic tumors with strategies for minimizing risk of recurrence. *J Surg Oncol* 2000; 73(1): 47-58.

[17] Laurent C, Nobili S, Rullier A, Vendrely V, Saric J, Rullier E. Efforts to improve local control in rectal cancer compromise survival by the potential morbidity of optimal mesorectal excision. *J Am Coll Surg* 2006; 203(5):684-691.

[18] Visser O, Bakx R, Zoetmulder FA, Levering CC, Meijer S, Slors JF, van Lanschot JJ. The influence of total mesorectal excision on local recurrence and survival in rectal canc Dig Surg. 2006;23(1-2):51-9.dy in greater Amsterdam. *J Surg Oncol* 2006 Oct 17; [Epub ahead of print]

[19] Bernardshaw SV, Ovrebo K, Eide GE, Skarstein A, Rokke O. Treatment of rectal cancer: reduction of local recurrence after the introduction of TME - experience from one University Hospital. *Dig Surg* 2006; 23(1-2):51-59.

[20] Luna-Perez P, Bustos-Cholico E, Alvarado I, Maffuz A, Rodriguez-Ramirez S, Gutierrez de la Barrera M, Labastida S. Prognostic significance of circumferential margin involvement in rectal adenocarcinoma treated with preoperative chemoradiotherapy and low anterior resection. *J Surg Oncol* 2005; 90(1): 20-25.

[21] Nagtegaal ID, Marijnen CA, Kranenbarg EK, van de Velde CJ, van Krieken JH; Pathology Review Committee; Cooperative Clinical Investigators. Circumferential margin involvement is still an important predictor of local recurrence in rectal carcinoma: not one millimeter but two millimeters is the limit. *Am J Surg Pathol* 2002; 26(3): 350-357.

[22] Laurent C, Nobili S, Rullier A, Vendrely V, Saric J, Rullier E. Efforts to improve local control in rectal cancer compromise survival by the potential morbidity of optimal mesorectal excision. *J Am Coll Surg* 2006; 203(5): 684-691.

[23] Heald RJ, Moran BJ, Ryall RD, Sexton R, MacFarlane JK. Rectal cancer: the Basingstoke experience of total mesorectal excision, 1978-1997. *Arch Surg* 1998; 133(8): 894-899.

[24] Wan J, Wu ZY, Du JL, Yao Y, Wang ZD, Lin HH, Luo XL, Zhang W. Mesorectal metastasis of middle and lower rectal cancer. *Zhonghua Wai Ke Za Zh* 2006; 44(13): 894-896.

[25] Sugihara K, Kobayashi H, Kato T, Mori T, Mochizuki H, Kameoka S, Shirouzu K, Muto T. Indication and benefit of pelvic sidewall dissection for rectal cancer. *Dis Colon Rectum* 2006; 49(11):1663-1672.

[26] Das P, Skibber JM, Rodriguez-Bigas MA, Feig BW, Chang GJ, Hoff PM, Eng C, Wolff RA, Janjan NA, Delclos ME, Krishnan S, Levy LB, Ellis LM, Crane CH. Clinical and pathologic predictors of locoregional recurrence, distant metastasis, and

overall survival in patients treated with chemoradiation and mesorectal excision for rectal cancer. *Am J Clin Oncol* 2006; 29(3):219-224.

[27] Park YA, Lee KY, Kim NK, Baik SH, Sohn SK, Cho CW. Prognostic effect of perioperative change of serum carcinoembryonic antigen level: a useful tool for detection of systemic recurrence in rectal cancer. *Ann Surg Oncol* 2006; 13(5):645-650.

[28] Oh YT, Kim MJ, Lim JS, Kim JH, Lee KY, Kim NK, Kim WH, Kim KW. Assessment of the prognostic factors for a local recurrence of rectal cancer: the utility of preoperative MR imaging. *Korean J Radiol* 2005; 6(1):8-16.

In: Rectal Cancer: Etiology, Pathogenesis and Treatment
Editors: Paula Wells and Regina Halstead

ISBN 978-1-60692-563-8
© 2009 Nova Science Publishers, Inc.

Short Communication B

CT-GUIDED INTERSTITIAL BRACHYTHERAPY AS AN INNOVATIVE ADJUNCT TO CURRENT THERAPEUTIC STRATEGIES IN THE TREATMENT OF COLORECTAL LIVER METASTASES

Christian Grieser, Dirk Schnapauff and Timm Denecke[*]
Klinik für Strahlenheilkunde, Berlin, Germany.

ABSTRACT

Beside surgical resection and systemic chemotherapy locally ablative treatment has gained a broad acceptance in multimodal treatment concepts of colorectal liver metastases over the past decade. Limitations of the thermodestructive ablation modalities such as radiofrequency ablation and laser induced thermotherapy are number, size, and location of target lesions. Combining technical features derived from locally ablative treatment in interventional radiology and from radiation therapy, these limitations can be overcome to a great part. After CT-guided percutaneous implantation of catheters into the hepatic tumor, the irradiation is performed via afterloading following a 3D-radiation plan based on CT images. This minimally invasive procedure allows circumscriptive high dose rate irradiation of the target lesion in a single session, independent of breathing motion or potential cooling effects of neighboring vessels. By modifying the dwell locations and dwell times of the radiation source (Iridium-192), the ablation zone can be adjusted to the shape and size of the lesion without repositioning of catheters. This enables sufficient dosing even of large tumors or lesions close to risk structures, such as liver hilum or adjacent bowel, in which thermoablation is not favored. Good local control rates have been achieved in colorectal liver metastases, and promising clinical indications

---

[*] Correspondence concerning this article should be addressed to: Dr. med. Timm Denecke, Klinik für Strahlenheilkunde, Campus Virchow-Klinikum, Charité – Universitätsmedizin Berlin, Augustenburger Platz 1, 13353 Berlin, Germany. Tel.: 0049 / (0)30 / 450-557001; Fax: 0049 / (0)30 / 450-557909; e-Mail: timm.denecke@charite.de.

are currently elaborated. This article gives an overview of the application technique and the possible fields of indication in the multimodal treatment setting of patients with colorectal liver metastases.

Keywords: Radiation therapy, brachytherapy, afterloading, liver metastases, local ablative therapy, interventional radiology, colorectal cancer.

INTRODUCTION

For patients with liver-only metastases of colorectal cancer, hepatic resection is the only option that offers a curative chance and thus is regarded as the treatment of choice [1]. However, the majority of patients do not fulfill the criteria for curative hepatic surgery. For those patients drug therapy is regarded as standard treatment and great achievements have been made through the last decade, almost doubling the survival rates of metastasized colorectal cancer patients [2,3,4]. This results in a growing number of heavily pretreated patients having used up all chemotherapeutic options but still present with a limited number of metastases.

As adjuncts to surgery and chemotherapy, interstitial locally ablative treatment is an interesting option as it eradicates single tumor lesions while sparing liver parenchyma. The majority of these procedures is performed by applying thermal ablation, such as radiofrequency ablation (RFA) or laser induced thermotherapy (LITT) with the aim of complete ablation of all hepatic lesions [5,6,7]. However, these procedures have limitations concerning number, localization as well as size and shape of the target lesions [8]. Therefore, especially in the palliative setting, there are great efforts to develop effective alternatives to thermoablative methods in order to achieve local control in those patients who are not suitable to undergo RFA, such as locoregional transarterial chemo- or radioembolization or infusion chemotherapy.

More recently, there is growing interest in applying external beam radiotherapy to hepatic metastases of colorectal cancer. However, therapeutic efficacy of percutaneous irradiation interferes with the mandatory maintenance of a sufficient liver function since the tolerance dose of liver parenchyma is lower than that of most tumor tissues. A relatively high radiation exposure of the normal hepatic parenchyma is achieved because of the breathing excursion of the liver and the flat dose shoulder surrounding the target volume. Even with triggered irradiation, stereotactic irradiation or tomotherapy devices, these problems are not generally solved to date [9]. Intraoperative radiotherapy in a high single dose has been used to treat unresectable liver metastases. Safety and efficacy have been shown in previous studies [10,11,12]. However, the invasiveness is not appropriate for a predominantly palliative treatment.

However, with the combination of irradiation and the CT-guided percutaneous access of thermoablation, the drawbacks of either method can be overcome. This combination can be realized using interstitial brachytherapy in afterloading technique, with the use of a radiation source (Iridium-192), which is inserted into catheters positioned inside or next to the tumor under CT-guidance [13]. With this technique, a novel treatment option for hepatic malignomas is available and it's unique characteristics open new fields of indication for minimal invasive local tumor destruction.

FIELDS OF INDICATION

In colorectal cancer patients, CT-guided brachytherapy of liver metastases can be used in different scenarios, predominantly in the palliative setting. It can be used to extent the time to progression and thus the chemotherapy free interval; this is a valuable approach especially in patients who develop serious side effects to the established treatment agents. Furthermore CT-guided brachytherapy can be applied followed by adjuvant chemotherapy for local tumor reduction and to retard systemic progression. Finally, it can be used in progressive disease when all effective chemotherapy agents have been used up. There are activities to introduce CT-guided brachytherapy even in the curative setting adjunctive to surgery.

These opportunities extend the therapeutic armamentarium in many patients. On the other hand, local overtreatment without the chance to influence the actual course of the disease should be avoided as an unnecessary risk. These considerations require individual interdisciplinary patient evaluation.

In this context, imaging procedures are necessary to allow for sufficient restaging and therapy planning. Whole body staging should be performed using CT of the chest and abdomen to search for extrahepatic disease. Additional FDG-PET scans or combined PET-CT has been shown to be very useful [14]. Beside imaging studies, clinical and paraclinical parameters such as comorbidity, liver function, and blood coagulation have to be taken into consideration [15].

FEATURES OF CT-GUIDED BRACHYTHERAPY

For accurate assessment of the actual status of disease inside the liver and topography of the lesions, liver MRI with hepatospecific contrast material is the optimal imaging modality to assort the patient to the appropriate treatment, and, if indicated, to plan the CT-intervention. Whether surgery, thermoablative treatment, CT-guided brachytherapy or regional/systemic treatment should be applied depends on a variety of factors.

Regarding the selection of the appropriate locally ablative modality, there are several specific characteristics to be taken into consideration. Depending on the probe configuration, complete tumor destruction by RFA is limited to lesions with a maximum diameter of approximately 5 cm, when the tumor is spherical. In large tumors, the RFA-probe has to be repositioned during the ablation procedure, and with increasing size, the local control rate decreases. In contrast to thermal ablation procedures, CT-guided brachytherapy is largely independent from complex geometric configurations of the lesions as dwell times and dwell locations of the source within the applicators can be adjusted to fit the dose coverage to the outlines of the tumor. By increasing the number of catheters or the dwell duration of the source, even very large tumors of up to 9-12 cm can be covered by tumor-destructive radation doses. Moreover, adjacent ducts and vessels do not influence the ablation zone as brachytherapy is not prone to disturbing cooling effects, which have been identified as potential causes of inadequate heating and local tumor progression in thermal ablation techniques.

In the opposite to external beam radiation breathing motions are not a problem because the catheters move with the tumor.

CT-guided brachytherapy does not immediately destroy tissue as radiation effects induce cell damages, such as apoptosis or inability of mitosis, that occur days to weeks later. This results in an extremely small rate of abscesses, which are known as a typical complication after thermoablation, especially in cases with biliodigestive anastomosis or bile duct stenosis. While being a major cause of complications after RFA, major bile ducts and blood vessels seem to be resistant to the applied doses of irradiation during brachytherapy. Other risk structures, such as bowel, even if directly adjacent to the target volume, can be reliably spared in the CT-based radiation plan.

THERAPY APPLICATION

The application of CT-guided interstitial brachytherapy consists of five steps. The first step is planning of number and position of the afterloading catheters depending on size, shape and location of the target lesions, followed by CT-guided catheter implantation, radiation planning, actual irradiation via afterloading, and, finally, removal of the catheters.

Catheter implantation is performed under aseptic conditions. The intervention is well tolerated by the patients under intravenous sedation and local anesthesia. The puncture is monitored by CT-fluoroscopy. Upon completion of catheter placement, a contrast enhanced CT-scan is acquired for documentation of the exact catheter location in relation to the tumor. This 3D-data set is the basis for computer assisted radiation planning. The afterloading plan is generated by outlining the clinical target volume (CTV), the catheters, and the surrounding tissues at risk (e.g. bowel, stomach wall, gall bladder, kidney, myelon, skin). Stop locations and dwell durations for the Iridium-192 source inside the afterloading catheters are calculated automatically, followed by approval and, if necessary, manual adjustment. This technique with retrospective registration of the catheter positions is highly accurate and less complex as compared to prospectively arranged catheter positions with templates or intraoperative raster placement [16]. After the afterloading procedure is performed, the catheters are carefully retracted while sealing the puncture channels with thrombogenic material to prevent bleeding.

RISK

Complications can be subdivided into acute complications, occurring during or immediately after treatment, and late complications.

The inadvertent acute events (e.g., bleeding, perforation of bowel, stomach, or gall bladder) are mostly due to mechanical alterations caused by the puncture and catheter placement. However, as CT-guided puncture of the liver is a safe way to avoid severe injuries of adjacent tissues, these inadvertent events occur very rarely. Another rare complication is hepatic bleeding which can be prevented by sufficient sealing of the puncture channel during retraction of the catheter sheaths. Other acute unspecific or radiation induced side effects are emesis, pain, and shivers, which are treated medically.

Potential late effects are mainly related to radiation exposure of non-target tissues. A sufficient hepatic reserve has to be ensured before treating hepatic malignomas, particularly in patients with large and/or multiple lesions, preexisting liver disease, previously irradiated liver (dose accumulation), or otherwise impaired liver function. The tolerance dose of the liver ranges from 30 Gy for the whole organ to 50 Gy for approximately one third of the liver volume. Ricke et al. showed, that in interstitial brachytherapy with Iridium192, the tolerance dose causing an early function loss of hepatocytes as determined in MRI with hepatotrope contrast material 6 weeks after irradiation was 9.9 Gy (±2.3 standard deviation) [17]. This and the careful assessment of the hepatic reserve have to be taken into consideration when planning the treatment in order to avoid posttherapeutic hepatic failure. Other tissues at risk are e.g. bile ducts, gall bladder, gastrointestinal tract, skin, kidney and spinal cord. Previously described complications have included strictures of the common bile duct at very high doses (>20-30 Gy) or gastric ulcers [18,19]. Concerning gastric complications, a threshold dose of 15.5 Gy/ml tissue for the clinical endpoint ulceration of gastric mucosa has been estimated [19].

Overall, however, early and late relevant inadvertent events are rare [17,18]. However, in all cases, a careful evaluation of risk/benefit ratio has to be performed before treatment initiation and during radiation planning.

CLINICAL OUTCOME

Initial data suggest that applying minimal doses of 12–20 Gy, local tumor control is as high as 87% after 6 months [20]. An analysis of 200 colorectal liver metastases between 1 and 11 cm (median 4 cm) revealed a local tumor control rate of 96% after 12 months when applying 25 Gy and 67% when applying 20 Gy as the minimal tumor dose (with larger lesions in the 20 Gy group) [21]. CT-guided brachytherapy can be repeated up to 10 times depending on clinical necessity. However, the use of interstitial brachytherapy is not only limited to its application inside the liver, as treatment of lung malignancies has also demonstrated promising results with respect to local tumor control and side effects [18].

CONCLUSION

CT-guided interstitial brachytherapy of colorectal hepatic metastases is a novel modality in radiation oncology and interventional radiology. This therapeutic instrument enables effective treatment even in those patients, who are not suitable to undergo surgery or thermal ablation such as RFA because of an impaired clinical condition or the extent of hepatic tumor load. The procedure is minimal invasive and save. There are promising results for the treatment of colorectal liver metastases, and further studies are upcoming. CT-guided brachytherapy has the necessary prerequisites to become a powerful tool in modern multimodal treatment concepts for colorectal cancer patients.

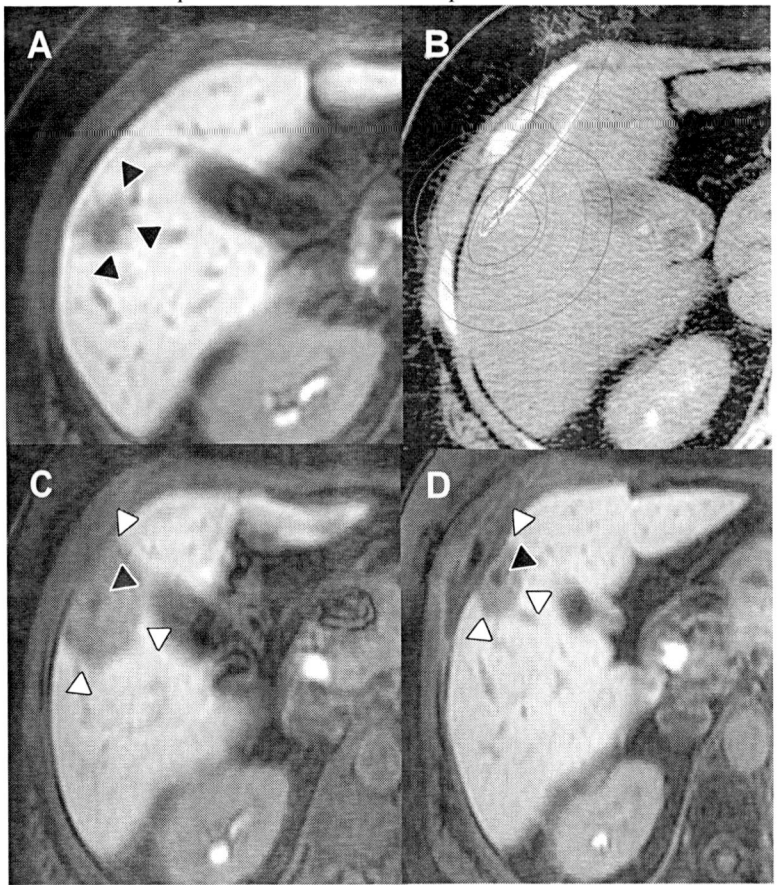

Figure. In this patient, with bilobar liver metatases from colorectal cancer and progression under third line chemotherapy CT-guided afterloading therapy was performed at several target lesions, one of which is displayed here (A). Therapy (B) was planned with a minimal dose of 25 Gy (red line) around the target volume (blue line). MRI of the liver using hepatocyte specific contrast material (C, after 12 weeks; D, after 6 month) demonstrates shrinkage of the lesion (black arrow heads) and the development of therapy induced inactivation of surrounding liver tissue (white arrow heads) as a safety margin.

REFERENCES

[1] Lambert LA, Colacchio TA, Barth RJ. Interval hepatic resection of colorectal metastases improves patient selection*. *Current surgery*. 2000 Sep 1;57(5):504.

[2] Saltz LB, Cox JV, Blanke C, Rosen LS, Fehrenbacher L, Moore MJ, et al. Irinotecan plus fluorouracil and leucovorin for metastatic colorectal cancer. Irinotecan Study Group. *The New England journal of medicine*. 2000 Sep 28;343(13):905-14.

[3] Hurwitz H, Fehrenbacher L, Novotny W, Cartwright T, Hainsworth J, Heim W, et al. Bevacizumab plus irinotecan, fluorouracil, and leucovorin for metastatic colorectal cancer. *The New England journal of medicine*. 2004 Jun 3;350(23):2335-42.

[4] Douillard JY, Cunningham D, Roth AD, Navarro M, James RD, Karasek P, et al. Irinotecan combined with fluorouracil compared with fluorouracil alone as first-line treatment for metastatic colorectal cancer: a multicentre randomised trial. *Lancet.* 2000 Mar 25;355(9209):1041-7.

[5] Solbiati L, Livraghi T, Goldberg SN, Ierace T, Meloni F, Dellanoce M, et al. Percutaneous radio-frequency ablation of hepatic metastases from colorectal cancer: long-term results in 117 patients. *Radiology.* 2001 Oct;221(1):159-66.

[6] Vogl TJ, Muller PK, Mack MG, Straub R, Engelmann K, Neuhaus P. Liver metastases: interventional therapeutic techniques and results, state of the art. *European radiology.* 1999;9(4):675-84.

[7] Denecke T, Steffen I, Hildebrandt B, Ruhl R, Streitparth F, Lehmkuhl L, et al. Assessment of local control after laser-induced thermotherapy of liver metastases from colorectal cancer: contribution of FDG-PET in patients with clinical suspicion of progressive disease. *Acta Radiol.* 2007 Oct;48(8):821-30.

[8] Ricke J, Wust P, Wieners G, Beck A, Cho CH, Seidensticker M, et al. Liver malignancies: CT-guided interstitial brachytherapy in patients with unfavorable lesions for thermal ablation. *J Vasc Interv Radiol.* 2004 Nov;15(11):1279-86.

[9] Herfarth KK, Debus J, Wannenmacher M. Stereotactic radiation therapy of liver metastases: update of the initial phase-I/II trial. *Frontiers of radiation therapy and oncology.* 2004;38:100-5.

[10] Thomas DS, Nauta RJ, Rodgers JE, Popescu GF, Nguyen H, Lee TC, et al. Intraoperative high-dose rate interstitial irradiation of hepatic metastases from colorectal carcinoma. Results of a phase I-II trial. *Cancer.* 1993 Mar 15;71(6):1977-81.

[11] Nauta RJ, Heres EK, Thomas DS, Harter KW, Rodgers JE, Holt RW, et al. Intraoperative single-dose radiotherapy. Observations on staging and interstitial treatment of unresectable liver metastases. *Arch Surg.* 1987 Dec;122(12):1392-5.

[12] Dritschilo A, Harter KW, Thomas D, Nauta R, Holt R, Lee TC, et al. Intraoperative radiation therapy of hepatic metastases: technical aspects and report of a pilot study. *International journal of radiation oncology, biology, physics.* 1988 May;14(5):1007-11.

[13] Ricke J, Wust P, Stohlmann A, Beck A, Cho CH, Pech M, et al. [CT-Guided brachytherapy. A novel percutaneous technique for interstitial ablation of liver metastases]. *Strahlenther Onkol.* 2004 May;180(5):274-80.

[14] Amthauer H, Denecke T, Hildebrandt B, Ruhl R, Miersch A, Nicolaou A, et al. Evaluation of patients with liver metastases from colorectal cancer for locally ablative treatment with laser induced thermotherapy. Impact of PET with 18F-fluorodeoxyglucose on therapeutic decisions. *Nuklearmedizin.* 2006;45(4):177-84.

[15] Denecke T, Lopez Hanninen E. Brachytherapy of liver metastases. Recent results in cancer research *Fortschritte der Krebsforschung.* 2008;177:95-104.

[16] Tonus C, Debertshauser D, Strassmann G, Kolotas C, Walter S, Zamboglou N, et al. CT-based navigation systems for intraoperative radiotherapy using the afterloading-flab technique. *Digestive surgery.* 2001;18(6):470-4.

[17] Ricke J, Seidensticker M, Ludemann L, Pech M, Wieners G, Hengst S, et al. In vivo assessment of the tolerance dose of small liver volumes after single-fraction HDR

irradiation. *International journal of radiation oncology, biology, physics*. 2005 Jul 1;62(3):776-84.

[18] Ricke J, Wust P, Wieners G, Hengst S, Pech M, Lopez Hanninen E, et al. CT-guided interstitial single-fraction brachytherapy of lung tumors: phase I results of a novel technique. *Chest*. 2005 Jun;127(6):2237-42.

[19] Streitparth F, Pech M, Bohmig M, Ruehl R, Peters N, Wieners G, et al. In vivo assessment of the gastric mucosal tolerance dose after single fraction, small volume irradiation of liver malignancies by computed tomography-guided, high-dose-rate brachytherapy. *International journal of radiation oncology, biology, physics*. 2006 Aug 1;65(5):1479-86.

[20] Ricke J, Wust P, Stohlmann A, Beck A, Cho CH, Pech M, et al. CT-guided interstitial brachytherapy of liver malignancies alone or in combination with thermal ablation: phase I-II results of a novel technique. *International journal of radiation oncology, biology, physics*. 2004 Apr 1;58(5):1496-505.

[21] Ruhl R, Ricke J. Image-guided micro-therapy for tumor ablation: from thermal coagulation to advanced irradiation techniques. *Onkologie*. 2006 May;29(5):219-24.

INDEX

A

AAA, 179
AAC, 177
ABC, 163
abdomen, 201, 204, 235
aberrant crypt foci, 212
aberrant crypt foci (ACF), 212
absorption, 170
ACC, 183
accumulation, 181, 182, 185
accuracy, ix, 4, 5, 28, 29, 30, 33, 62, 65, 66, 69, 81, 83, 84, 85, 86, 87, 91, 92, 104, 106, 117, 119, 120, 121, 122, 130, 138
acetate, 161, 162
acid, x, xi, 159, 160, 161, 162, 163, 164, 165, 168, 169, 177, 195, 212, 213, 215, 216, 217, 218, 219, 221, 222
acidosis, 168
acoustic, 67, 70
activation, 182, 184, 213, 214, 216, 218, 219
actuation, 68
acute, 27, 32, 43, 55, 89, 128, 129, 203, 236
acylation, 214, 215
Adams, 76, 90, 186
adenocarcinoma, 8, 33, 35, 36, 38, 59, 63, 64, 93, 123, 133, 137, 138, 139, 142, 208, 219, 226, 227, 229, 230
adenocarcinomas, 63, 192
adenoma, x, 76, 77, 78, 104, 107, 108, 120, 125, 138, 139, 145, 146, 147, 153, 155, 157, 158, 174, 183, 185, 188, 193, 205, 212
adenomas, x, xi, 86, 90, 91, 92, 110, 115, 117, 120, 122, 123, 124, 125, 126, 127, 128, 130, 131, 138, 139, 140, 145, 146, 154, 155, 156, 174, 185, 193, 196, 205, 206, 212
adenovirus, 56
adjustment, 236
administration, xi, 160, 162, 166, 167, 168, 169, 170, 200
Adrenaline, 96
adverse event, 55
AE, 108, 140, 221
age, xii, 16, 17, 52, 114, 127, 128, 135, 136, 150, 161, 163, 174, 175, 178, 193, 195, 196, 197, 203, 216, 224, 225
agent, 56
agents, viii, 41, 42, 49, 50, 53, 54, 56, 194, 195, 200, 235
aggregates, 220
aid, 126
AIM, xii, 223
air, 96, 119, 122, 123, 127
AJ, 157
AKT, 219
AL, 171, 230
Alberta, 197
alcohol, 193, 194, 196
algorithm, 68
allele, xi, 173, 179
alleles, 181, 188, 216, 217
allergic reaction, 168
alpha, 205
alpha-tocopherol, 205
alternative, ix, 21, 28, 44, 51, 54, 95, 107, 111, 133, 134, 145, 146, 155, 178, 184
alternatives, 115, 234
American Cancer Society, 88, 204
amino, 177
amino acid, 177

ammonia, 168, 169
Amsterdam, 175, 177, 196, 230
analgesia, 125, 154, 202, 208
analgesic, 99
anastomoses, 48, 202, 208
anastomosis, 2, 11, 12, 13, 14, 15, 16, 17, 19, 20, 21, 22, 25, 34, 35, 36, 89, 201, 202, 208, 236
anatomy, 90, 119, 192
anemia, 197, 217
angulation, 81, 83
animals, 217
anorexia, 204
antibiotic, 128
antibody, 163
anticancer, 167, 169
anticancer drug, 167, 169
anticoagulant, 124
anticoagulants, 139
antigen, 92, 231
anti-inflammatory drugs, 195
antioxidant, 205
anti-tumor, 166, 167, 169
Anti-tumor, 170
anus, 12, 34, 138, 154, 201
Anxiety, 105
AP, 157, 230
APC, xi, 173, 174, 176, 182, 183, 185, 188, 190, 212, 217
apoptosis, xi, xii, 174, 185, 211, 213, 214, 215, 216, 218, 219, 220, 222, 236
apoptotic, 54, 182, 215
appendix, 148
application, xiii, 66, 67, 140, 169, 170, 233, 236, 237
arachidonic acid, 216, 219
argon, 131, 140
argument, 26
arousal, 203
arrest, 181
artery, viii, 2, 12, 23, 28, 30, 31, 38
ascending colon, 200
aseptic, 236
Asian, 31
aspiration, 85
aspirin, 195, 206
assessment, ix, 3, 4, 5, 15, 19, 21, 33, 36, 46, 49, 51, 54, 78, 85, 86, 89, 91, 92, 95, 97, 98, 100, 105, 106, 117, 138, 139, 140, 235, 237, 239, 240
assessment tools, 105
association, 186
asymptomatic, 197, 205

Atlantic, 170
Atlas, 67, 89, 90
ATP, 168, 214
attachment, 218
atypical, 186
autosomal dominant, 174, 185, 212
availability, 197
avoidance, 154, 194
awareness, ix, 95, 203
azoxymethane, 217, 221

B

barium, 44, 93, 197, 198
barium enema, 44, 93, 197, 198
barrier, 197, 207
base pair, 180
Bax, 63
BD, 59, 62, 63, 93, 142, 154, 219, 229
beam radiation, 236
behavior, 92, 192, 219
benefits, 35, 44, 45, 46, 48, 49, 50, 52, 57, 87, 200, 207, 219
benign, 74, 84, 86, 87, 92, 115, 116, 120, 123, 131, 145, 155, 156, 200
beta-carotene, 205
bevacizumab, 55, 56, 199, 200
Bevacizumab, 56, 64, 238
bias, 86, 92, 98
bile, 236, 237
bile duct, 236, 237
binding, 162, 187, 218, 219
bioinformatics, 222
biologic agents, 200
biopsies, 77, 115, 122, 131, 218
biopsy, 3, 7, 77, 85, 86, 119, 122, 125, 131, 138, 149
biosynthesis, 219
bladder, 6, 23, 37, 83, 114, 117, 135, 236, 237
bleeding, 96, 100, 107, 125, 126, 128, 197, 236
BLM, xi, 174, 176, 181, 185, 188
blood, 7, 10, 24, 71, 85, 99, 100, 127, 136, 152, 153, 169, 175, 196, 200, 235, 236
blood transfusion, 152, 153
blood vessels, 71, 85, 200, 236
blot, 175, 176, 177
body image, xi, 96, 191, 202, 203, 204
body weight, 194
bolus, 42, 50, 132, 170
bowel, xiii, 12, 17, 21, 22, 24, 25, 42, 58, 78, 108, 124, 125, 127, 128, 140, 152, 175, 192, 193, 197, 201, 202, 203, 204, 208, 217, 233, 236

bowel obstruction, 17, 197
brachytherapy, 50, 234, 235, 236, 237, 239, 240
brain, 175, 178
branching, 85
Brazil, 53
breast cancer, 28, 191, 197, 221
breathing, xiii, 233, 234, 236
Britain, 50
bubbles, 67
budding, 106, 118, 120
buffer, 161, 162, 163, 175, 176
burn, 77

C

calcium, 194, 196, 206, 213
caliber, 10
calorie, 193
Canada, 192, 197, 206
cancer cells, 132, 163, 182, 187, 219
cancer progression, 182
cancer screening, ix, 95, 192, 196, 197, 206, 207
cancer treatment, vii, ix, 1, 16, 27, 95, 96, 107, 136, 150
candidates, 48, 127, 134, 203
capacity, 115
capillary, 162
capital cost, 107, 154
capital expenditure, 107
carbohydrate, 217
carcinoembryonic antigen, 92, 231
carcinogen, 217
carcinogenesis, xii, 174, 181, 182, 184, 185, 186, 188, 212, 214, 216, 217, 218, 219, 221, 222
carcinoid tumor, 148, 156, 193
carcinoma, vi, vii, xii, xiii, 22, 31, 34, 35, 36, 37, 42, 44, 45, 47, 49, 51, 52, 53, 54, 55, 57, 58, 59, 60, 61, 63, 77, 85, 86, 88, 89, 90, 91, 92, 93, 97, 104, 107, 108, 134, 138, 139, 146, 149, 155, 156, 157, 167, 169, 170, 171, 174, 185, 188, 189, 207, 208, 212, 213, 223, 224, 225, 226, 227, 228, 229, 230, 239
carcinomas, ix, x, 31, 42, 44, 45, 47, 50, 52, 55, 58, 65, 66, 77, 90, 91, 93, 108, 145, 149, 155, 157, 188, 205, 225, 226, 227
cardiovascular risk, 194
carotene, 205
caspase, 182, 216
caspases, 218
catabolic, 169

catabolism, 169
category a, 60
catheter, 86, 92, 133, 168, 202, 236
catheterization, 152
catheters, xiii, 233, 234, 235, 236
C-C, xi, 160, 165
CD95, 218, 220
cDNA, 176, 177
CE, 140, 209
CEA, xii, 198, 204, 223, 224, 225, 227, 228
cell, 7, 10, 166, 181, 182, 193, 213, 215, 218, 222, 236
cell cycle, 181
cell death, 182
cell growth, 222
cell line, 182, 218
cell lines, 182, 218
cell surface, 215
cellulose, 161
centralized, 134
cervical cancer, 197
cervix, 83
CGC, 179
CGT, 179, 184
channels, 28, 29, 122, 123, 125, 127, 215, 222, 236
chemoprevention, 194, 195
chemotherapeutic agent, 42, 54, 200
chemotherapy, viii, xiii, 2, 13, 41, 42, 45, 46, 47, 49, 50, 51, 54, 55, 56, 57, 58, 59, 60, 62, 63, 106, 121, 123, 133, 134, 149, 151, 169, 198, 199, 201, 203, 204, 207, 225, 227, 233, 234, 235, 238
Chemotherapy, 57, 60, 141, 160, 169, 170, 171, 200
chicken, 193, 194
China, 31, 223, 226
Chi-square, 225
chloride, 163
chloroform, 161, 162, 175
cholesterol, 195, 217
chromatography, 161, 162, 169
chromosomal instability, 185
chromosome, 199, 222
chromosomes, xi, 174, 185
cigarette smoking, 193, 205
circadian, 169
Cisplatin, 171
Citric, 171
CK, 33
CL, 207
classes, 42

Index

classification, xii, 15, 26, 27, 51, 73, 77, 79, 163, 224, 226, 228
clinical assessment, 49
clinical examination, 115, 116, 117
clinical symptoms, 169
clinical trial, 55, 57, 89, 199, 205, 207
clinical trials, 55, 199
clinically significant, 124
clinics, 141
cloning, 216
closure, 2, 12, 16, 126, 146, 154
clustering, 22
c-myc, 182
C-N, xi, 160, 165
Co, 49
coagulation, 140, 235, 240
Cochrane, 203, 205, 206, 207, 208, 209
Cochrane Database of Systematic Reviews, 205, 206, 207, 208, 209
coding, xi, 174, 175, 176, 180, 185, 188, 213
codon, 177, 183, 184
codons, 179, 180, 182, 183
coenzyme, 214
cohort, 62, 83, 193, 194, 195, 206
coil, 87, 90
colectomy, 24, 195, 200, 207
colic, viii, 2, 27
colitis, 193
collaboration, 23
Collaboration, 203, 207
colloid particles, 122
colon, xi, xii, 19, 34, 54, 55, 57, 58, 63, 64, 89, 93, 119, 124, 125, 131, 138, 140, 154, 156, 163, 164, 168, 169, 173, 180, 181, 184, 185, 186, 187, 188, 190, 192, 196, 197, 198, 199, 200, 201, 202, 203, 205, 206, 207, 208, 211, 216, 219, 221, 222
colon cancer, xi, xii, 54, 63, 64, 89, 93, 163, 164, 168, 169, 173, 180, 181, 185, 186, 187, 188, 190, 192, 196, 198, 199, 200, 201, 202, 203, 205, 206, 207, 208, 211, 216, 219, 222
colonoscopy, 115, 123, 134, 145, 196, 197, 198
colorectal, x, xi, 159, 160, 161, 163, 167, 169, 170, 171
colorectal adenocarcinoma, 37
colorectal surgeon, 135, 198
colorectum, 140
colostomy, 2, 9, 11, 12, 16, 17, 19, 21, 22, 32, 146, 154, 201, 208
common bile duct, 237
community, 99, 200

co-morbidities, 17, 53, 54
comorbidity, 130, 235
complete remission, 133, 134
compliance, 49, 99, 114, 135, 152, 197
complications, vii, ix, 10, 16, 17, 22, 32, 36, 47, 95, 96, 99, 100, 107, 108, 114, 123, 126, 128, 130, 135, 136, 141, 150, 151, 152, 236, 237
components, 54, 69, 182, 185, 217
composition, xii, 212, 213
compounds, 169, 220
computed tomography, ix, 4, 65, 66, 90, 92, 93, 240
computer technology, 67
concentration, 161, 162, 167
conception, 170
concrete, 162
condom, 119
conduction, 115
configuration, 235
conflict, 137
Congress, 57
consciousness, 169
consensus, 57, 96, 127
consent, 4, 11, 32, 162, 175
constipation, 21, 151
construction, vii, 1
consultants, 229
consumption, 205
contamination, 22
continuity, 12, 17
control, ix, xiii, 12, 13, 16, 18, 23, 28, 31, 37, 42, 43, 44, 46, 57, 60, 66, 69, 95, 96, 99, 110, 133, 150, 152, 193, 202, 205, 230, 233, 234, 235, 237, 239
control group, 28
controlled trials, 107, 196, 206, 207
conversion, 154, 188, 215
cooling, xiii, 233, 235
correlation, x, xi, 90, 91, 105, 160, 164, 165, 167, 226, 227
correlations, vii, x, xii, 159, 160, 163, 164, 165, 167, 169, 223, 224, 225, 227
cost-effective, 107
costs, 45, 107, 136
counseling, 196
coupling, 67
covalent, 218
coverage, 235
COX-2, 194, 216, 217, 221
CRC, 191, 192, 193, 194, 195, 196, 197, 199, 202, 204, 212, 216, 217, 218
CRM, ix, 65, 66, 82, 85

Index

Crohn's disease, 193
cross-sectional, ix, 65, 66, 85
CRT, ix, 60, 65, 66, 81, 84, 85, 100, 104, 106
cryosurgery, 3
crystals, 119
CT, vi, xiii, 4, 5, 33, 60, 66, 71, 87, 92, 106, 115, 117, 119, 121, 139, 197, 198, 201, 204, 233, 234, 235, 236, 237, 238, 239, 240
CT scan, 71, 121, 198, 204
Cuba, 145
culture, 169, 170, 221
current limit, 47, 52
cycles, 67, 175, 176
cyclin D1, 182
cyclooxygenase, 216, 221
cyclooxygenase-2, 216
cystectomy, 23
cysteine, 218
cytoplasm, 184, 213

D

dairy, 194, 195
damage, 201, 203
data analysis, 119
data set, 69, 236
database, 52
de novo, 214, 215, 218
death, ix, 95, 96, 102, 136, 137, 153, 182, 196, 201, 204, 220
deaths, xi, 114, 136, 191, 192
decision making, 106
decisions, 42, 239
defecation, 106, 135
defects, 15, 76, 96, 105, 126, 129, 152, 184, 221
deficiency, 168
definition, 78, 85
degradation, 167, 169, 182
dehiscence, 107
dehydrogenase, 170
delivery, 42, 50, 51
Denmark, 66, 67, 113, 137
deposits, 13
depressed, 91, 115
depression, 96
derivatives, xii, 211, 213, 214, 215, 218
descending colon, 200
destruction, 3, 149, 150, 235
detection, ix, 65, 66, 86, 90, 92, 187, 192, 196, 204, 231

developed countries, 136
deviation, 98, 104
diarrhoea, 114
Dicks, 189
diet, 193, 205, 212, 217
dietary, 193, 194, 212, 213, 215, 217, 219, 220
dietary fat, 213
dietary fiber, 193, 194
dietary intake, 194
diets, 193
differentiation, xii, 3, 6, 7, 10, 27, 47, 106, 131, 199, 216, 224, 225, 227, 228
digestive tract, 12, 167
diploid, 185
dipole, 219
discrimination, 118, 119
disease free survival, 18, 24, 25, 30
disease-free survival, 46, 49, 51, 52, 53, 62, 199
diseases, 200, 217
Disease-specific, 44
disorder, 168
dissociation, 7, 10
distribution, 198, 215, 216
division, 200
DNA, xi, 166, 167, 168, 173, 174, 175, 176, 177, 179, 180, 181, 182, 183, 184, 185, 186, 188, 189, 216, 220
DNA polymerase, 180
DNA repair, 181, 182, 185, 188
domain, 182, 183
donor, xi, 173, 177, 179
dose-response relationship, 133
dosing, xiii, 167, 233
downsizing, 46, 48
DPD, x, xi, 159, 160, 162, 163, 164, 165, 166, 167, 168, 169
drainage, 12
drug reactions, 160
drug therapy, 234
drugs, 42, 124, 167, 169, 195
durability, 35
duration, 10, 24, 105, 152, 153, 235
dyhydropyridine, x, 159
dyhydropyridine (DPD), x, 159
dyspareunia, 203
dysplasia, 123, 124, 139

E

eating, 195

EB, 140, 230
elasticity, 119
elderly, ix, 95, 96, 98, 109, 134, 136
elderly population, ix, 95
elective surgery, 201
EM, 89, 93, 139, 219
emboli, xii, 224, 225, 227, 228
embryo, 221
endometrial cancer, 178, 179, 180, 189
endometrium, 174, 185
endoplasmic reticulum, 213
endoscope, 10, 122
endoscopy, 123, 148, 151, 200
end-to-end, 21
energy, 84, 206
England, 17, 205, 206, 208
environment, 216
environmental conditions, 217
enzyme, x, xi, 159, 160, 161, 162, 165, 167, 168, 169
enzymes, x, xii, 159, 160, 161, 163, 164, 165, 166, 167, 168, 169, 177, 212, 213, 214, 216, 218
epidemiologic studies, 194
epidermal growth factor, 54
epidermal growth factor receptor, 54
epigenetic, 212
epinephrine, 123, 125, 126, 128
epithelia, xii, 211, 215
epithelial cell, 181, 184, 217, 221
epithelial cells, 181, 184, 217, 221
ER, 205, 213, 220
ESR, 126
estrogens, 203
ethanol, 161, 162
ethyl acetate, 161, 162
etiology, iv
Europe, 17, 42, 43, 44, 53, 169
evacuation, 21, 36, 202
evidence, 169, 194, 196, 199, 202, 203, 204, 206
examinations, 86
excitation, 138
exclusion, 42, 184
execution, 212, 215, 216
exercise, 194, 196
exons, 175, 177
expert, 57, 134
expertise, 51, 128, 129
exposure, 50, 108, 141, 153, 234, 237
extra help, 202

F

FA, 37, 221, 230
factorial, 105
faecal, 19, 100
failure, viii, 15, 16, 21, 32, 41, 59, 63, 80, 93, 128, 130, 132, 142, 153, 229
familial, 174, 186, 187, 188, 189, 194, 196, 212, 220
family, xii, 150, 177, 178, 182, 184, 187, 193, 196, 206, 213, 214, 215, 221, 223, 224, 225, 227
family history, xii, 193, 196, 206, 223, 224, 225, 227
family members, 178, 196
fascia, 5, 13, 14, 15, 16, 33, 71, 72, 73, 81, 82, 83, 85, 88, 106, 117, 128, 135
fasting, 217
fat, 19, 28, 74, 75, 80, 81, 85, 88, 106, 128, 193, 195, 205, 213
fatty acids, xii, 211, 212, 213, 214, 215, 217, 218, 220
fax, 113
FDG, 235, 239
feeding, 12, 217
females, 31, 37
fever, 129, 152
fiber, 126, 128, 193, 194, 196, 202, 205
fibrosis, 21
fidelity, 180
film, 175, 176
Finland, 205
first degree relative, 196
fish, 193, 194
fistulas, 129, 130, 151
fixation, 69
FL, 37
fluid, 70
fluoride, 169
fluoroscopy, 236
focusing, x, 159
folate, 193, 194, 196, 205, 221
Folate, 195
food, 154, 205
forceps, 122, 127
formamide, 175, 176
FP, 110
frameshift mutation, xi, 174, 177, 180, 181, 184, 185, 188
France, 55
fruits, 193, 195
FS, 218
functional changes, 36

fusion, 213

G

gall bladder, 236, 237
gas, 129, 162, 169
gas chromatograph, 162, 169
gastric, 170, 178, 179, 180, 237, 240
gastric mucosa, 237, 240
gastric ulcer, 237
gastrointestinal, vii, ix, 28, 38, 95, 96, 99, 104, 107, 119, 148, 187, 188, 193, 217, 237
gastrointestinal tract, 119, 148, 217, 237
GC, 32, 92, 141, 162, 183, 205
GCC, 183
GE, 205, 230
gel, 162, 175, 176
gender, xii, 16, 27, 197, 224, 225
gene, xi, xii, 54, 63, 173, 174, 175, 177, 179, 181, 182, 183, 184, 185, 186, 187, 188, 189, 190, 211, 212, 213, 216, 217, 219, 221, 222
gene expression, xii, 63, 211, 217
general anesthesia, 49
general surgeon, 198
generation, 121, 154, 168
genes, xi, 173, 174, 175, 176, 177, 179, 180, 181, 182, 183, 185, 188, 189, 212, 216, 217, 220
genetic instability, xi, 174
genetic marker, 54
genetic testing, 196, 206
genome, 180, 216
genomic, xi, 173, 175, 176, 177, 179, 180, 182, 187, 189
genomic instability, 180, 182
genotype, 57, 220
Georgia, 211
Germany, 104, 211, 233
germline mutations, xi, 173, 174, 175, 176, 177, 178, 179, 185, 189
GH, 207
Gibbs, 34
GL, 90, 93, 109, 170, 206, 207
glass, 163
glioma, 222
gliomas, 222
glucose, 219
glycerol, 175, 213, 218
gold, 17, 24, 42, 96, 99, 121, 201
gold standard, 17, 24, 42, 96, 121, 201
grading, 120, 131, 212

grains, 196
Great Britain, 135
groups, ix, x, xii, 31, 42, 43, 44, 48, 50, 53, 54, 55, 78, 84, 95, 98, 100, 106, 149, 150, 151, 159, 161, 199, 203, 224, 226, 227
growth, xi, 54, 87, 174, 181, 184, 185, 187, 212, 222
growth factor, 54, 181, 185, 187
growth hormone, 54
Guangdong, xii, 223, 224, 225
Guangzhou, 223
guidance, 234
guidelines, 91, 110, 122, 139
Guinea, 171

H

haemostasis, 129
half-life, 167
handling, 114, 131
harbour, 131
hardness, 119
harm, 125
harvest, 38
HE, 137, 141, 155, 158, 206, 229
health, ix, 95, 96, 135, 137, 194, 197, 198, 204
health care, ix, 95, 137, 197
health care workers, 137
health insurance, 197
health status, 198
heat, 215
heating, 236
height, 3, 130
helix, 217
hemorrhoids, 197
hepatic failure, 237
hepatocyte, 238
hepatocytes, 217, 237
heterogeneous, 49, 87, 149, 212, 213
high resolution, 117, 121
high risk, 14, 30, 97, 114, 122, 124, 128, 130, 131, 132, 136, 137, 195
higher education, 197
high-risk, 5, 7, 16, 47, 49, 98, 118, 194, 199
Hispanic, 197
histological, 52, 123, 146
histology, 3, 123, 131
histopathology, 86
HK, 33, 37, 92, 138
homogeneity, 116
homogenized, 161, 162

homolog, 186
Honda, 37
Hong Kong, 110, 158
hormone, 54
hospital, 16, 24, 44, 99, 100, 107, 129, 134, 137, 153, 202, 207
hospitalization, 200
hospitals, 86, 107, 134, 137, 202, 207
hot water, 161
housing, 68
HPLC, 162
human, 67, 169, 170, 175, 180, 184, 186, 187, 188, 189, 190, 216, 217, 219, 220, 221, 222
human genome, 180
humans, 217
hybridization, 175, 176, 177
hydro, 214
hydrochloric acid, 162
hydrogen, 163
hydrogen peroxide, 163
hydrolysis, 219
hydrolyzed, 162
hydrophilic, 214
hydrophobic, 213
hydroxide, 162
hypomethylation, 220
hypothesis, 50, 55, 203, 216, 217

I

iatrogenic, 19
ice, 161, 162
identification, viii, 1, 28, 29, 30, 52, 84, 123, 216, 220
IgG, 163
ileostomy, 16, 201
image analysis, 91
images, ix, xiii, 65, 66, 67, 68, 87, 233
imaging, 4, 5, 62, 66, 70, 71, 85, 88, 90, 92, 93, 106, 109, 138, 139, 231, 235
imaging modalities, 5, 88, 106
immune response, 24
impairments, 167
implementation, 226, 227
impotency, 114
in situ, 77
in vitro, 91
in vivo, 29, 168, 169, 221
inactivation, xi, 167, 173, 174, 180, 181, 185, 238

incidence, xi, 10, 16, 17, 18, 31, 43, 81, 147, 160, 165, 169, 192, 205
incubation, 161, 162
indication, xiii, 3, 4, 5, 6, 9, 10, 16, 23, 29, 31, 33, 93, 124, 126, 146, 234, 235
indicators, 122
indirect measure, 118
individual differences, 217
induction, 55, 56, 151, 217, 222
induction chemotherapy, 55, 56
infection, 126, 128, 129
Infiltration, 126
inflammation, 27, 79, 80, 83, 85, 106, 213
inflammatory, 80, 84, 87, 193, 195, 218, 220
inflammatory bowel disease, 193
informed consent, 4, 11, 32, 162, 175
infusions, 133
inheritance, 174, 185
inherited, 193, 196
inhibition, x, 159, 166, 169, 212, 218, 219, 221
inhibitor, 194, 216
inhibitors, 195, 215
inhibitory, 216
inhomogeneity, 58, 84
initiation, 212, 214, 217, 237
injection, x, 28, 29, 38, 125, 132, 138, 159, 160, 161, 167, 168
injuries, 212, 236
injury, 201
innominate, 116
inspection, 115, 116
Inspection, 115
instability, xi, 173, 174, 176, 177, 180, 182, 185, 187, 188, 199
institutions, 53, 154
instruments, 115, 125, 126, 127, 128, 146, 154
insulin, 187, 219
insulin-like growth factor, 187
insulin-like growth factor I, 187
insurance, 197
intensity, 69, 133
interaction, 52, 182, 213
interactions, 216
interdisciplinary, 235
interest, 199
interface, 71, 73, 74, 75, 76, 77, 80, 81, 82, 83, 88
interference, 215, 216
interpretation, 43, 76
interstitial, 234, 236, 237, 239, 240
interval, 48, 51, 60, 235

Index

intervention, 17, 21, 152, 199, 235, 236
intestinal obstruction, 217
intestinal tract, 169
intestine, xi, 160, 168, 174, 192, 200, 201
intracellular signaling, 221
intraoperative, 14, 20, 50, 157, 208, 236, 239
intraperitoneal, 96, 108
intravenous, 167, 169, 236
intrinsic, 162
invasive, xiii, 7, 24, 33, 76, 78, 86, 90, 91, 92, 98, 110, 111, 131, 139, 146, 154, 156, 199, 212, 233, 235, 237
invasive adenocarcinoma, 78, 90
invasive cancer, 76, 78, 199
investment, 10
ion transport, 213
IP, 220
IR, 93
Ireland, 135
Irinotecan, 170, 238
iron, 122
irradiation, xiii, 3, 16, 33, 58, 61, 62, 143, 215, 233, 234, 236, 237, 239, 240
ischemia, 15
isoforms, 215, 217, 220
ISS, 105
Italy, 55, 65, 69, 70, 111, 151

J

JAMA, 206, 208
Japan, 31, 159, 168, 173
Japanese, xi, 77, 79, 169, 170, 173, 175, 177, 178, 189
JI, 142
JNK, 219
JT, 207
judgment, 124
Jun, 110, 238, 240
Jung, 16, 33, 35, 38, 63, 90, 142, 220

K

kidney, 236, 237
King, 109, 158
knockout, 221
knowledge, 196
KOH, 161
Korea, 31

Korean, 231

L

LA, 238
lactic acid, 168
lamina, 116, 125
laparoscopic, viii, 2, 24, 25, 37, 66, 89, 100, 109, 134, 143, 154, 200, 207, 229
laparoscopic surgery, viii, 2, 24, 25, 37, 200
laparotomy, 100, 125, 129
large colon, 140
large intestine, xi, 140, 160, 168, 200, 216
laser, xiii, 3, 131, 233, 234, 239
latency, 194
latex, 67
LC, 138
leakage, 14, 15, 16, 35, 96, 107, 146, 202
leaks, 96
learning, 10, 86, 92, 107, 200
legume, 193
Lesion, 76, 147
lesions, viii, xiii, 2, 6, 25, 53, 74, 75, 76, 77, 78, 80, 83, 84, 85, 86, 87, 88, 90, 92, 108, 111, 115, 126, 131, 140, 141, 145, 147, 150, 155, 160, 212, 233, 234, 235, 236, 237, 238, 239
levator, 13, 16, 18, 19, 48
libido, 203
life expectancy, 199
life span, 3
lifestyle, xi, 191, 193, 195, 202, 204
lifetime, 191
ligands, 220, 221
likelihood, 197, 200, 201
limitation, 104
limitations, xiii, 5, 21, 47, 52, 99, 106, 233, 234
linkage, 216
lipid, 213, 215, 216
Lipid, 221
lipid metabolism, 215, 216
lipids, 212, 213, 220
liquids, 127, 202
liver, xiii, 32, 134, 169, 193, 198, 199, 217, 220, 233, 234, 235, 236, 237, 238, 239, 240
liver disease, 237
liver metastases, xiii, 199, 233, 234, 235, 237, 239
LM, 108, 219, 230
local anesthesia, 236
localization, 148, 234

Index

location, viii, xiii, 2, 6, 10, 34, 69, 86, 106, 107, 116, 146, 192, 198, 201, 233, 236
locus, 187, 217, 220, 221
London, 108
long distance, 32
loss of heterozygosity, xi, 173, 199, 217
loss of libido, 203
low risk, 47, 96, 97, 114, 121, 128, 130, 131, 136, 137, 199, 201, 203
low-dose aspirin, 195
LPS, 157
lubrication, 203
lumen, 71, 81
luminal, 122
lung, 134, 191, 199, 237, 240
lung cancer, 191
lung metastases, 199
lungs, 134
LV, 55, 63, 171
lying, 132
lymphadenectomy, viii, 2, 18, 28, 29, 31, 32, 38
lymphadenopathy, 201
lymphatic, 3, 4, 6, 7, 10, 12, 18, 26, 28, 30, 84, 106, 133, 149, 192
lymphomas, 193
lysine, 177

M

M1, 199
magnetic, ix, 4, 62, 65, 66, 93, 122, 138
magnetic resonance, ix, 4, 62, 65, 66, 93, 138
magnetic resonance imaging, 4, 62, 66, 93, 138
Magnetic Resonance Imaging, 106, 110
maintenance, 234
maize, 221, 222
males, 193
malignancy, 90, 116, 120, 122, 123, 124, 131, 146
malignant, 28, 76, 78, 80, 83, 84, 85, 87, 88, 91, 116, 119, 121, 122, 123, 132, 139, 145, 149, 169, 196, 212, 222
malignant melanoma, 28, 139
malignant tumors, 169
mammalian cell, 221
mammalian cells, 221
mammogram, 197
management, 32, 34, 37, 42, 44, 57, 60, 62, 85, 88, 91, 92, 108, 109, 139, 140, 151, 155, 156, 158, 200, 227
manipulation, 154

MAPK, 219
mapping, 28, 38
masking, 151
mass, 204
mass spectrometry, 162, 169
matrix, 67
maturation, xii, 211
measurement, 204
measures, 10, 97, 99, 118
meat, 193, 195, 205
median, 12, 27, 44, 45, 46, 50, 51, 53, 57, 99, 100, 202, 237
medication, 202
medications, 194, 195
medicine, 202, 238
Medline, x, 145
melanoma, 123, 193
membranes, 122, 123, 214, 215, 220, 222
men, xi, 19, 21, 23, 25, 96, 161, 191, 196, 197, 205, 206, 225
mesenchyme, 217
mesentery, 12, 25
meta-analysis, 92, 139, 207, 208
metabolic, x, xi, 159, 160, 163, 164, 165, 167, 168, 169, 215
metabolism, xi, 160, 167, 168, 169, 170, 212, 213, 214, 215, 216, 218, 219, 221, 222
metabolites, 162, 214, 221
metabolizing, x, 159, 161
metastases, viii, ix, xii, xiii, 44, 47, 52, 62, 65, 66, 78, 80, 81, 84, 85, 88, 90, 93, 100, 133, 134, 150, 198, 199, 207, 224, 226, 227, 233, 234, 235, 237, 238, 239
metastasis, vii, xii, xiii, 1, 6, 7, 13, 22, 26, 30, 31, 32, 33, 38, 39, 78, 87, 90, 91, 121, 122, 134, 139, 148, 165, 166, 198, 200, 220, 223, 224, 225, 226, 227, 228, 230
metastatic, 54, 62, 84, 87, 93, 130, 170, 199, 207, 209, 238, 239
metastatic disease, 199
methylene, 28, 29, 30
mice, 170, 212, 216, 217, 221
microarray, 222
micrometastasis, 26, 29
microscope, 127, 128
microsurgery, v, ix, x, 3, 9, 34, 53, 62, 66, 88, 95, 108, 109, 110, 111, 112, 114, 127, 137, 139, 140, 141, 143, 145, 146, 147, 148, 153, 154, 155, 156, 157, 158
microwave, 163

migration, ix, 95
milk, 163, 194
minimal residual disease, 61
minority, 204
MIP, 69
misconception, 191
misinterpretation, 87
mitochondria, 213, 215, 216, 218, 219
mitochondrial, xii, 168, 211, 214, 215, 219, 220, 222
mitochondrial membrane, 214
mitosis, 236
ML, 61, 109, 158
modalities, ix, xiii, 2, 5, 47, 48, 50, 51, 65, 66, 87, 88, 106, 121, 122, 135, 136, 166, 233
modality, viii, 2, 21, 41, 47, 61, 82, 85, 91, 135, 142, 157, 208, 235, 237
mode, 174
models, 52, 136, 216, 219, 221, 222
modifier gene, 212, 216, 217, 219, 220
modulation, 213, 215
modulus, 138
molecular changes, 212
molecular markers, 199
molecular mechanisms, 213
molecular structure, 215
molecules, 213, 215, 221
monoclonal, 56, 163
monoclonal antibodies, 56
monoclonal antibody, 163
Moon, 38
morbidity, vii, ix, 3, 9, 14, 17, 18, 20, 21, 23, 24, 31, 32, 35, 48, 51, 52, 55, 95, 96, 97, 98, 99, 107, 114, 123, 130, 133, 134, 136, 146, 148, 150, 151, 154, 155, 226, 230
morphological, 87
morphology, 27, 69, 212
mortality, vii, ix, 17, 18, 21, 23, 24, 32, 95, 96, 99, 107, 114, 126, 127, 130, 135, 136, 137, 143, 146, 148, 150, 151, 154, 196, 205, 226
mortality rate, 130
mortality risk, 136
moths, 100
motion, xiii, 233
mouse, 163, 169, 170, 216, 219, 220, 222
mouse model, 216, 219
MRI, 4, 5, 16, 33, 35, 47, 54, 66, 81, 87, 106, 115, 117, 119, 121, 122, 198, 201, 235, 237, 238
mRNA, 215
MS, 38, 63, 92, 162
MSI, 199

MSS, 169
mucosa, xii, 71, 76, 78, 114, 116, 117, 120, 124, 152, 177, 211, 212, 215, 216, 237
mucous membrane, 167
mucus, 197
multidisciplinary, 66, 85, 114, 115, 199
multiple regression, 27
multiple regression analysis, 27
multiplicity, 217
multivariate, 18, 36, 78, 82, 133, 138, 139
muscles, 13
mutant, 182
mutants, 221
mutation, xi, 173, 177, 178, 179, 181, 182, 183, 184, 185, 186, 188, 189, 190, 196, 217
mutations, xi, 173, 174, 175, 176, 177, 178, 179, 180, 181, 182, 183, 184, 185, 186, 187, 188, 189, 190, 212
myocardial infarction, 129, 152

N

NA, 60, 61, 230
NAD, 215
narcotic, 202
Nash, 62
natural, 169, 170, 212
navigation system, 239
NC, 111
ND, 101, 110
neck, 78
necrosis, 115
needle aspiration, 85
neoplasia, 138, 139, 140, 205, 212, 220, 222
neoplasias, 86
neoplasm, 28, 37, 148
neoplasms, 34, 38, 111, 140, 146, 154, 156, 157
Neoplasms, iv
neoplastic, 87, 115
nerve, 11, 13, 14, 21, 192, 201, 203
nerves, viii, 1, 71, 201
neuroendocrine, 148
neuroprotective, 200
neurotoxicity, 168, 200
New England, 205, 206, 208, 238
New York, 37, 154, 191, 205
Ni, 159
NIH, 42, 57
nitrogen, 162

nodal involvement, 5, 6, 7, 25, 26, 27, 31, 86, 87, 106
nodes, viii, 2, 27, 28, 29, 30, 31, 33, 74, 78, 81, 84, 85, 87, 122, 198, 200, 201, 227
nodules, 216
noise, 69, 119
non-invasive, 86
non-random, 98, 129
normal, xi, xii, 69, 71, 72, 74, 76, 83, 88, 105, 119, 121, 169, 173, 175, 176, 177, 179, 180, 181, 182, 184, 201, 202, 204, 211, 234
North America, 191, 200, 201, 204
Norway, 113
nuclear, 182, 217
nuclei, 182, 184
nucleic acid, x, xi, 159, 160, 161, 162, 163, 164, 165, 169
nucleus, 213
nurse, 202
nurses, 128
nutrition, 212, 219
nylon, 176

O

obese, 25
obesity, 193, 194, 206
observations, 139, 227
obsolete, 126
obstruction, 99, 128, 198, 207
occult blood, 196
office-based, ix, 65, 88
old age, 16
old-fashioned, 154
oncogene, 188
Oncogene, 222
oncogenes, 174, 190
oncological, ix, 22, 32, 61, 95, 96, 114, 124, 127, 130, 135, 136, 137, 141, 151, 153
oncology, 37, 141, 152, 237, 239, 240
Oncology, 43, 53, 58, 59, 64, 142, 170, 204, 207, 208, 209
online, 33
opacity, 69, 88
operator, 68, 86, 87, 115, 126
OPRT, x, 159, 160, 161, 163, 164, 165, 166, 167, 168
optical, 96
optics, 128
oral, 42, 55, 133, 142, 170, 200

organ, 22, 23, 52, 76, 83, 153, 237
organization, 216
orgasm, 203
orientation, 129
orotate phosphoribosyl transferase, x, 159
orotate phosphoribosyl transferase (OPRT), x, 159
ovaries, 174
ovary, 175
overweight, 116
oxide, 122

P

p38, 219
p53, xi, 173, 174, 176, 182, 184, 188
PA, 60, 109, 141, 148, 156, 157, 221
pain, 24, 128, 134, 151, 152, 154, 197, 200, 202, 204, 237
palliative, 3, 10, 11, 98, 107, 128, 150, 157, 200, 234, 235
palpation, 115
Pancreatic cancer, 178
Pap, 197
paper, 54, 161
parameter, 9, 69, 137
parenchyma, 234
paresis, 135
Paris, 32
particles, 122
pathogenesis, iv, 140, 178, 186
pathogenic, 178, 184
pathologist, 20, 27, 28, 123, 129, 130, 200
pathologists, 45, 77, 225
pathology, 43, 44, 45, 46, 86, 202
pathophysiological, 215
pathways, xii, 70, 107, 167, 211, 212, 213, 214, 215, 217, 218, 221
PCA, 202
PCR, 175, 176, 177, 179
PD, 206, 221
pelvic, vii, viii, 1, 2, 11, 12, 13, 15, 23, 24, 25, 29, 30, 31, 32, 34, 35, 37, 38, 39, 58, 72, 89, 119, 152, 192, 198, 201, 203, 208, 229, 230
pelvic pain, 152
pelvis, 19, 21, 25, 47, 133, 175, 198, 203, 204
penetrance, 216
perception, 152, 197
perforation, xii, 19, 107, 124, 125, 129, 130, 152, 153, 224, 225, 227, 228, 236

Index

performance, 87, 90, 92, 117, 127, 128, 132, 135, 136, 137, 169, 216
perineum, 201
periodic, 163
peripheral blood, 175
peritoneal, 20, 22, 29, 36, 39, 74, 129, 141
peritoneal cavity, 22, 129, 141
peritoneum, 29, 129, 130
peritonitis, 25
permeation, 165, 166
permit, vii, 1, 11, 19, 25, 29, 32, 63
peroxide, 163
personal, 193
personal history, 193
PET, 122, 134, 198, 235, 239
PET scan, 198, 235
PET-CT, 122, 134, 235
PF, 108
PG, 90, 109, 111, 138, 140, 157, 205
P-glycoprotein, 222
pH, 161, 162, 216
pharmacological, 142
pharmacotherapy, 200
phenol, 175
phenotype, 188, 217, 220
Philadelphia, 34, 37
phosphate, 163, 214, 215, 218, 221
phospholipids, 213
Phosphorylase, 171
phosphorylation, 166, 170
physical activity, 193, 194
physical exercise, 196
physicians, 207
physics, 239, 240
physiological, xii, 135, 161, 211, 215
physiology, 104, 105, 208
pilot study, 239
planning, 35, 55, 85, 235, 236, 237
plasma, 133, 140, 169
plasma levels, 169
plasmids, 176
play, xi, 6, 32, 106, 151, 166, 174, 185, 222
plexus, vii, viii, 1
PM, 92, 230
PMS, 186
PN, 219
Poland, 46
politicians, 137
polyacrylamide, 175, 176
polymerase, 26, 175, 176, 180

polymerase chain reaction, 26
polymorphism, 217
polyp, 77, 123, 140, 146, 194, 195, 199
polypectomy, 78, 90, 91, 123, 148
polyps, 18, 78, 90, 123, 139, 140, 146, 154, 155, 156, 158, 174, 192, 193, 194, 195, 196, 198, 205, 206, 207, 217
polyunsaturated fat, 212
polyunsaturated fatty acid, 212
polyunsaturated fatty acids, 212
poor, 7, 10, 15, 16, 19, 21, 26, 43, 48, 49, 65, 84, 86, 105, 106, 122, 127, 130, 199, 203
poor performance, 127
population, ix, 27, 38, 95, 98, 104, 196, 201, 206, 216
population group, ix, 95
ports, 96
positive correlation, 167
postoperative, vii, viii, 1, 5, 9, 10, 13, 14, 15, 16, 17, 18, 20, 21, 22, 23, 24, 26, 27, 29, 32, 37, 42, 43, 46, 47, 49, 50, 51, 52, 53, 54, 56, 57, 58, 60, 63, 119, 129, 131, 132, 134, 146, 147, 150, 152, 154, 169, 200, 202, 203, 208, 227
potassium, 162
power, 98, 212
precipitation, 162
prediction, ix, 63, 65, 66, 87, 88, 106, 160
predictive marker, 63
predictors, 7, 27, 93, 98, 139, 207, 227, 230
preference, 117, 197, 207
pressure, 105, 123, 127, 128, 154
prevention, 34, 194, 195, 205, 206, 212, 216
primary tumor, vii, 1, 3, 4, 12, 22, 26, 48, 74, 84, 85, 87, 198, 199, 224
probability, ix, 84, 95, 96, 101, 102
probe, 66, 67, 68, 70, 71, 81, 83, 85, 86, 92, 119, 120, 175, 177, 235
proctoscopy, 115, 117
production, 168
prognosis, xi, 14, 15, 26, 31, 42, 49, 51, 52, 65, 84, 85, 115, 160, 169, 212
prognostic factors, xi, 62, 107, 138, 160, 169, 231
prognostic value, 31, 51
program, 90, 124, 128
proliferation, 61, 213, 218
promoter, 57, 189
prophylactic, 196
prostate, 6, 83, 120, 128, 178, 189
prostate cancer, 189
Prostate cancer, 138, 142, 178

protection, 35, 205
protein, xii, 161, 162, 170, 177, 180, 181, 182, 184, 193, 212, 213, 215, 216, 218, 219, 221
protein function, 180
proteinase, 175
proteins, xi, 173, 177, 179, 180, 181, 216, 218, 220
protocol, viii, 1, 7, 9, 16, 17, 22, 23, 27, 53, 57, 98, 99, 104, 124, 129, 135
protocols, 22, 132, 134
proto-oncogene, 188
proximal, 68, 74, 81, 84, 85, 86, 104
public, 204
public health, 204
purification, 175
pyrimidine, 169

Q

QOL, 105
quality of life, vii, viii, ix, 2, 12, 17, 20, 21, 24, 32, 36, 59, 66, 95, 96, 99, 104, 105, 108, 109, 134, 137, 150, 152, 200, 202, 203, 204, 207, 208
Quality of life, xi, 109, 191, 201, 208
questionnaire, 104
questionnaires, 105

R

RA, 93, 109, 220, 221, 230
race, 169
radiation, xiii, 2, 11, 14, 21, 41, 42, 44, 45, 46, 48, 50, 51, 55, 56, 57, 58, 59, 60, 61, 62, 63, 64, 96, 110, 114, 121, 133, 141, 142, 154, 199, 201, 202, 203, 204, 208, 229, 233, 234, 236, 237, 239, 240
Radiation, 41, 43, 53, 58, 59, 142, 201, 208, 234
radiation therapy, xiii, 2, 14, 21, 41, 42, 50, 51, 56, 57, 59, 61, 64, 141, 142, 154, 201, 203, 204, 208, 233, 239
radical, ix, x, 3, 4, 5, 7, 9, 10, 11, 18, 33, 34, 39, 41, 47, 52, 54, 65, 77, 78, 88, 95, 96, 97, 98, 100, 106, 107, 108, 114, 123, 124, 127, 130, 131, 136, 137, 141, 142, 145, 146, 148, 149, 150, 151, 153, 156, 157, 201, 208, 224
radio, 121, 239
radioactive tracer, 28, 38
radiofrequency, xiii, 199, 233, 234
radiofrequency ablation, xiii, 199, 233, 234
radiological, 106, 134

radiotherapy, viii, 13, 16, 17, 34, 35, 41, 42, 43, 44, 45, 46, 47, 48, 49, 50, 51, 53, 55, 56, 57, 58, 59, 60, 64, 89, 99, 109, 111, 123, 132, 133, 137, 141, 142, 149, 151, 155, 157, 198, 201, 202, 204, 208, 225, 234, 239
Radiotherapy, 142, 151
range, 54, 66, 85, 86, 153
rapamycin, 57
ras, 174, 176, 184, 190
RAS, 184, 190
rat, 217, 220
rats, 217, 222
RB, 61, 62, 169
RC, 33, 90, 204
reaction rate, 161, 162
reaction time, 161
reactivity, xii, 211
reality, 98, 99
receptors, 185, 216, 221
recognition, 81
reconstruction, 21, 23, 67, 68, 72, 82, 85, 119, 201, 202, 207
recovery, 104, 105, 202, 203
rectal examination, 4, 69, 115, 116, 119, 134, 197
rectosigmoid, 2, 25, 58, 89, 192
rectum, vii, viii, x, 1, 2, 3, 10, 11, 12, 13, 17, 18, 19, 23, 25, 32, 34, 35, 36, 37, 42, 47, 57, 58, 61, 63, 67, 69, 71, 78, 86, 87, 88, 90, 91, 92, 96, 104, 107, 108, 109, 110, 114, 115, 116, 119, 120, 122, 123, 124, 125, 126, 127, 128, 129, 130, 131, 132, 134, 135, 137, 138, 139, 140, 141, 142, 145, 146, 148, 149, 154, 156, 192, 201, 208
recurrence, vi, vii, viii, ix, xii, 3, 4, 5, 7, 8, 9, 10, 11, 13, 14, 15, 16, 17, 18, 21, 22, 24, 25, 26, 30, 31, 34, 35, 36, 37, 38, 41, 43, 44, 45, 46, 47, 50, 51, 52, 54, 56, 57, 58, 61, 65, 66, 82, 89, 91, 95, 96, 97, 98, 99, 100, 101, 107, 110, 114, 121, 125, 126, 130, 132, 134, 136, 139, 140, 141, 146, 147, 148, 150, 151, 153, 154, 155, 157, 201, 203, 205, 206, 223, 224, 225, 226, 227, 228, 229, 230, 231
red meat, 193, 195
reduction, 13, 43, 46, 48, 152, 167, 195, 196, 215, 216, 230, 235
refining, 114
reflection, 20, 29, 36, 39, 74, 84, 87, 117, 118, 119
regional, 81, 85, 87, 151, 198, 235
regression, 51, 52, 61, 62, 133
regular, 195, 218
regulation, 217, 219
rejection, 146

relapse, 51, 58, 169
relationship, x, 33, 50, 51, 62, 87, 133, 159, 168, 193, 200, 220
relationships, vii, xii, 168, 193, 223, 224
relatives, 175, 196
reliability, 92
remission, 132, 133, 134, 151, 203
renal, 169, 175
renal function, 169
repair, xi, 153, 173, 174, 179, 180, 181, 182, 184, 185, 186, 188, 189, 190, 212
repair system, 185
replacement, 195
replication, 174, 180, 182
reproductive organs, 201
research, 19, 93, 159, 173, 191, 199, 203, 211, 212, 239
researchers, 31
reservation, 46
reservoir, vii, 1, 12, 21, 89
residual disease, 5, 8, 10, 27, 61
resolution, ix, 16, 35, 65, 66, 67, 68, 80, 87, 88, 93, 115, 117, 121, 138, 139
resource availability, 197
restriction enzyme, 176, 177
retention, 130, 151, 152
reticulum, 213
RF, 89, 109, 138
RFA, 234, 235, 236, 237
risk, vii, viii, ix, xi, xii, xiii, 3, 4, 5, 6, 7, 9, 10, 11, 13, 14, 15, 16, 21, 23, 27, 30, 31, 33, 41, 42, 47, 49, 50, 53, 62, 78, 90, 91, 95, 96, 97, 98, 100, 102, 104, 105, 114, 118, 122, 123, 124, 126, 128, 129, 130, 131, 132, 133, 134, 136, 137, 139, 146, 149, 152, 153, 155, 191, 193, 194, 195, 196, 197, 199, 201, 203, 204, 205, 206, 211, 217, 221, 223, 224, 230, 233, 235, 236, 237
risk assessment, 137
risk factors, vii, xii, 5, 7, 16, 21, 33, 78, 123, 152, 155, 193, 194, 205, 223, 224
risks, ix, 47, 52, 53, 95, 96, 194, 197
RNA, x, 159, 160, 162, 166, 167, 168, 169, 170, 175, 178
road map, 222
Romania, 1
room temperature, 161, 163

S

safety, 54, 63, 97, 99, 238

saline, 123, 125, 126, 161, 163
sample, xiii, 50, 52, 175, 224, 227
sampling, 67
saturated fat, xii, 193, 211, 212
saturated fatty acids, xii, 211, 212
savings, 107
scar tissue, 106
Schmid, 108
scores, 99, 104, 105
SCP, 176, 177, 179
SD, 101, 109, 110, 208, 221
SDS, 175, 220
search, x, 29, 54, 145, 216, 235
security, 20
sedation, 236
seeding, 43, 132
selecting, ix, 4, 6, 65, 88
self-report, 49
seminal vesicle, 83
senescence, 216
sensitivity, 76, 119, 120, 121, 122, 169, 170, 197
separation, 69
sepsis, 25
septic shock, 153
sequencing, 176, 177, 179
series, 4, 37, 49, 50, 51, 52, 53, 78, 84, 86, 87, 89, 111, 116, 117, 129, 130, 131, 132, 134, 146, 151, 154
serine, 215
serum, 227, 231
services, 202
severity, 22, 55, 99, 202
SH, 33, 35, 38, 61, 110, 112, 138, 231
shape, xiii, 87, 233, 234, 236
shock, 153, 215
short-term, 46, 59, 108, 133, 194, 202, 207
Short-term, 46, 200
shoulder, 234
side effects, 58, 99, 114, 135, 168, 169, 235, 237
sigmoid, 12, 119, 127, 192, 200
sigmoid colon, 119, 192
sigmoidoscopy, 196, 204
sign, 120
signal transduction, 213, 221
signaling, xi, xii, 174, 181, 182, 184, 185, 190, 211, 212, 216, 220
signaling pathway, xi, 174, 181, 182, 184, 185
signalling, 218, 221
signals, 184, 219
signal-to-noise ratio, 119

signs, 197, 204
silica, 162
sites, x, 27, 159, 160, 161, 163, 164, 165, 167
skin, 175, 178, 236, 237
small intestine, 148, 168, 174, 192, 216, 220
smoke, 126, 127, 128
smoking, 193, 196, 205
sodium, 138, 139, 140
software, 67, 87, 90, 119
solvent, 161
somatic mutations, xi, 173, 174, 176, 177, 179, 185, 186
Southern blot, 175, 176, 177
SP, 63, 93, 139, 169
spatial, 87, 88, 93, 139, 215, 216
specialization, 19
species, 215
specificity, 5, 76, 86, 119, 122
spectrum, 216, 221
speed, 119
sphincter, vii, 1, 11, 12, 16, 17, 18, 19, 21, 22, 32, 35, 36, 43, 46, 48, 50, 51, 52, 59, 60, 66, 70, 89, 104, 105, 109, 125, 126, 132, 133, 142, 146, 151, 152, 158, 229
sphingolipids, 214, 215, 222
sphingosine, 214, 215
spinal cord, 237
sporadic, 174, 184, 185, 187, 188, 212
squamous cell, 193
SR, 33, 58, 92, 102, 104, 222, 229
stages, viii, 2, 22, 38, 44, 45, 46, 47, 49, 50, 161, 163, 227
standard deviation, 237
standardization, 44, 45, 140
standards, 44
Statins, 195, 206
statistical analysis, 162
statistics, 191, 204
stenosis, 96, 126, 129, 236
stenotic lesions, 86
stoma, vii, ix, 16, 35, 95, 96, 99, 104, 107, 129, 133, 135, 153
stomach, 174, 175, 221, 236
storage, 119
strain, 116, 119, 217
strains, 170
strategies, xi, 109, 115, 191, 197, 206, 209, 230
stratification, 42, 45, 50
strength, 206
stress, 120, 168, 203, 215

strictures, 126, 140, 237
stromal, 193
Subcellular, 219
subgroups, 135, 213
subjective, 49
submucosa, 7, 71, 74, 75, 76, 77, 78, 81, 88, 96, 117, 123, 124, 125, 134, 149
substances, 167, 213
substitution, 177
sucrose, 217
Sun, 157, 187
superiority, 21, 87, 99, 199
supernatant, 161, 162
supplemental, 205, 206
supply, 200, 217
suppository, 21
suppression, 181
suppressor, xi, 173, 174, 180, 181, 185, 188
surgeons, 3, 24, 31, 42, 45, 48, 53, 86, 98, 128, 135, 137, 154, 200, 207
Surgeons, 48, 53
Surgery, viii, xii, 25, 32, 34, 41, 43, 60, 113, 138, 139, 150, 155, 159, 173, 191, 200, 201, 207, 223, 224, 225
surgical, vii, viii, ix, xiii, 2, 3, 4, 10, 12, 14, 15, 17, 18, 19, 21, 22, 23, 25, 27, 32, 35, 36, 37, 38, 41, 42, 44, 45, 46, 47, 48, 49, 50, 52, 54, 56, 58, 60, 65, 66, 85, 88, 90, 95, 104, 107, 114, 122, 123, 131, 132, 133, 137, 139, 146, 147, 148, 150, 152, 156, 198, 199, 200, 201, 202, 204, 230, 233
surgical intervention, 17, 21, 152, 199
surgical pathology, 202
surgical resection, xiii, 4, 10, 35, 47, 50, 54, 56, 60, 150, 199, 200, 233
surveillance, 203, 204, 207, 209
survival, viii, x, xi, 2, 4, 9, 14, 15, 16, 17, 18, 21, 24, 25, 26, 27, 30, 31, 32, 35, 36, 37, 38, 42, 43, 44, 45, 46, 49, 51, 52, 53, 55, 57, 58, 59, 61, 62, 63, 78, 82, 91, 97, 98, 99, 101, 102, 104, 106, 114, 123, 127, 130, 132, 133, 134, 135, 136, 137, 142, 145, 148, 149, 150, 151, 157, 160, 165, 166, 198, 199, 201, 204, 208, 213, 226, 227, 229, 230, 231, 234
survival rate, x, xi, 4, 9, 16, 17, 18, 25, 31, 38, 46, 98, 136, 137, 145, 149, 150, 151, 160, 165, 166, 234
survivors, 32, 203, 208
susceptibility, xii, 211, 216, 217, 219, 221
susceptibility genes, 216
suture, 22, 107, 129, 146, 154

Index

symptom, 150
symptoms, 22, 32, 169, 197, 204
synchronous, 122, 198, 199
syndrome, 187, 188, 196
synthesis, ix, xii, 65, 66, 67, 68, 211, 213, 214, 215, 218
systems, 215

T

TE, 150
technology, 87, 106
telephone, 113
TEM, v, ix, x, 3, 9, 10, 11, 53, 95, 96, 97, 98, 99, 100, 101, 104, 105, 106, 107, 110, 111, 112, 114, 122, 123, 124, 126, 127, 128, 129, 130, 131, 132, 133, 134, 136, 137, 145, 146, 147, 148, 149, 150, 151, 152, 153, 154, 156, 157
temperature, 161, 163
territory, 3, 12
Tesla, 121, 138
TGA, 177
TGF, xi, 174, 181, 185, 187
theory, 50
therapeutic benefits, 52
therapeutic interventions, 203
therapy, iv, 2, 3, 14, 27, 38, 43, 47, 50, 51, 52, 56, 57, 58, 59, 61, 62, 63, 64, 82, 91, 104, 111, 115, 130, 132, 136, 142, 143, 148, 154, 156, 168, 169, 170, 195, 199, 200, 201, 203, 204, 207, 208, 229, 234, 235, 238, 239, 240
thermal ablation, 234, 235, 237, 239, 240
Thomson, 137
thoracic, 208
three-dimensional, ix, 65, 66, 87, 90
three-dimensional representation, 87
threshold, 69, 237
thresholds, 47
thrombosis, 124
thymidine, x, 159, 169, 171
time, x, 11, 13, 14, 22, 24, 25, 26, 27, 28, 42, 43, 45, 48, 50, 51, 54, 55, 59, 60, 68, 99, 100, 104, 107, 110, 119, 121, 122, 136, 138, 142, 145, 148, 152, 154, 161, 162, 195, 202, 203, 212, 235
time consuming, 28, 121, 122
time factors, 60, 142
time frame, 195
timing, viii, 41, 42, 199

tissue, 3, 4, 6, 10, 13, 19, 26, 50, 67, 68, 71, 80, 84, 96, 106, 120, 138, 162, 167, 169, 175, 178, 180, 181, 217, 236, 237, 238
TJ, 33, 62, 110, 111, 155, 157, 229, 239
TM, 219, 220
Tokyo, 159, 173
tolerance, 133, 234, 237, 239, 240
toxic, 104
toxicity, 43, 44, 46, 50, 55, 89, 132, 202, 203
traction, 128, 154
trainees, 229
training, 19, 24, 25, 154, 230
trans, 96, 114, 130, 141, 146, 201, 204, 215
transcription, xii, 182, 212, 217
transcription factor, 182, 217
transcriptional, 213
transducer, 67, 85, 86
transfer, 215
transformation, 88
transfusion, 129
transition, 119, 125, 212
translation, 200
transparency, 69
transparent, 69, 129
transport, 170, 214, 221
transportation, 213
transverse colon, 200
trauma, 100
travel, 69, 134
trend, 10, 43, 48, 226
trial, ix, 10, 16, 35, 36, 43, 44, 45, 46, 47, 48, 49, 50, 51, 53, 54, 55, 56, 57, 58, 59, 60, 62, 64, 89, 95, 97, 98, 99, 108, 109, 110, 129, 133, 140, 141, 142, 143, 151, 170, 194, 195, 200, 205, 206, 207, 208, 239
trichloroacetic acid, 162
triggers, xi, 173, 174, 215
triglycerides, 213, 218
trust, 20
TT, 177, 221, 222
T-test, 162
tumor cells, 170, 182, 225
tumor depth, 33, 139
tumor invasion, xii, 15, 33, 35, 58, 73, 75, 76, 77, 78, 79, 80, 86, 224, 226, 227
tumor progression, 236
tumorigenesis, 182, 187, 220, 221
tumors, viii, xi, xiii, 2, 5, 6, 9, 10, 16, 22, 31, 32, 45, 47, 49, 52, 63, 66, 74, 76, 78, 80, 81, 83, 85, 86, 87, 88, 89, 90, 91, 92, 108, 109, 110, 111, 123,

124, 128, 140, 146, 148, 149, 151, 155, 156, 157, 158, 169, 173, 174, 176, 177, 179, 180, 182, 183, 185, 187, 188, 189, 193, 198, 199, 200, 201, 204, 224, 225, 227, 230, 233, 235, 240
tumour, 98, 99, 106, 107, 115, 116, 117, 119, 123, 126, 130, 131, 133, 134, 135, 136, 192, 212, 215, 216, 217
tumour growth, 212
tumours, 89, 98, 100, 104, 105, 106, 107, 108, 109, 110, 115, 116, 117, 119, 121, 122, 123, 126, 130, 131, 132, 133, 134, 138, 139, 140, 141, 155, 158, 212, 217
turnover, 217
two-dimensional, ix, 65, 66
tymidylate synthetase inhibition, x, 159

U

UG, 109
UK, 111, 130, 154
ulceration, 237
ulcerative colitis, 193
ultrasonography, ix, 61, 65, 67, 89, 90, 91, 92, 93, 117, 118, 138, 139
ultrasound, 4, 5, 47, 66, 67, 69, 71, 84, 86, 89, 90, 91, 92, 93, 108, 115, 116, 117, 118, 119, 120, 121, 122, 134, 138, 149, 151, 157, 198, 201
ultraviolet, 161
uniform, 76, 84, 216
United Kingdom, 95, 96, 111, 155
United States, 17, 34, 42, 43, 44, 45, 46, 50, 51, 52, 55, 62, 65, 206
univariate, 7
UP, x, 159, 160, 161, 163, 164, 165, 166, 167, 168
urea, 168, 176
ureter, 175
uridine, x, 159
uridine phosphorylase, x, 159
urinary, vii, viii, 1, 2, 11, 13, 17, 31, 100, 114, 117, 130, 135, 146, 151, 174, 178
urinary bladder, 114, 117, 135
urinary dysfunction, 11
urinary retention, 130, 151
urinary tract, 174, 178
urologist, 23
uterus, 23, 83

V

vagina, 83, 128, 203
validity, 13, 53, 92
values, 46, 69, 124
variability, 48
variable, 43, 86, 104, 107, 148, 217, 228
variables, xii, 48, 224, 225
variation, 120, 169, 170, 202, 220
vascular endothelial growth factor, 54
vessels, xiii, 7, 71, 72, 85, 200, 233, 235
villus, 215, 216, 220
visible, 14, 15, 28, 84, 118, 125
vision, 126, 128
visual perception, 69
visualization, 69, 87, 119
vitamin A, 193
vitamin D, 196, 206
Vitamin D, 194, 195
vitamins, 194, 205

W

water, 67, 119, 120, 161, 162, 175
weight loss, 197, 204
Weinberg, 220
whole grain, 196
women, xi, 23, 92, 96, 161, 191, 192, 193, 194, 195, 197, 203, 204, 205, 206, 207, 208, 225
workers, 137
worry, 134
wound dehiscence, 107
writing, 55

Y

yeast, 162, 189